sex Rx

ALSO BY LAUREN STREICHER, MD

The Essential Guide to Hysterectomy:
Advice from a Gynecologist on Your Choices
Before, During, and After Surgery

sex Rx

HORMONES, HEALTH, AND YOUR BEST SEX EVER

Lauren Streicher, MD

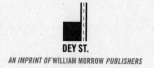

DEY ST.

AN IMPRINT OF WILLIAM MORROW *PUBLISHERS*

DEY ST.

Illustrations by Ashley Halsey © 2014 by Lauren F. Streicher.
Used by permission.

HarperCollins books may be purchased for educational, business, or sales promotional use. For information please e-mail the Special Markets Department at SPsales@harpercollins.com.

A hardcover edition of this book was published under the title *Love Sex Again* in 2014 by It Books, an imprint of HarperCollins Publishers.

FIRST DEY STREET BOOKS PAPERBACK EDITION PUBLISHED 2015.

Designed by Ashley Halsey

Library of Congress Cataloging-in-Publication Data has been applied for.

ISBN 978-0-06-230152-9

15 16 17 18 19 DIX/RRD 10 9 8 7 6 5 4 3 2 1

In memory of my parents,
Lyle Bass Streicher and Dr. Daniel Streicher

contents

Introduction   1

PART ONE
SexAbility: A View from My Side of the Stirrups   7

1   Taboo Topics: Let's Talk
    Who's having sex? Who's not? And if not, why not?   9

2   The Science of SexAbility
    How normal sexual response can morph into
    NO sexual response   30

3   An Up-Close View of Your Genitals
    Your private parts should be a little less private—
    at least to yourself   47

4   When Your Vagina Is in a Phunk
    What your vaginal pH should be—and why it matters   60

PART TWO
SexAbilitators: Essentials to Fix What's Broken   73

5   Slip-Sliding Away: Lubricants and Moisturizers
    The right product makes all the difference between
    sandpaper sex and slippery sex   75

6 Kegels with a Kick
*A trip to the gym for your pelvic floor and the ergonomics
of sex (who knew?)* 92

7 Say Yes to Drugs
*Sometimes a prescription doesn't just make sex better,
it makes it possible* 110

PART THREE
SexAbility Saboteurs 121

8 It Hurts!
Turn vaginal agony into vaginal ecstasy 123

9 A Real Pain in the Pelvis
*Some sexual pain can be an indicator of
a deeper problem* 148

10 Lost My Mojo
Want to find your mojo? Here's how 171

11 Nothing's Happening
*I'd like to buy a vowel—the key to getting
the big O back* 199

PART FOUR
Hormone Havoc 233

12 I Am Woman—Hear Me ROAR
*PMS, pregnancy, postpartum, infertility, contraception—
strap in, it's going to be a bumpy ride* 235

13 Hormone Hell
*How to turn back the clock on your vagina when your
estrogen tank is on empty* 257

14 The Cold Truth About Hot Flashes
*Vaginal dryness is not the only issue that sabotages
your SexAbility* 280

PART FIVE
You're Special   297

15   Medical Conditions
         Add low SexAbility to your list of symptoms   *299*

16   I'm Glad to Be Alive but . . .
         The impact of cancer on SexAbility   *323*

PART SIX
Other People   349

17   Finding a Clinician Who Will Actually Listen
         Let's talk vagina   *351*

18   Dating Dangers
         Have a positive sexual experience without testing positive   *367*

PART SEVEN
Taking Your New SexAbility to the Next Level   385

19   Vaginal Vanity
         Why some opt for an upgrade   *387*

20   Toys You Don't Want to Share with Your Children
         How toys can add pleasure and novelty to your sex life   *402*

Resources   *415*
Acknowledgments   *435*
Index   *439*

introduction

This book is about SexAbility. I coined that phrase a few years ago when I realized that too many of my patients had quietly given up or drastically compromised their expectations of having enjoyable, fun, satisfying sex ever again. This didn't happen because they stopped caring about sex.

Women like sex. The truth is that too many women no longer have the ability to have sexual pleasure. They haven't been given the information or the tools to alleviate the pain, the lack of feeling, or the dryness. In most cases they are not even aware that solutions exist. They have lost their SexAbility.

Most women have a gynecologist they trust. He or she delivered their kids, diagnosed their cancer, and maybe performed major surgery. So of course, when a woman goes to that trusted person with sexual problems (assuming she is one of the minority who actually discusses sex with a doctor) and is not offered solutions, it never occurs to her that there are answers out there. This woman doesn't assume that actual remedies exist, or that her doctor, who is an expert in all things relating to her female organs, is simply not knowledgeable about diagnosing and treating sexual pain and libido and arousal disorders. So without fanfare, without discussion, she quietly gives up on pleasure or drastically compromises her expectations about having a sex life.

Here's why. Typically, medical students attend only one lecture on sexual health during medical school. Unless they train at one of the few medical centers with a sexual dysfunction clinic, there is rarely any formal training in sexual health beyond that one lecture. Taking that into consideration, it's not all that surprising that your otherwise excellent doctor would not be knowledgeable about the impact of your medical condition on your ability to have a healthy, pleasurable sex life.

I know because up until ten years ago I was one of those doctors. I went to a superb medical school and did my ob-gyn residency at one of the finest programs in the country. I honestly don't think I ever attended a formal lecture on normal human sexuality, much less a lecture on sexual dysfunction. After I stopped delivering babies, I devoted my time to becoming an expert in minimally invasive surgery for women. I also developed an interest in menopause. It soon became obvious to me that many of the women who came to see me were less concerned about temporary hot flashes than they were about the permanent loss of their sex lives. Soon I became quite expert at treating postmenopausal sexual problems. I started to write what I affectionately called my "dry giney book." But along the way, I found that sexual dysfunction issues were not limited to problems caused by a lack of estrogen, or a lack of ability to get wet. I began to appreciate that it wasn't just women who have turned that menopausal corner but women as young as twenty who had serious sexual problems. So I dove in and immersed myself in the complex world of sexual health—a world that is alive, well, and packed with solutions and ongoing research.

I wrote *Sex Rx* because there was no comprehensive book about dealing with the *physical* side of maintaining sexual health. This book is for both the woman who never had a satisfying sex life and the woman who once had a good sex life but has been robbed of it by the ravages of menopause, surgery, pregnancy, cancer, medication, or other illness and wants to reclaim that part of her life. If you are one of these women, know that you are not alone. One of the reasons I surveyed thousands of women about their sexual behaviors and attitudes (my SexAbility Survey) was to be able to tell you what other women like you are thinking, doing, and experiencing. You will see answers to the survey throughout the book.

My goal is to tackle these taboo topics that desperately need to be out in the open.

I am going to give you the language, the knowledge, and, yes, the permission to talk about your vagina, your orgasms, and your sexual concerns, not only with your partner, your husband, and your doctor but also with yourself as you honestly explore what you need, what you want, and what brings you pleasure. My goal is to give you the tools and information about your sexual health that will empower you to take control.

If you are looking for a quick, definitive solution to your particular sexual health issue, I can tell you right now that it's not always that simple. I have found that four things are essential to achieving sexual health and sexual pleasure—what I call SexAbility.

1. **Motivation:** You would not have bought this book if you were not motivated to take control of a situation that has been frustrating and distressful and may have created a problem in your relationship.
2. **SexAbilitators:** Chapters 5–7 will introduce you to many of the tools you will need to reclaim your sex life. The world of lubricants, moisturizers, and medications is complicated and often confusing. There are also an increasing number of devices and therapies that will facilitate your sexual health recovery, and I'll explain them to you. Sexual ergonomics is an exciting new field that addresses the physical mechanics of having sex. I call all of these helpers "Sex-Abilitators."

3. **SexAbilitation:** It's not enough to have the right tools. You need to know which of the tools to use, how to use the tools, and when to use those tools. You can have the best hammer and drill that money can buy, but you can't build a house unless you understand the basics of the foundation, why your foundation has crumbled, and how to put it together again. Once you understand how and why things went wrong, you can get into the specifics of how to "rebuild."

4. **Patience:** I would love to give you an instant fix, and in many cases the fix can be pretty quick. But for the majority of women the road to reclaiming fulfilling, enjoyable sexual health takes some time. If you broke your hip, you would not expect to go for a pain-free run the day after surgery. There would be months of healing, strengthening, and physical therapy. I can't promise that a bottle of lube is going to make your sex life amazing the first time you use it. If so, good for you, but in most cases there is going to be more involved.

How to Navigate This Book

The best way to use this book and get the best result is to read it from beginning to end, though you can certainly skip the discussions of specific situations that do not apply to you, such as the effects of cancer or diabetes on sexual health. You may say, "But my only problem is vaginal dryness! That is the only section I need to read." Well, you may think the only reason you are having painful intercourse is because of vaginal dryness, but you may also have a hypertonic pelvic floor or a vulvar dermatologic condition. You won't know that unless you read those sections so that you have the vocabulary to talk to your doctor.

Not to mention that it's the rare person who has only one isolated sexual problem. Pain leads to decreased desire. Decreased desire leads to lack of arousal. And so on. I think you get the idea why I think your best bet is to read the whole book. Besides, you don't want to miss the answers to my SexAbility Survey—the responses from more than 3,000 men and women about their sexual practices and preferences that are sprinkled throughout the book.

Still, for many of you it may be useful to try to pinpoint which parts of the book are most relevant to you by taking my SexAbility Screen. The following ten questions will help you decide whether you should focus on issues relating to pain, decreased arousal, decreased desire, or decreased response and will also help you identify which chapters are the most important to get you on the right road to sexual health and pleasure.

SexAbility Screen

1. *I have pain at the outside of the vagina when my partner is inserting his penis or when I attempt to insert a toy.*
   If you answer yes to this question, the following chapters are essential: 1, 2, 3, 4, 5, 6, 7, 8, 9, 12, and 14.

2. *My vagina is so dry that if I put a penis or toy inside me, it hurts.*
   If you answer yes to this question, the following chapters are essential: 1, 2, 3, 4, 5, 6, 7, 8, 9, 12, and 14.

3. *My partner gets in just fine, but the minute he moves I have pain deep in my pelvis.*
   If you answer yes to this question, the following chapters are essential: 1, 2, 3, 4, 5, 6, 7, 8, 9, and 14.

4. *I'm not dry, but intercourse still hurts.*
   If you answer yes to this question, the following chapters are essential: 1, 2, 3, 4, 5, 6, 7, 8, 9, and 14.

5. *When I attempt intercourse, the pain in my pelvis lasts for hours or even days.*
   If you answer yes to this question, the following chapters are essential: 1, 2, 3, 4, 5, 6, 7, 8, 9, and 14.

6. *I have difficulty achieving or am unable to have an orgasm.*
   If you answer yes to this question, the following chapters are essential: 1, 2, 3, 4, 5, 6, 7, 8, and 11.

7. *My vagina is always irritated and sometimes has an odor.*
   If you answer yes to this question, the following chapters are essential: 1, 2, 3, 4, 5, 6, 7, 8, 12, and 13.

8. *I have no pain and am able to have an orgasm. I just never think about having sex and don't really care if I never have sex again.*
   If you answer yes to this question, the following chapters are essential: 1, 2, 3, 4, 5, 6, 7, 8, 10, and 11.

9. *Everything was fine until I went through menopause.*
   If you answer yes to this question, the following chapters are essential: 1, 2, 3, 4, 5, 6, 7, 8, 9, 10, 11, 13, and 14.

10. *I don't have pain, and I do have pleasure. I just want my sex life to be like it was when I was twenty!*
    If you answer yes to this question, the following chapters are essential: 1, 2, 3, 4, 5, 6, 7, 8, 20, and 21.

This book does not focus on the emotional and relationship aspects of maintaining a healthy sex life. There are plenty of books and therapists out there who can help you fix your relationship. What I can do is fix your vagina. So, yes, this book is about salvaging your sexual health. It is also about empowerment and enabling you to have the information to take charge of a problem that for many women has an impact not only on their pleasure but on their happiness, levels of anxiety, relationships, and experience of intimacy. This is what I tell my patients. This is what works. This is what will empower you to enhance (or reclaim) your SexAbility.

part one

SEXABILITY:

A VIEW FROM MY SIDE OF THE STIRRUPS

1

TABOO TOPICS: LET'S TALK

Who's having sex? Who's not?
And if not, why not?

No one hesitates to say to a friend, "I have a cough I'm concerned about," "I'm not sleeping very well lately," or, "I'm a little worried about my swollen ankles." But when was the last time you admitted to a coworker, "My vagina smells funny," or, "I have a terrible headache every time I have an orgasm," or, "My vulvar itch doesn't go away no matter how many times I get treated for a yeast infection"?

Exactly.

And because no one, *no one,* is talking about her sexual health, you would never know that 40 percent of your friends are likely to have experienced some sexual difficulty. You would think from what is presented in books and magazines, in films and TV shows, on the Internet and billboards, that the whole world is erotically charged and every single person (other than you) is having *amazing,* passionate sex and earth-shattering orgasms on a daily basis.

Even the postmenopausal character played by Meryl Streep in the movie *Hope Springs,* despite a sexual hiatus of years, was able to have fantastic sex without so much as a bottle of lubricant in sight.

I can pretty much guarantee that every gynecologist (and about half the women) in the audience thought, *Really? I don't think so.* Just because Meryl's character's relationship was suddenly passionate doesn't mean her vagina and clitoris were cooperating.

Painful sex, difficult sex, and the lack of sex have always been at the top of the list of taboo topics for women. Many women can't even comfortably say the *word* "vagina," much less talk about a vagina that is dry, painful, bleeding, or the source of incredible agony—all conditions that make intercourse pretty much out of the question. Even really close girlfriends rarely have the courage to say, "Jenny, my vagina has been really dry lately. How's yours?"

Women rarely even talk to their sexual partner or husband about this topic, not just because they are embarrassed, but because of the shame and fear associated with perhaps no longer being perceived as "sexy." Indeed, in the 2013 *Revive* survey of sexual behavior among postmenopausal couples, 53 percent of women experienced at least one sexual problem, an astounding 61 percent hid their symptoms from their partner, and a shocking 73 percent admitted that they silently endured painful intercourse to please their partner. The other 40 percent solved the problem by simply avoiding sex altogether. The majority of women who used a vaginal product had a "secret ritual" behind a closed door to insert or apply it because they didn't want their partner or husband to know they were not as naturally moist and sexy as when they were twenty.

What is this hiding really about?

Sexual Problems Are Even Taboo in the Doctor's Office

In spite of the fact that almost 50 percent of women have sexual issues significant enough to interfere with or put a screeching halt to intercourse and intimacy, few doctors ask about this, and if the topic does come up, many doctors have very little to offer beyond, "Relax," "Try some lubricant," or even worse, "Don't worry, it's a natural part of aging." Studies also confirm that it is the rare woman who brings it up to her doctor.

Dr. Streicher's SexAbility Survey

Women were asked how often their doctor inquired about their sexual health:

26.2 percent said "routinely"
31.9 percent said "sometimes"
41.8 percent said "never"

My experience is different. Because I am a gynecologist who specializes in sexual health, I see women every day who specifically come to me to get treatment for painful intercourse or a lapse in libido. But even I see plenty of patients who have a hard time spitting out the real reason for their visit.

A typical scenario goes something like this: A patient comes in for her annual visit. Before the exam, we chat about her irregular periods, the occasional hot flash, and her daughter's new boyfriend. I generally ask, "What's going on in your sex life?"

All too often, the response is, "Sex life? I don't have one."

"Do you want to talk about it?"

She assuredly says, "No, that's all right."

So I move on to the breast exam, Pap, and pelvic. Before I leave the room, I ask, "Is there anything else you'd like to discuss?"

Then, with an embarrassed look on her face, she finally brings it up. "Is there anything you can do about my lack of libido? I really want my sex life back."

I call this very common moment the "hand on the door question." Those questions that women—regardless of their age—have been too uncomfortable, too defeated, to ask earlier.

Every year millions of women make that annual trek to their gynecologist's office and usually leave *without* asking that question, even though it is on a lot of women's minds. That "hand on the door question" is more often than not the reason the patient came to see me in the first place.

And even though most women are more comfortable discussing their sexual issues with me than with other doctors, I can count on one hand the number of patients who spontaneously tell me that it hurts when they masturbate or they are no longer able to have an orgasm. Sadly, for the majority of women, there is shame in admitting that they self-stimulate, enjoy orgasms, miss orgasms, and would like to have orgasms again.

A lot more is broken here than vaginas.

The whys and why-nots of who's sexually active, who's not, and who cares are incredibly complex. At the risk of oversimplifying, I can say that it almost always comes down to two questions: is there the opportunity, and is there pleasure?

There are really three groups of women:

- Women who enjoy a great deal of gratification from self-stimulation and/or partnered sex
- Women for whom there is little or no pleasure in sexual activity and for whom sex represents an obligation exclusively for the purpose of procreation and fulfillment of their marital or relationship expectations
- Women for whom sex represents intimacy and relationship far more than physical release and for whom the cuddling is great, the act itself is superfluous, and the orgasms are generally absent

I, of course, maintain that all women can and should enjoy sex. But sadly, once a medical barrier presents itself, women who never particularly enjoyed sex are often relieved to have a legitimate excuse to cross intercourse and sexual activity off their "to-do" list. Being nonsexual becomes the new normal. And women who enjoyed sex, when faced with a medical barrier, are, if not devastated, at a minimum saddened by the loss.

Here's what this book is intended to do: give you the information you need about how your body is working or not working to decide yourself what needs fixing.

Big Pharma to the Rescue?

Nevertheless, our reluctance to talk about sexual health is changing. It used to be that I was one of the few people to talk about problems with vaginas in public (my family is used to it), but now there are ads everywhere—in magazines, on radio and TV, online—all touting solutions for sexual pain or low libido. Those ads inevitably have pictures of sad-looking midlife couples lying on opposite sides of the bed.

What is emerging is a push to give women permission to address sexual dysfunction too. Of course, this change is not driven by gynecologists like me who have been trying to start the conversation for years, but by the pharmaceutical industry, which appreciates the magnitude of female sexual dysfunction in women and knows there is a lot of money to make from vaginas that have lost the ability to have pleasurable, slippery intercourse. But because the topic is still a cultural taboo, and the majority of women are not asking for or getting the help they need, companies are now spending millions in marketing dollars to encourage women to talk to their doctors about getting a prescription or, in the case of products that don't require a prescription, go shopping.

This is not a bad thing, nor is this a new phenomenon. For the guys this happened years ago. Indeed, it was the pharmaceutical industry that gave men the "permission" and the language to talk about their sexual problems. Without a doubt one of the most brilliant marketing successes of the 20th century was the introduction of the phrase "erectile dysfunction." That's right—marketing gurus, not medical doctors, popularized the term that is now part of the lexicon. Prior to 1998, men who were unable to maintain an erection suffered from *impotency*. Think about it. It's bad enough to have a penis that won't cooperate, but then to have a diagnosis that implies you are also weak, incompetent, and powerless is too much to expect any man to deal with. What self-respecting guy is going to say to a woman, "Sorry, honey, not tonight, I'm impotent"?

A guy who was impotent didn't just have a medical problem. He was a personal failure. No way was he going to make an appointment to discuss his impotency with his medical doctor. The poor guy had to suffer in silence.

Suddenly, in 1998, the impotent man disappeared. Enter the man with erectile dysfunction, or ED. The man with ED was handsome, successful, and sexy. The man with ED was so powerful that he could even run for president—he'd lose (remember Bob Dole?), but he could still run. So who commercialized the term "erectile dysfunction"? The people who had a lot to gain from men admitting they had a problem. I think you know where I'm going.

Yes, it was the inventors of Viagra who also popularized the term ED. And I give them a lot of credit. Pfizer launched Viagra and at the same time launched a marketing campaign that redefined impotency as erectile dysfunction. Not only was the condition normalized, but the marketing campaign gave men the language to talk to their doctors about it so they could comfortably ask for a prescription.

And now it is starting to happen for the women.

Because the reality is that for every man who suffers from erectile dysfunction, there is a woman who suffers from sexual dysfunction. Women who suffer from painful sex, who have no libido, or who are unable to have an orgasm are just as common as men with erectile dysfunction.

Guys Have ED, Women Have GD

So while the guys had the language and the permission for years, women are just now finally getting permission to talk about sexual dysfunction. The language, though, is still an obstacle. The medical term for thin, dry vaginal tissue is "vaginal atrophy." But like being impotent, no women (even if they are familiar with the term) want to have vaginal *atrophy!* Talk about a buzz kill. "Honey, my vagina is atrophied, wasting away. Minimized. Sick. I can't have sex tonight. Or ever."

Since the pharmaceutical marketing gurus haven't come up with a term to replace "vaginal atrophy," I decided to coin the term GD, for "genital dryness," to describe the changes that occur not only around the time of menopause but from a number of other medical conditions as well, including diabetes, heart disease, cancer treatments, and more—all of which you will learn about in the pages ahead.

Your physician may not know the term GD (not yet anyway), but he or she will understand what you mean when you say you have "genital dryness" and you need a solution. You also need a solution to the many other conditions that can affect your sexual health and therefore your right to experience pleasurable sex, a healthy libido, and a gratifying orgasm!

How Many People Are Really Having Sex?

Let's go back to one of my original questions: how many people in this country are routinely sexually active and how often? These are not easy numbers to come by. Most studies are based on surveys and past recollection as opposed to a camera in every bedroom in America. In addition, in the scientific literature, sexual activity is often defined only as heterosexual vaginal-penile intercourse. (As discussed in chapter 2, that is not the case with many, if not most, men and women.)

One of the largest and most interesting surveys looking at frequency of sexual activity was conducted by the sociologists

Dr. Pepper Schwartz and Dr. James Witte, who surveyed more than 100,000 individuals from around the world about every detail of their romantic lives for their 2013 book *The Normal Bar*. Their sample included women from across racial, ethnic, and educational lines. Roughly half the respondents were 45 or older, but the results included all ages (18 and up) combined. Among their sample, Schwartz and Witte found that:

7.5 percent had sex daily
40 percent had sex three to four times a week
27 percent had sex three to four times a month
8 percent had sex once a month
13 percent had sex rarely
4.5 percent never had sex

Since frequency is known to decrease as age and medical issues intervene, as expected, the numbers look very different when divided by age. A telephone survey of 2,000 US women between the ages of 18 and 94 was conducted in 2003 by randomly dialing individuals and inquiring about their sexual activity, including oral (active or receptive), vaginal, or anal intercourse, in the past three months. (One has to wonder about *who* would give this information to a stranger over the phone.) The percentage of sexually active women overall was 53 percent, and the results broke down by age as follows:

66 percent of women ages 18 to 29 years
70 percent of women ages 30 to 39 years
65 percent of women ages 40 to 49 years
46 percent of women ages 50 to 59 years
20 percent of women ages 60 to 94 years

Clearly something is happening at age 60, and it's not good. But is it simply age? Or is it other variables that go along with age, such as lack of a partner or medical illness?

In the most comprehensive study of sexual activity in older adults, published in the *New England Journal of Medicine* in 2007, Dr. Stacy Lindau conducted extensive face-to-face interviews with 3,000 men and women between the ages of 57 and 85 and reassuringly found that most of them had remained sexually active into their sixties. Nearly half continued to have sex (not necessarily intercourse) regularly into their early seventies, but women were far more likely than men to not be sexually active, either because they had no partner or because sexual activity was no longer pleasurable. Here's a breakdown of the numbers:

Ages 57 to 64
62 percent of women reported sexual contact
15 percent rated sex as "not at all important"

Ages 65 to 74
40 percent of women reported sexual contact
25 percent rated sex as "not at all important"

Ages 75 and Older
17 percent of women reported sexual contact
41 percent rated sex as "not at all important"

Of the women who stated that sex was no longer important, 48 percent were in the "not sexually active" group. This study was important because it looked not only at age but at medical illness as a predictor of sexual activity and found that, while sexual activity did decline with age, the drop was much more significant in people with medical problems. In other words, healthy old people are far more likely to have sex than sick old people. In fact, among healthy adults who were sexually active, about two-thirds had sex at least twice a month into their seventies, and more than half continued at that pace into their eighties.

How Real Is Sexual Dysfunction? Very.

There is a movement, more political than scientific, that asserts that sexual dysfunction in women does not exist but is in fact a "normal" experience made medical by profit-motivated pharmaceutical companies. As a physician and a woman, I find this argument offensive. The notion that pain, an inability to have an orgasm, and loss of libido are not "real" conditions but are manufactured so that pharmaceutical companies can sell drugs is clearly entertained by people who have never spent time in my office. Not to mention that they give pharmaceutical companies way too much credit. Sexual problems in women have been recognized by the medical community as specific conditions for over thirty years, long before Big Pharma entered the picture of what happens in people's bedrooms. The potential negative impact of this movement is huge and could destroy women's hard-won entitlement to have their experience validated. Female sexual dysfunction deserves appropriate research and treatment options. Hypoactive sexual desire syndrome (low libido) is not the pharmaceutical equivalent of a Hallmark holiday manufactured to sell more greeting cards any more than Viagra was developed to treat fake erectile dysfunction.

So yes, in spite of the fact that the pharmaceutical companies are motivated by profits, their research and development of new drugs have validated that female sexual health problems are real and desperately deserving of the attention they are finally getting.

Although it is true that the majority of women with sexual problems are in midlife or beyond, the problem is not limited to the over-40 crowd. For some women, the problems started with their first sexual encounter. Others did not have issues until something like pregnancy, medication, illness, or surgery sabotaged their sex life.

The Benefits of Having Sex

I am obviously a consistent proponent of trying to make sex an active part of your life. However, I would be remiss as a physician if

I didn't share a bit of healthy skepticism about the ever-expanding list of purported physical, psychological, and social benefits of good sex. So here goes. Let's take a look at why people have sex to begin with—starting, of course, with the fact that it's supposed to feel good. There are three main reasons why people have sex:

Pleasure: *People like to do things that feel good. The release of endorphins and neurotransmitters, the physical pleasure, and the intimacy and connection that occur with sexual activity all result in pleasure. The biological reason that sex feels good is so people will have sex a lot and procreate.*

Partner: *People have sex because it enhances their relationship with their partner. Biologically, of course, partnered sex is necessary for procreation.*

Procreation: *So yes, procreation is biologically why people have sex. Period. From an evolutionary viewpoint, it also makes sense for healthy people to procreate, which is why people who are sick, weak, or dying (the biologically unsuitable) are less likely to be sexually active.*

While everyone agrees that healthy people have more sex, on the flip side, does having sex *make* you healthier? Google "health benefits of sex" and you will learn that regular sex prevents cancer, boosts your immune system, improves heart health, cures arthritis, eliminates PMS, lowers blood pressure, eliminates headaches, prevents wrinkles, makes your hair thicker, whitens your teeth . . . the list goes on and on.

There is no doubt that pleasurable sexual activity has psychological benefits, but when it comes to physical benefits, which of the many claims out there has an actual scientific basis? What's cause and what's effect? Does having a lot of sex make your heart healthier? Or is it just that people who have better heart health have more sex? Correlation and causation are not the same thing, so let's separate the hype from the facts.

Sex Promotes Weight Loss?

There is no question that having sex burns more calories than, say, sitting in front of the television and eating Twizzlers. But do women who have regular sex actually lose weight? Sex burns around five calories a minute. Most people have sex for about ten to fifteen minutes. Tops. The average person burns around two hundred calories a week having sex, less than the number of calories in the two glasses of wine you drank before you had sex. Don't cancel the gym membership.

Sex Reduces Pain?

Sexual activity releases endorphins. High endorphin levels are associated with less pain. There are many claims that increased endorphins from sexual activity relieves headache pain, back pain, muscle pain, you-name-it pain. There are actually very few scientific studies that look at pain reduction as a direct result of sexual activity. One study conducted at the Headache Clinic at Southern Illinois University did find that half of female migraine sufferers reported relief after orgasm. So much for the "I have a headache" excuse.

Sex Reduces Menstrual Cramps?

This claim is based on pain reduction from increased endorphins along with the uterine contractions that occur with orgasm. Uterine contractions get the menstrual blood out faster. Shorter periods reduce the amount of time you are in pain. While there are a lot of anecdotal reports of pain-free periods as a result of sexual activity, there are no scientific studies that prove this to be true.

Sex Eases Depression?

High levels of dopamine are associated with decreased depression. Sexual activity increases dopamine. Depression (accompanied by low levels of dopamine) is associated with decreased sexual activity. So again, is it cause or correlation? One interesting study claims that the components of semen, including prostaglandins, testosterone, and oxytocin, are absorbed through the vaginal tissues and improve mood in women. Obviously, only women who do not use condoms potentially benefit from this effect. One can't help but wonder if this hypothesis (never proven, by the way) was construed by a condom-hating scientist.

Sex Prevents Infection?

This one pops up a lot and is based on a small study that measured postcoital salivary levels of immunoglobulins, our body's defense against infection. In that study, intercourse transiently boosted immunoglobulins by about 30 percent. As a result of that one tiny study, there are countless claims that sex fights off infection. So do people who have lots of sex have fewer colds? Who knows? This has also never been proven. Since kissing and heavy breathing tend to spread colds, it may be a wash. And we're not even talking about STDs.

Sex Leads to Better Heart Health?

In one often-cited British study, men who had at least three orgasms per week had 50 percent fewer heart attacks than men who did not. The theory is that sex causes an increase in DHEA (didehydroepiandrosterone), which in turn helps circulation. Another is the assumption that the exercise of sex builds heart health. Having sex takes about the same amount of effort as climbing two to three flights of stairs. Now, if you were to climb about twenty flights of stairs and then have sex . . .

Sex Improves Sleep?

Orgasm causes a transient rise in prolactin and oxytocin, hormones that increase during sleep. But having higher prolactin levels *during* sleep is not the same thing as *inducing* sleep. In fact, it is sleep that induces elevated prolactin levels. This is a perfect example of upside-down science being used to make a point. An elevation in oxytocin is associated with emotional bonding and sexual pleasure, but it doesn't directly help you fall asleep. The physical activity of sex may make you tired, but again, we're talking two to three flights of stairs. Does sex make you feel relaxed and satisfied? I'll go for that.

Sex Lowers the Risk of Cancer?

A 2004 study in the *Journal of the American Medical Association* showed that men who had at least twenty-one ejaculations a month had a significantly lower risk of developing prostate cancer than men who ejaculated fewer than seven times a month. The validity of this study has been questioned, particularly since the study was based on men's recollections of how much sex they'd had at different times in their life, and as you know, men *never* exaggerate about how much sex they have. A 1989 French study showed that women who never had sex were three times as likely to develop breast cancer as women who regularly had sex.

Sex Prevents Incontinence?

Not only does a long session of sex supposedly tone your thighs and butt, but there are claims that strong orgasms, which induce pelvic floor contractions, may also help tone your pelvic floor, which in turn prevents incontinence. There is no question that a strong pelvic floor prevents involuntary loss of urine. But it is also known that women who are incontinent avoid having sex and are also likely to have difficulty reaching orgasm. (See chapter 15 on medical issues.) So, does sex prevent incontinence, or do women who don't leak urine just have more sex?

Sex Reduces Wrinkles?

Wrinkles are caused by loss of collagen. Estrogen increases collagen formation. In fact, women in the 1950s were encouraged to put estrogen cream on their face to keep their youthful appearance. But sexual activity doesn't increase estrogen; estrogen increases the ability and desire to have sex. Are you confused? I'm confused. In the meantime, stick with your sunscreen, which *is* proven to prevent wrinkles.

Sex Prevents Tooth Decay?

Semen has calcium, zinc, and other minerals needed to fight tooth decay. Women who swallow semen should therefore have healthier teeth. This is a stretch. A very big stretch, unless you are using semen as toothpaste.

Sex Increases and Sustains Vaginal Lubrication and Elasticity?

This is the old "use it or lose it" issue, which happens to be very true. Regular intercourse increases blood flow to the vaginal walls, which in turn increases lubrication and elasticity. So, if things are working fine, having intercourse on a regular basis does help to sustain vaginal health. On the other hand, once the tissues are thin and dry, "using it" more times than not only causes more pain and more dryness. Fix it and then use it.

Sex Makes You Happier?

A National Bureau of Economic Research study calculated that regular sexual activity brings the same levels of happiness as earning an extra $100,000 annually. I can't vouch for the $100,000 claim, but I can tell you that satisfying, pain-free sex does tend to make people happier.

Sex Prolongs Life?

Do people who have sex live longer *because* they have sex, or are healthier people who are the most likely to live longer also more likely (and able) to have sex? A study in the *British Medical Journal* found that men who had sex less than once a month were twice as likely to die in the next ten years as those who had sex once a week. A 25-year study of 270 men and women age 60 to 96, conducted at Duke University, found that the more men had sex, the longer they lived. Women who said they enjoyed their sex lives lived seven to eight years longer than those who were not interested in having sex. Cause or correlation? In either case, it's easy to make the argument that having good sex gives you an incentive to live longer.

So What's the Verdict?

Call me a skeptic, but the jury is still out on most of these claims. However, it doesn't matter. What is known is that sex is *associated* with the elevation of "feel-good" hormones and neurotransmitters, sex is not bad for you, and the *correlation* between good health and pleasurable sex is proven. Get your sexual health together and your general health is likely to benefit as well. Besides, sex feels good. And while the *only* biological reason to have sex is procreation, we live longer now, well beyond the years of childbearing. Therefore, sexual activity has taken on a different role: in short, sex enhances the quality of life.

So why then do women start avoiding sex?

It's Not Always Physical

If you have painful sex—whether you have a partner, don't have a partner, or don't want a partner—you are likely to avoid situations that lead to sex. And while your ability to have pleasurable sex and the frequency of your sexual activity are influenced by your physical ability to do so, clearly there are many nonmedical considerations that impact your sexual activity as well. Before launching into the myriad of medical, physical, and hormonal issues behind sexual dysfunction (the next 15 chapters are devoted to those subjects!), let's take a look at some of the nonmedical factors that negatively influence not just how good sex is but how frequent (or infrequent) it is.

Cultural Factors

Every society has behaviors that are unique to that culture, and sexual behavior is no exception. Homosexuality is acceptable in some cultures, but not in others. Women baring their breasts on the beach is the norm in France, while in some cultures even nudity in the bedroom isn't allowable. Some cultural sexual behaviors, such as female genital mutilation, are not only hazardous to health, but can eliminate or reduce pleasure. Dry sex (preferred by men, not women!) in some cultures, as opposed to the American preference for slippery, lubricated intercourse, may also pose health risks for women beyond pain.

Sexual practices and attitudes vary not only from culture to culture but within cultures. In the United States, there are plenty of people who would never consider anything other than male-female intercourse in the missionary position, while their next-door neighbor routinely has mixed-gender threesomes that involve light bondage and strap-on dildos.

The Length of the Relationship

Even with a really strong couple, the longer the relationship the less frequent the sex. There are exceptions, of course, but virtually every study shows that new sex is not only hotter but also more frequent.

Partner Issues

Relationship issues aside, not having a partner, or a functional partner, is the most common issue for women. While erectile dysfunction is frequently discussed, another common problem that is talked about less is premature ejaculation.

Lack-of-partner issues are particularly common among aging women, since age disparities at the time of marriage leave women often outliving their husbands or having a significantly older husband. It is also a reality that divorced or widowed men are more likely to remarry than divorced or widowed women. Even when a functional partner is available, there may be a disconnect when it comes to sexual interest. Women are not the only ones who have varying levels of libido.

Age Issues

The perception that older people do not have sex is not based in reality. More than half of women continue to be sexually active after menopause. Having said that, even if there are no medical or partner issues, women's interest in sex and the type and frequency of their sexual activity eventually decline as part of the normal aging process.

Religious Factors

Women from strict religious upbringings who have an engrained belief that premarital sex is evil are sometimes unable to shake that belief and continue to feel that sex is "wrong" even after they marry and are expected to become sexually active. While most religions encourage sexual activity (within marriage) for procreation, some place restrictions on either the type of sexual activity or the timing. Almost every religion forbids intercourse during menstruation. Why bother if the chance of pregnancy is almost nil?

Observant Jews take it a step further and forbid intimacy (including hand-holding, kissing, or touching of any sort) for days after the flow has stopped. My Orthodox friends tell me that this forced abstinence results in an anticipation that enhances enjoyment of sex. On the other hand, Orthodox Jews are not only permitted to be intimate but are *obligated* to have intercourse at certain times. Having sex on the Sabbath is a *mitzvah*—meaning that God gives you extra credit. As an extra perk for Jewish women, the traditional marriage contract states that a husband has the *obligation* to make sure his wife is sexually satisfied and cannot force her to have sex if she doesn't want to.

For Muslims, pretty much anything goes as long as it's in the marital bed, it's not happening during menstruation, and it's not sodomy. Islam actually sees sex (in the proper setting) as *ibadah,* or an act of worship. While modesty and chastity in public are the hallmarks of a Muslim woman, there is nothing wrong with that woman being active and responsive during sex. In fact, foreplay by both partners is strongly encouraged—those who skip straight to penetration are said to be behaving like animals.

Mormons are bound by the "law of chastity," which says that they are "to stay morally clean in their thoughts, words, and actions." But there aren't many restrictions when it comes to what a Mormon couple can do after they tie the knot. And there's no "till death do us part" in Mormon wedding vows: since Mormon marriages are "celestial," they continue into the afterlife. Although Mormonism has been associated with polygamy in the past, this is now a touchy subject, and any Mormon who enters into a polygamous relationship will be excommunicated from the Church of Latter-Day Saints. There's one loophole: a widowed man (but not a widowed woman) *is* allowed to marry again and thus have multiple wives—and sexual partners—in the afterlife. Now that would make for a very awkward celestial reunion.

For Catholics, sex is all about procreation, so using it for a reason other than that is considered a sin. That's not to say that sex shouldn't be pleasurable for Catholics, but that it should happen within marriage, without birth control, and definitely not with someone of the same sex. Masturbation is also a no-no. In fact, even if there is no chance of the woman getting pregnant (she is already pregnant, postmenopausal, etc.), Catholic men must only ejaculate into a woman's vagina.

Excluding monks and nuns, the Buddhists get the gold ribbon for sexual leniency. After all, they are the inventors of tantric sex and sexual yoga, which, according to some Tibetan authorities, are necessary practices in order to attain Buddhahood (the state of complete enlightenment). Buddhism teaches that cravings—including sexual cravings—lead to suffering, so acknowledging those desires is strongly encouraged. The only restrictions are very vague: followers are to "refrain from sexual misconduct," but what that actually means is open for interpretation. And there's no mention of homosexuality in ancient Buddhist texts, so that's up for interpretation too.

Having a History of Sexual Abuse

A history of rape or sexual abuse increases the likelihood that consensual sexual activity may be problematic, even if the issues surrounding the trauma have been resolved. The experience of early and repeated sexual abuse is highly associated with adult issues of low libido, low arousal, sexual pain, and inability to orgasm. One study showed that 75 percent of women with a history of coercion had sexual dysfunction.

Fear of Infection or Pregnancy

It's hard to "let go" if you think you might get a sexually transmitted infection or are worried about becoming pregnant. Fear of pregnancy goes both ways: you may not want to get pregnant and are having sex without contraception, or you may desperately want to become pregnant and have not been able to.

Body Image and Self-Esteem Issues

He is not looking at your cellulite—he is too worried about the size of his penis—but you are. Studies consistently show that women who feel physically undesirable avoid sex. Even if there are underlying self-esteem issues that have nothing to do with body image, sexual intimacy may be problematic.

Stress

While men may try to convince women that sex is a stress reliever, that is generally not the case, and in fact the endless list of stresses— financial issues, work, caretaking of parents, unemployment, life— has a negative influence on frequency of sexual activity.

Sleep Patterns/Schedule

If your husband works nights and you work days, the likelihood of your having sex is going to decrease. Ditto if you get up at the crack of dawn to get an exercise session in before you get the kids up and off to school, run around like a crazy person all day, and then collapse into bed right after the dishes go into the dishwasher. Snoring that leads to separate bedrooms can also be a real sexual sabotage.

Privacy

If your kids are bursting into the bedroom unannounced every time they have a question (or more likely every time they hear the bed squeaking), it's hard to be "in the moment." This may also be an issue if you live in really cramped quarters.

So yes, cultural factors, religious beliefs, social issues, general health, and age all influence the frequency of sexual activity. More than any other factor, though, the frequency of sex is determined by pleasure. Most people don't want to do things that don't bring them pleasure.

If there is a physical, hormonal, or medical condition that has sabotaged your sex life, you are far from alone, and that is what the next 19 chapters are all about: comprehensive, up-to-date, accurate information about improving your SexAbility—*minus* the speculum, Pap smear, and stirrups.

2

THE SCIENCE OF SEXABILITY

*How normal sexual response can
morph into NO sexual response*

Brad Pitt (substitute the fantasy partner of your choice) walks toward you, and you think, *I wonder what he looks like naked?*

He walks up to you, brushes up against you, and looks longingly into your eyes. Suddenly, there is increased blood flow to your breasts and genitals. Your nipples get hard, your breasts get engorged, and there is definite moisture and "fullness" in your vagina. Your heart rate speeds up, and you breathe a little faster.

Minutes later, you rendezvous in the bathroom, and before you know it he is passionately kissing you and touching your engorged nipples with one hand and caressing your clitoris with the other. Of course, you have conveniently forgotten to put on panties to avoid an unsightly underwear line with your little black dress.

Your brain fires, resulting in a widespread rhythmic pelvic muscle contraction, your heart races, and a euphoric feeling of pleasure, release, and satisfaction streams through your body.

You then return to your unstimulated state, quickly pull down your dress, and walk back out to the party and casually pop a shrimp into your mouth. Hopefully he wrote down your number before he disappeared into the crowd.

Okay, this may not be the most realistic scenario, but as fantasies go, it gets the point across. Fantasy or not, this is how women with normal sexual health should experience their sexual response cycle.

Here's what's happening physiologically:

When Brad Pitt is walking toward you, you experience *desire*.

When your blood starts to flow and your body begins to respond, you are becoming *aroused*.

When you're in the bathroom locked in a passionate tango, there is a buildup of muscle tension known as the pre-orgasmic or *plateau* phase.

When your brain fires and your body convulses in delicious contractions, you climax or *orgasm*.

As you take a breath and gather your wits about you, your body returns to its unstimulated state and you have reached *resolution*.

Sexual Orientation Does Not Define What Normal Is

Today when most people define sexuality, they think not in terms of *what* someone is doing but in terms of *whom* they are doing it with. And though sexual orientation has nothing to do with what's normal—in both behavior and health—most women are *heterosexual*, meaning they are attracted to men and prefer to have sex with men. *Homosexuality* is when women are attracted to and prefer to have sex with women; such women identify as lesbians. *Bisexual* women are attracted to and have sex with both men and women.

The largest group of normal is what I refer to as self-sexual. Whether someone is heterosexual, homosexual, or bisexual, pretty much everyone has engaged at some point, if not on a regular basis, in self-stimulation for sexual satisfaction and release.

It's interesting how every guy has no problem admitting or acknowledging that he masturbates, yet women are generally secretive and embarrassed to acknowledge that they do too.

So the bottom line is that normal sexuality includes heterosexuality, homosexuality, bisexuality, and self-sexuality, and even though it is very popular for celebrities and sports figures to publicly announce which gender they are having sex with, it's not necessary to declare that you identify with one group or another. For the purposes of this book, the focus (and language used) is on heterosexuality and self-sexuality, not because they are *more* normal but simply because they are more common. So if I am talking about intercourse and you are a woman who has sex with women or who is primarily self-sexual, please know that while I might mention a penis, the same discussion holds for women who enjoy vaginal penetration with an inanimate, penis-like object. (More on that subject in chapter 20!) If I refer to a male partner, know that I have no intention of excluding lesbians.

William Masters and Virginia Johnson gave us the classic description of sexual response in 1966. They identified four phases:

- Excitement
- Plateau
- Orgasm
- Resolution

In the 1970s, Helen Singer expanded on Masters and Johnson's description of sexual response and divided the excitement stage into two phases:

- Excitement
  Desire
  Arousal
- Plateau
- Orgasm
- Resolution

What about relationship? Or emotional intimacy? To answer these questions Dr. Rosemary Basson came up with a different paradigm for "normal" sexual response. Basson acknowledges that, first of all, sexual response is more than just a biologic firing of muscles and nerves. In addition, for most women, sexual desire, arousal, and climax are not linear. In other words, it is normal to not be in the mood but, in the spirit of "I want to make my partner/boyfriend/husband happy," to let him initiate sex and find that, lo and behold, it actually feels good when he touches your breasts, and suddenly you are having a jolly good time.

Basson emphasizes that for many women it is normal to start from a point of sexual neutrality and for desire to actually come after arousal. However, Basson also points out, receptivity is essential to initiating intimacy—as in "well he *did* make dinner tonight and put the kids to bed." If you feel adequate emotional intimacy with your partner, you will seek or be receptive to sexual stimuli. Receptivity to sexual stimuli allows you to move from sexual neutrality to arousal. If your mind continues to process the stimuli and proceeds to further arousal and sexual desire, and if everything is intact hormonally and physically, you will be able to move forward to sexual satisfaction and orgasm. This positive outcome fosters intimacy and reinforces sexual motivation, so that *you* may even be the one initiating sex the next time.

From Dr. Streicher's History Files

The supreme law for husbands is: Remember that each act of union must be tenderly wooed for and won, and that no union should ever take place unless the woman also desires it and is made physically ready for it.

—Married Love, 1918

Acknowledging sexual neutrality as real and as not a problem is an important concept in sexual health. So is appreciating that even if your sex drive appears to be gone, you are still a sexual being. Here's why:

You've heard it a million times in magazine articles and books:

Have sex even if you are not in the mood. Make a date. Put it on a schedule. And even if you are not in the mood, once he is kissing you, touching your breasts, and stimulating your clitoris, the flame of interest will flicker and five minutes later you'll be totally ready to go. The desire comes *after* the arousal. It works. And if you "schedule" sex often enough, your body will come to anticipate it, becoming aroused at the memory of what happened two nights ago and the anticipation of what's about to happen again. So yes, it does work to have sex even if you are not in the mood. The physical act of having sex will *put* you in the mood.

It's like going to the gym. You aren't in the mood to exercise, but you know you should and you have already paid your personal trainer for the session. You show up and ten minutes into the workout you realize that you are actually enjoying it, and by the time you finish you feel satisfied and are glad you went. Then you sign up for another training session.

What is key here is that sexual encounters should ultimately result in sexual satisfaction. If there is no pleasure—or worse yet, if the sex hurts or is impossible—the likelihood of there being a "next time" quickly diminishes.

Are you shaking your head, wondering when was the last time you even imagined, much less enjoyed, a bedroom scenario like the one described above? You are not alone. The fact is that if this whole sex-begets-more-sex thing is going to work, a number of things need to be in place.

Dr. Streicher's SexAbility Survey

Asked which movie best describes their usual sex experience,

> 10.6 percent said *Les Misérables*
> 33.9 percent said *It's a Wonderful Life*
> 32.7 percent said *Paradise Lost*
> 6.2 percent said *Rush Hour*
> 16.6 percent said *Are We There Yet?*

Female Sexual Dysfunction

Normal sexual function is so complex that it's *amazing* how often things go right. Its complexity also makes it easier to appreciate that many, many things can go wrong. All the things that can go wrong are grouped under the large heading of "female sexual dysfunction," or FSD.

FSD can manifest itself as low libido—just not having any interest in sex. Other women with FSD may have a desire for sex but experience intense pain when they do have intercourse. Still other women may experience desire but cannot become aroused.

Sexual problems are generally divided into four categories:

- Decreased libido (not feeling desire)
- Impaired arousal (being unable to lubricate and become excited)
- Problems with orgasm (having no orgasm or taking a really long time to climax)
- Dyspareunia (sex hurts)

The largest study in this area is called the Preside Study. Conducted in 2008 by Harvard gynecologist Dr. Jan Shifren, this study surveyed over 30,000 women age 18 to 102 to determine the frequency and impact of sexual dysfunction. Overall, 43 percent of women identified having at least one of the above dysfunctions, 39 percent reported low desire, 26 percent low arousal, and 21 percent orgasm difficulties. Sexual pain was not specifically examined in the Preside Study but has been identified in other studies as occurring about 15 percent of the time in the general population and over 50 percent of the time in postmenopausal women.

To further complicate matters, it is extraordinarily rare for any of these problems to stand alone. They inevitably overlap. If you don't become aroused, you won't lubricate and sex will hurt. If sex hurts, you will have no desire to do it again anytime soon. Additionally, psychological issues such as depression, anxiety, and fear are obviously going to affect your ability to feel desire or become aroused. Your ability to have a normal sexual response cycle is also affected by medical conditions such as diabetes and heart disease. The following chapters will look at all these conditions specifically.

And finally, while this book is not about relationships, I do need to emphasize that unless you are primarily self-sexual (most people have an excellent relationship with themselves!), your partner has an enormous impact on your sexual receptivity and ultimately your response. In other words, if you have no desire to have sex with your husband, or if you have a partner who is cruel to you, belittles you in the bedroom, or can't be bothered to shower, you do not have a sexual dysfunction disorder. Your lack of response is an absolutely normal response to your situation.

It All Starts in the Brain: Hormones and Neurotransmitters

While our life situations need to be safe, comfortable, and loving and our bodies need to be functioning, one of the most important prerequisites for normal, healthy sexual response begins in the brain. Perhaps you are aware that estrogen and testosterone are necessary before you can feel desire and arousal (more on that in chapters 12 and 13), but triggering sexual response involves many other factors, especially in the brain. MRI studies of women while they are sexually stimulated have shown the specific areas of the brain that are active during arousal and orgasm. Beyond hormones, neurotransmitters like epinephrine, dopamine, and oxytocin are also required. For example, too much serotonin squashes desire, which is why some women who take serotonin-stimulating antidepressants have low libido. Prolactin, the hormone that allows the production of milk in a nursing mother, also decreases desire. Our brains create a balance so that we want to have sex, but not all the time.

Here's a breakdown of the key hormones and neurotransmitters: some need to be present in order to have a normal sexual response, while others are increased by having sex.

Hormones and Neurotransmitters That Promote Sex

Dopamine *is associated with the reward portion of the brain. Think of things that you like experiencing—that's elevated dopamine. Sexual desire, pleasure, motivation, craving. High dopamine levels make you feel not only attracted to someone but maybe slightly obsessed. Dopey with love? That's all dopamine.*

Nitric oxide *is a neurotransmitter that is required for physical sexual responses, such as vaginal lubrication and the relaxation of smooth muscle fibers that allows the vagina to expand.*

Adrenaline *is one everybody knows. The release of adrenaline causes that sense of excitement and exhilaration that you feel when on a roller coaster or in the throes of a new relationship. It is also what makes you run really fast if a lion happens to be chasing you. A surge of adrenaline in the so-called fight-or-flight response is your body's automatic way of alerting you and getting your attention: your heart rate increases, your pupils dilate, your blood flow increases, and often you lose your appetite. (Who feels hungry when madly in love or being chased by a lion?!)*

Endorphins *come from the pituitary gland and hypothalamus. These are the feel-good chemicals that are also natural painkillers. That euphoric feeling that runners get during a race is the same euphoric feeling that occurs during orgasm, which might explain why millions of women run in marathons every year.*

Norepinephrine *is very similar to adrenaline and essentially causes a racing heart and that feeling of excitement. It also promotes the ability to orgasm.*

Oxytocin, *as every woman who has ever been in labor knows, is the hormone that causes uterine contractions; its synthetic version is Pitocin, which women are sometimes given to stimulate labor. Oxytocin is also responsible for bonding with your baby. Think of all the feelings that you have toward a newborn baby—the gushing affection, the love, the need to touch, hold, and cradle him. These feelings are reinforced through the release of oxytocin and help build long-term attachment and unconditional love in spite of the fact that this same baby may* have caused you 20 hours of excruciating pain and a large tear in your vagina. Oxytocin is also secreted during sexual touching and orgasm, resulting in the same kind of bonding and affection toward your partner that you feel toward your newborn baby.

Testosterone is a key hormone that not only is responsible for libido but also contributes to vaginal lubrication and arousal. Studies on the role of testosterone in female sexuality have been inconsistent, and while it is not clear how much testosterone a woman needs, we know she needs some!

Estrogen is not only the hormone associated with desire and excitement but also the primary hormone required for the physical changes that make sex pleasurable. Estrogen increases blood flow to the genitals and is responsible for vaginal lubrication.

Neurotransmitters That Put the Brakes On

Serotonin balances out the "I want to have sex all the time" feeling that comes from dopamine. This is why antidepressants that increase levels of serotonin can sometimes decrease libido.

Prolactin is increased in a nursing mother. In addition to stimulating milk production, elevated prolactin also decreases the desire to have more sex. Biologically, prolactin gives the new mother a break before she goes on to the next pregnancy.

So with these hormones and neurotransmitters in mind, let's revisit the four phases of sexual response. Here's how it all fits in:

Desire

Increased dopamine, norepinephrine, testosterone, and estrogen
Decreased serotonin and prolactin

Arousal

Increased dopamine, norepinephrine, nitric oxide, acetylcholine, estrogen, and testosterone
Decreased serotonin and prolactin

Orgasm
Increased norepinephrine, oxytocin, serotonin, and prolactin

Resolution
Increased serotonin
Decreased dopamine

And, while all of that is happening, your body is *also* going through the physical changes that are required for intercourse!

The vagina is not normally prepared for intercourse. During the excitement phase, the presence of estrogen and the increase in neurotransmitters not only increase lubrication but allow the vagina to lengthen and expand in preparation for "receiving" a penis. These physical changes require a complex cascade of events.

Normally, moisture and lubrication result from a combination of secretions. While some of these secretions come from tiny vaginal glands (the Bartholin's and Skene's glands, described in chapter 3), the majority of the required moisture for sex comes directly from the vaginal walls.

What happens is that neurotransmitters during arousal cause the capillaries—the tiny vessels that supply blood to the vaginal walls—to dilate and fill with blood. The watery part of the blood (called the transudate) seeps out of the cells and provides moisture to the surrounding tissue. Estrogen also stimulates production of glycogen and acid mucopolysaccharides, substances that keep vaginal tissue slippery. Estrogen increases not only the number of capillaries in the vaginal wall but also the thickness of the tissue, allowing multiple accordion-like folds known as rugae to form. All of these physical properties are needed in order for the walls to lubricate and expand.

Estrogen is not the only hormone required for a normal physical response. There is now an increasing appreciation that testosterone is needed as well, since there are receptors in the vagina for testosterone that increase glycoprotein and mucous synthesis.

All those hormones and neurotransmitters need to get to the right place, which is why healthy blood flow throughout your body is essential. This is why many medical conditions, such as heart disease, hypertension, arteriosclerosis, stroke, venous insufficiency, sickle cell disorder, and diabetes, can have an impact on vaginal health and sexual function. Anything that alters hormones, such as hypothyroidism, adrenal dysfunction, diabetes mellitus, or menopause, can be problematic too.

In addition, your nerves need to fire and your muscles need to contract (and relax!) A medical illness, extreme fatigue, medication, or certain neurologic problems such as spinal cord injury, neuropathy, herniated disc, and multiple sclerosis can affect neuromuscular function and, in turn, your sex life (see chapter 15).

So Back to What's "Normal" When It Comes to Your Sexual Response

"Normal" is the coordination of hormones, neurotransmitters, blood flow, neurons, and muscles that allows you to feel desire, get aroused, and ultimately have a satisfying sexual experience. Again, when I talk about what's "normal," I'm not talking about what constitutes normal in terms of sexual behavior, what turns people on, or what activities they engage in. I'm speaking about normal in terms of physiological response, as in the way the body is supposed to work . . . if all is working the right way.

What Are People Really Up To?

Having said that, there is always a curiosity about what other people are doing to "light their fire," so here it is:

82 percent of women masturbate

96 percent of men masturbate

91 percent of women give oral sex (52 percent swallow)

79 percent of men give oral sex

65 percent of men find it important for their partner to have an orgasm

67 percent of women find it important for their partner to have an
orgasm

Source: Pepper Schwartz and James Witte, *The Normal Bar* (2013)

Masturbation: "Dancing with Myself"

Self-sexuality is normal human sexual behavior. Masturbation, or self-stimulation, is often solo, but in many cases also enjoyed by couples. While self-stimulation has no doubt been a reality since Eve found her clitoris and Adam discovered his penis (a far easier task), societal and medical views of masturbation have been far from accepting for a long time.

In 1916, Winfield Scott Hall, a professor of physiology at Northwestern University Medical School, published *Sexual Knowledge* for "the instruction of young wives and young husbands." He wrote:

> *Nature's plan for development of radiant womanhood may be defeated, if she plays with these organs. This act is usually called "self abuse" . . . the destructive and loathsome habit of self abuse is occasionally acquired by girls quite accidently (or) learned from older, low-minded, vulgar girls who seem to delight in teaching their own bad habits to younger girls. Whether this habit is learned accidently or through evil associations, it is in every case not only subversive of Nature's plan for the development of the girl into beautiful woman hood, but it also serves as a serious shock to her nervous system, and if persisted in, will cause a wreck of that system.*

Phew!

So while masturbation is hardly a new phenomenon, a number of factors have influenced the frequency of masturbation among women, and it is now likely that the number of women who self-stimulate is higher than ever. Why are more women self-stimulating today? Here are some possible answers:

Women live longer than men, as a rule. If they don't have partners later in life, masturbation may play a role in their sexuality.

Much more information on self-stimulation is now available to women, especially on the Internet.

It has become less taboo to buy and use vibrators and other sex toys.

With greater concern about sexually transmitted infection, self-stimulation becomes a safe option.

And like every other sexual behavior, masturbation frequency changes over the course of someone's life span. In 2006 the Kinsey Institute conducted the National Survey of Sexual Health and Behavior via the Internet. Over 2,000 women, age 18 to 92, were polled. This survey determined, among other things, the number of women who self-stimulated on a regular basis according to age, general health, and relationship status. Both women who masturbated when alone and those who did so with a partner were included.

The frequency of self-stimulation was different by age group (and most common in the 18 to 39 age group), but it was not related to relationship status or general health. Overall, about one-third of women included in the survey self-stimulated on a regular basis.

Here's the breakdown according to age:

Age	Solo	Partnered
18–24	50.0%	26.7%
25–29	61.4	34.7
30–39	49.5	29.9
40–49	50.1	19.7
50–59	39.6	12.1
60–69	33.1	8.1
70–100	16.1	3.2

These numbers are considerably lower than the 82 percent reported by Dr. Pepper Schwartz in *The Normal Bar*. The interesting point here, however, is that while it is commonly accepted that every red-blooded healthy young man masturbates, there is a shame and silence about young women doing the same. Many of them don't even know *how,* since it is unlikely that most mothers give their daughters instructions! No wonder women often make it to middle age without ever having an orgasm!

Make no mistake: women who self-stimulate are more orgasmic, more sexually satisfied, and more likely to have healthy partnered sex than women who don't. After all, how can a woman direct a partner in what to do if she doesn't even know how to do it herself?

From Dr. Streicher's History Files: What Doesn't Cause Sexual Problems

It wasn't very long ago that masturbation was perceived to be a potentially life-threatening activity, and the belief was that anything other than the missionary position during intercourse was immoral. This started in 1712 with the publication of *Onania: The Heinous Sin of Self Pollution and all its Frightful consequences in both Sexes considered with spiritual and physical advice to those who have already injured themselves by this abominable practice.* The title (possibly the world's longest) says it all. In 1758 the Swiss physician Samuel-Auguste Tissot published a popular textbook with the same theme entitled *Onanism, Treatise on the Diseases caused by Masturbation, Self Pollution and Other excesses;* in it he outlines the scientific basis for why masturbation was not only responsible for multiple diseases but was often fatal!

Can You Have a Healthy Sex Life Without Vaginal Intercourse?

Ask any lesbian this question and she will answer, *"Of course!"* But what most heterosexual women want is penetrative vaginal-penile sex. Many women are reading this book because they are no longer able to have enjoyable penetrative sex and would like to do so.

There is no question that the majority of women will be able to solve whatever issues have been sabotaging their love life. But as much as I would like to promise that every woman who wants to have satisfying penetrative intercourse will in fact do so after reading this book, I can't. The truth is that some women, no matter how motivated, will find that their personal issues prevent them from having comfortable intercourse.

This may be the woman who has been treated for a pelvic cancer and suffered severe radiation changes, or the woman who loses the use of her vagina because of surgery. In a number of relatively rare but all too real circumstances, intercourse is out of the question, either temporarily or permanently. And that's where the concept of the "new normal" comes in. The new normal may be sexual satisfaction from external clitoral stimulation, oral sex, anal sex, or maybe just kissing and hugging.

Sadly, many couples expect any sexual overture to culminate in the grand finale of intercourse and assume that, if that's not going to be the case, it is best not to even start.

There are many ways to be sexual without intercourse, and many women (and men) find that without the pressure of intercourse, sexual activity can become even more satisfying. As more than one patient has told me, "We don't have intercourse, but we have great sex!"

The Perfect Ending? The Truth About Women and Anal Sex

Masturbation is not the only sexual activity that is considered by many to be taboo. The fact is that anal intercourse is part of the sexual repertoire of many couples. In some cases, anal intercourse becomes a welcome substitute if vaginal intercourse is out of the question. Indeed, according to some surveys, as many as 5 to 10 percent of sexually active women are estimated to engage in anal intercourse regularly. Another 2010 study of over 2,000 women reported a total of 10.3 to 14.4 percent of women in the 18 to 39 age range as having anal intercourse in the past 90 days.

The vagina is a two-way passage—the penis goes in, and the baby comes out. The rectum, on the other hand, is meant to be a one-way passage, so there are a number of health considerations to keep in mind if you want to engage in anal play:

- The anus lacks the natural lubrication of the vagina, which means that penetration can cause tearing inside, allowing bacteria and viruses to enter the bloodstream. When this happens, the body becomes vulnerable to sexually transmitted infections (see chapter 18).
- The anus was designed to hold in feces and is therefore full of bacteria, which can cause or transmit infection. A pre-session enema may make things appear "cleaner" but does not eliminate bacteria.
- Anal sex may weaken the anal sphincter, which may result in fecal incontinence.
- Oral contact with the anus can spread virus and bacteria and cause infection. If you do enjoy anal sex, make sure to use a condom.

You Can Find Your SexAbility!

As you work your way through the rest of the book, you will understand why you need to address every aspect of sexual function, not just one. So, if you have no libido, don't just flip to the libido chapter and expect your problem to be solved.

This book is not about fixing your relationship, though I do address (though only in passing) the fact that the inability to have sexual pleasure can sabotage a relationship and a problematic relationship can sabotage your sex life. Any bookstore, however, has shelves of excellent books on fixing your relationship, putting excitement back into your marriage, or feeling sexual about your partner again after the "magic" has evaporated. Some of those books are listed in the resources section at the end of this book.

The next 16 chapters are about dealing with physical, hormonal, and medical problems so that sex becomes enjoyable and, in some cases, possible. In other words, this book will help you find your SexAbility and help you love sex again!

3

AN UP-CLOSE VIEW OF YOUR GENITALS

*Your private parts should be a little
less private—at least to yourself*

The vagina is a dark and mysterious place. It is the passage by which most of us enter the world. As a child, we think that pee magically comes out of it. As an adult, the vagina becomes the place where our sexuality is housed, and regardless of our orientation (heterosexual, homosexual, or self-sexual), the vagina is associated with pleasure. Until, that is, something goes awry; then the vagina becomes a place associated with pain.

Men have always had the clear advantage of being able to inspect their genitals with very little effort. Women's genitals are not quite as accessible, resulting in a lot more uncertainty about what's normal and what's not. Most women simply rely on their annual gynecologic exam to ensure that all is well.

The Gynecologic Exam

Many women approach their yearly exam the way I approach yearly maintenance on my car. I honestly have no clue what the mechanic is checking for, but I routinely do it and am always relieved to hear that "everything's fine" without ever knowing or caring about the details. While there is nothing wrong with trusting your physician (or your mechanic!), if you are having issues, you really need to understand the specifics of what is being checked during the exam.

Basically, an annual exam includes a visual inspection of the external genitalia, a speculum exam to look inside the vagina, and then the bimanual exam in which the physician places one or two fingers in the vagina and the other hand on the abdomen in order to feel the uterus and ovaries and check for any pelvic masses. Most women aren't even aware that the external inspection is occurring unless your gynecologist comments on normal or abnormal findings. The bimanual exam may feel strange, but is usually painless. It's the speculum exam that many women dread, almost as much as the scale. Some women skip their annual checkup, deciding it is far more appealing to take a chance on dying from some unnamed, undiagnosed gynecologic disease than enduring a potentially painful speculum exam. This is particularly true for the woman who is experiencing sexual pain.

But speculums are not "one size fits all," and sometimes it's just a matter of using the right speculum to ensure that the exam is not agonizing. Just as many women are "hard to fit" types when it comes to jeans or bras, there are also "hard to fit" types when it comes to speculums. It's not just about length and width; it's also about how wide they open. The speculum I use for a 16-year-old virgin is a completely different instrument than the one I would use for a 40-year-old woman with three kids or a 70-year-old who is well into menopause, and it is unlikely that I would use the same speculum for a four foot ten woman as a six foot tall woman. My choice of speculum is dependent not only on the size of the vaginal opening but also on the length of the vagina, the elasticity of the vaginal walls, the position of the uterus, and what I need to accomplish while up there. For example, the amount of exposure I need to swab vaginal discharge is different from what I need to do a Pap test, a uterine sampling, or a major procedure. In some types of exams I don't need to use a speculum at all.

So if the speculum is pinching, it can be readjusted. If it hurts, your doctor might be able to use a different size. Your doctor has no way of knowing if you are uncomfortable unless he or she reads your face—so don't hesitate to speak up.

In addition, a family practitioner or internist is not going to be as experienced or have the wide selection of speculums that a gynecologist has, so if your annual exam has been painful in the past, you might want to see a specialist.

One last thing about your annual exam: At least once a day a patient apologizes to me for not having shaved her legs or had a pedicure before climbing into the stirrups. In addition to being worried that I am going to find some dread disease, these patients think I am judging their hairy legs, unwaxed crotch, or chipped toe polish. It reminds me that what is a very routine exam for me is anything but routine for the women who are experiencing it. But going for your annual gynecological exam is not like your annual dental checkup, where brushing and flossing are essential. Women need do nothing to prepare for an exam with their gynecologist. A trip to the gyno is a "come as you are" party. Truly, my only expectation is basic hygiene—a shower or bath within the previous 24 hours is always appreciated.

In fact, sometimes a woman's efforts to prepare for an exam could actually diminish my ability to accurately assess the situation or get accurate test results. It is impossible to evaluate an abnormal discharge or odor if the environment has been altered. That means no spermicide, no medications, no lubricants, no douching, and, ideally, no sex for 24 hours before your appointment.

Should you cancel your annual exam if you "forget" the night before and do have intercourse? Realistically, after waiting two months for an appointment, asking for the afternoon off work, and discovering that you're in desperate need of a refill on your hormone therapy, it may not be practical to take a pass. Usually it won't make a difference, but do be sure to mention to your gynecologist that you had sex and be aware that you may need to schedule a return visit if the evaluation is incomplete. If you are coming in specifically to check out an abnormal discharge or odor, you should probably reschedule. It's pretty much impossible to figure out what is going on if you had intercourse hours before your visit.

If you are bleeding as a result of intercourse, don't reschedule. It is actually ideal for me to see you within 24 hours so I can see if the blood is originating from the uterus, the cervix, or the walls of the vagina. Just don't "prepare" for your visit in my waiting room or bathroom.

And no, I swear that I really don't notice and don't care if you have shaved your legs and gotten a pedicure.

The Details of Down There: Anatomy 101

While it is tempting to rely on your gynecologist to ensure that all is well, understanding where things are and how they work will ultimately enable you to better understand the source of many sexual issues. And since for many women the last (maybe only) time they read about the sexual parts of the pelvis was in seventh grade, a review is in order. So here's my view from the other side of the stirrups.

External Genitalia

Your external genitalia, or vulva, include all the parts you can see without any special instruments. All you need is a decent-sized hand mirror with a long handle. The vulva specifically includes the mons pubis, labia, clitoris, vestibule, hymen, and perineum.

Pubic Hair

Mons pubis refers to the soft mound where the majority of pubic hair grows. The distribution of hair as well as its color and coarseness are genetically determined, with a wide range of what is considered normal. Of course, what I see is often not a reflection of what is really going on, since changing trends in hairstyles are not limited to the hair on your head. As a gynecologist, I get a firsthand view of what's fashionable. Today less is more, and many women I see alter their pubic hair in some way, whether it's just a trim or complete removal.

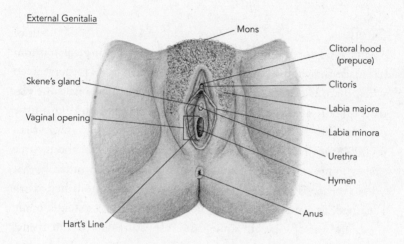

External Genitalia

Mons

Clitoral hood (prepuce)

Skene's gland

Clitoris

Labia majora

Vaginal opening

Labia minora

Urethra

Hymen

Anus

Hart's Line

But let's get back to what's normal. Left untouched, the pubic hair of most young women ranges in its thickness, texture, and degree of abundance; some women have a sprinkling of scant fine hair, while others have coarse, curly hair that not only covers the mons but also creeps up the abdomen and down the thighs. Loss of pubic hair can be an indication of illness, and sudden excessive growth can be an indication of a hormonal abnormality.

Hormones influence hair growth, so it makes sense that as women age and hormones decline, pubic hair thins out. It is not unusual for a woman in her seventies or eighties to have very little to no pubic hair. And yes, just like the hair on your head, genital hair can go gray, but strangely enough, not always at the same time. While some women dye their grays, I don't recommend it. I have seen a number of dying disasters, including one really nasty clitoral burn from peroxide that put my patient in the hospital.

Vulvar Skin

The skin on the vulva should appear similar to the skin everywhere else on your body. Any inflammation, rash, new growth, discoloration, ulceration, bleeding, burning, or very itchy area should be evaluated by your doctor.

Clitoris

Thank God for the clitoris. Even when pain or surgical removal has made the vagina completely unusable, the clitoris is there. Even when there is no penis available, the clitoris is there. And the clitoris is really a wondrous structure. While it just seems like a little pea, the clitoris is actually made up a bundle of nerves (more than 8,000!) that dives into the body and usually measures about three inches long, reaching just under the pubic bone. In other words, what you see is just the tip of the iceberg. I was astonished when I learned, as a medical student, how far the clitoris extends inside the body, out of view. In some cases it measures up to four inches in length. No wonder it is capable of giving such remarkable pleasure! Like a penis, the clitoris becomes engorged with blood when sexually stimulated, and it is the site that triggers most orgasms for women. (In my lecture on sex reassignment surgery—yes, I do that, but we'll save talking about it for the next book—I describe a procedure in which the clitoris is surgically dissected and used to make a penis for transgender women, because embryologically the clitoris and the penis develop from the same tissue.)

The part of the clitoris that is visible is called the glans. The glans is partially or completely covered by the prepuce, which looks like a little hood. While normal clitorises vary widely in size, a very small or very large clitoris is associated with hormonal abnormalities. The clitoris should be at least partially visible and the size, at a minimum, of a Q-tip.

Labia Majora

Yes, your vagina speaks Latin! The labia majora refer to the "large or outer lips" that surround the vagina. The labia majora are folds that include the skin and fatty tissue that start at the mons pubis and extend to about an inch above the anus. In young women they tend to be plump and full, and in older women less so.

Labia Minora

The labia minora are the "minor lips" that surround the "mouth" of the vagina. Unlike the labia majora, the labia minora have no fatty tissue and are very thin. The labia minora start at the clitoral hood and end right below the vaginal opening.

There is a wide variation of normal when it comes to the labia minora. They may be short and barely visible, or they may protrude outside of the labia majora and be very visible. Their color also varies—from rosy pink to dark brown. As women age and estrogen levels decline, the color tends to fade.

While we are on the subject of labia, it is worth noting that one of the side effects of sparse pubic hair is making the labia minora much more visible. No one is more self-critical than women, and in keeping with the popularity of surgical procedures to alter nose, breast, and butt size, women are more frequently asking to have their labia size altered. Take

Dr. Streicher's SexAbility Survey

From a list of descriptions, women identified their pubic hairstyles as:

> 22.8 percent said "an overgrown forest"
>
> 43.9 said "neat and trimmed"
>
> 9.7 percent said "a landing strip"
>
> 19.3 said "bald"
>
> 4.37 percent said "Vajazzled"

Men weighed in on their preferred pubic hairstyle for the ladies in their lives:

> 7.5 percent said "an overgrown forest"
>
> 32.3 percent said "neat and trimmed"
>
> 9.7 percent said "a landing strip"
>
> 20.3 percent said "bald"
>
> 32.3 percent said "I don't care, I'm just happy to be invited to the party"

a look at chapter 19 if you are interested in the details of that procedure!

Perineum
This soft, sensitive territory lies between the vagina and the anus and is sometimes quite short. This is the area that sometimes tears during childbirth and where an episiotomy (an intentional cut to facilitate delivery) is sometimes performed.

Vestibule
The vestibule refers to the area immediately outside of the vagina, from and including the hymen and ending with the labia minora. The vestibule has a rich nerve supply, which is why it is the area that is most likely to be painful, uncomfortable, or itchy if there is an infection or atrophy. When most women refer to their vagina, they are really referring to the vestibule. Within the vestibule are tiny lubricating glands—Skene's glands, which are located right next to the urethral opening, and Bartholin's glands, which are located at the bottom of the vaginal opening.

Urethra
The urethra is the tube that carries urine from the bladder to the outside. The urethra is actually about an inch long, but you only see the opening, known as the meatus, where the urine comes out. It is inside the vestibule.

Introitus
The introitus is the port of entry into the vagina and is marked by the hymen in virgins, or hymeneal remnants in someone who has had intercourse. That said, if a hymen is not "intact" it does not mean that someone is not a virgin. Hymens can be broken as a result of exercise or other activities. Contrary to popular belief, tampon use does not alter the appearance of a virginal hymen.

Hymens vary from very thin and flimsy to a virtual wall. (In such a case, first attempts at intercourse can be very painful and traumatic.) In some very rare cases, hymens have no opening and may require surgical excision. These girls are unaware of when they start to menstruate (because of the lack of flow), and the blood accumulates in the vagina. Usually after months of progressively painful cramps, a doctor figures this out and surgically opens the hymen to treat the problem.

In a young woman, the introitus is often not visible without separating the labia minora with fingers. A "relaxed" introitus refers to a vaginal opening that appears gaping or stretched out. This is typically seen in women who have had vaginal deliveries. In general, a gaping introitus is not a cause of pain or sexual dysfunction. In a postmenopausal woman, the appearance is even more variable, depending on whether she delivered vaginally, how much relaxation is present, the degree of atrophy, and whether she has remained sexually active.

Internal Genitalia
Vagina

Just inside the hymen (or the remnants of the hymen) is where the vestibule officially ends. The actual vagina is an internal tubelike organ that begins at the hymen and ends at the cervix. Unless you own a speculum, it is not something you can see on your own.

The health of your vagina is associated with several characteristics:

Color: *The color should be a rich, deep pink.*

Rugae: *These are accordion-like folds of the wall of the vagina that allow for maximum elasticity and stretchability. The more of these folds the better.*

Vaginal wall thickness: *A normal vaginal wall is about three to four millimeters thick. With age and lack of estrogen, the walls become very thin and pale.*

Lubrication: *The walls of the vagina should appear moist, not dry.*
Discharge: *A clear mucous discharge is normal.*

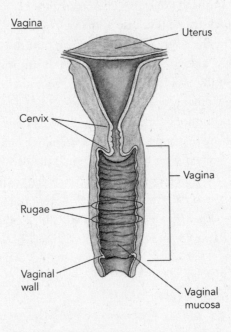

If you put the vaginal wall under a microscope, you would also see that the walls normally have a rich blood supply and lots of plump cells that make up the three layers. The vagina itself does not contain a lot of nerve endings. Most "vaginal" pain actually emanates from the areas that do have a rich nerve supply, such as the vestibule.

The length of a normal vagina is not only highly variable but changes throughout a woman's cycle and throughout her life. It also changes depending on the situation . . . childbirth, intercourse, and so on. There is a wide range of normal. The important thing is that a normal vagina is highly stretchable and can comfortably accommodate even the most substantial penis.

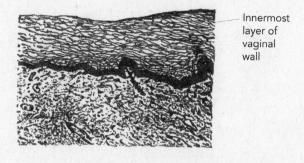

Innermost layer of vaginal wall

The G-Spot

A G-spot is not something you are ever going to see. Indeed, some researchers still doubt its existence. The existence of the G-spot is heatedly debated, and I have found that talking about the G-spot in a room full of sexual experts is like talking politics in a room full of Republicans and Democrats. Very few are going to let actual facts stand in the way of opinion.

First described in 1981 by a German gynecologist by the name of Grafenberg, the G-spot is an area approximately one to three inches from the vaginal opening under the urethra. G-spot stimulation, according to believers, results in powerful orgasms and ejaculation of fluid. One hypothesis is that the G-spot is actually just an extension of the clitoris. Others believe it to be a discrete, separate structure. Probably the best evidence that the G-spot actually exists was published in 2012 in an article in the *Journal of Sexual Medicine*. Dr. Adam Ostrzenski described the anatomical location of the G-spot as a distinguishable sac of erectile-type tissue, measuring eight millimeters by three millimeters, located a few millimeters from the urethra. (For the record, I do think there is a G-spot, but I do not believe every woman experiences pleasure from stimulation of that specific area.)

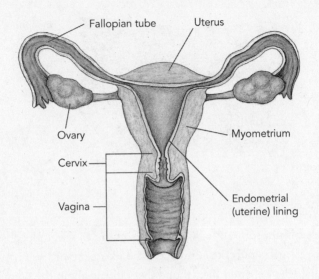

Fallopian tube Uterus

Ovary

Cervix

Vagina

Myometrium

Endometrial
(uterine) lining

Cervix

The cervix is the opening to the uterus. It lets menstrual blood out and sperm in. It is fused to the bottom of the uterus but is actually a separate structure, both anatomically and functionally. Normally, the cervix is a thick-walled tubular structure about three to four inches long; it shortens and thins out in labor to allow the baby to exit the uterus. The internal os (the opening) is the part that connects to the uterus; the external os is at the back of the vagina and is what the gynecologist sees when she uses a speculum during your pelvic exam.

Uterus

The uterus is a muscular organ, normally the size of a small pear. During pregnancy it expands to hold whatever it needs to, whether that is a six-pound baby or quadruplets. It normally weighs about two ounces and sits in the pelvis behind the pubic bone, nestled between the bladder and the rectum.

Prior to menopause, the lining of the uterine cavity sloughs off each month during menstruation, unless a woman becomes pregnant. If conception occurs, the uterus becomes a soft, cushy bed for the developing fetus. In a menopausal woman, the lining becomes thin and should be totally inactive, which is why postmenopausal bleeding always needs to be evaluated.

The uterus is such an interesting organ that I have written an entire book, *The Essential Guide to Hysterectomy,* about the controversies surrounding decisions to remove it.

Ovaries

The ovaries are next to the uterus. During the reproductive years, ovaries secrete the hormones estrogen and progesterone. Estrogen stimulates receptors in multiple locations throughout a woman's body, including the uterus, breasts, and vaginal walls. Among other things, estrogen is partially responsible for female sexual maturation, libido, sexual response, and initiation and regulation of the menstrual cycle. Progesterone is responsible for preparing the uterus for pregnancy and maintaining the pregnancy. Androgens such as testosterone are also secreted from the ovaries and are responsible, in part, for libido.

Now that you know what is down there, it's time to take a look at what is happening—or not.

4

WHEN YOUR VAGINA IS IN A PHUNK

What your vaginal pH should be— and why it matters

Any woman who has ever watched a celebrity flip her shiny hair in a TV commercial knows how vitally important it is to use a pH-balanced shampoo. No one knows why (I certainly don't), and I would refer you to your hairdresser for more information. When it comes to the importance of vaginal pH, however, I'm an expert. To have a healthy sex life, a woman has to have a healthy vagina. Making sure your vaginal pH is normal is a key component of your "tool box," since it is critical to almost every issue that will be discussed going forward—from vaginal dryness to vaginosis to pain in your pelvis.

What Is pH and Why Is It Important to My Vagina?

The term "pH" stands for "potential hydrogen" and is a measure of the acidity of the vaginal environment. (Yes, your vagina is an environment!) Your vaginal ecosystem is predominantly populated with beneficial bacteria called lactobacilli, the so-called good guys, which produce lactic acid and keep your pH in a healthy range.

But like most neighborhoods, the vagina houses just enough of the pathogenic (bad) bacteria to potentially cause trouble if allowed to get out of hand.

A low, acidic pH keeps the vagina healthy for a number of reasons:

- Low pH increases antibacterial activity to keep good and bad bacteria in balance and decrease the opportunities for bad bacteria to grow.
- Low pH allows lactobacilli to colonize vaginal tissue, which in turn allows vaginal walls to function as a protective barrier to infection.
- Low pH prevents the growth of the pathogenic bacteria, such as *Gardnerella,* that cause odor, irritation, and discharge.

Unless something tips the balance, reproductive-age women (after puberty and before menopause) can normally maintain a healthy vaginal pH between 3.5 and 5 on a scale of 0 to 14. The healthy range between 3.5 and 5 indicates that there is an abundance of lactobacilli, a minimum of pathogenic bacteria, and a generally acidic environment. The problems occur when this balance is thrown off.

Triggers That Upset Your pH Balance

A number of triggers can upset the vaginal ecosystem and elevate pH, causing a funky odor, an increase or change in vaginal discharge, or a bacterial infection.

- **Menstruation:** Blood has a pH of 7.4, so when you menstruate, vaginal pH becomes elevated. Many women who suffer from recurrent infections find that their period is often the event that sets them in motion. This is particularly a problem for the perimenopausal woman, who has the double whammy of fluctuating estrogen levels upsetting her ecosystem along with her periods.

- **Intercourse:** The pH of semen is 7.1 to 8. That funky "day after intercourse" odor happens not because he has smelly sperm, but because the elevation in pH caused by his semen allowed the pathogenic bacteria to quickly multiply, crowding out the "good guys."
- **Douching and Cleansers:** Any vaginal infusion of water or other fluids can affect pH. The pH of water is 7. Fragrances and perfumes can further tip the balance and be irritating to the vagina.
- **Medication:** Many medications, such as medicated douches, allergy and cold medications, and anti-estrogen chemotherapies, can dry out tissues and sometimes change vaginal pH.
- **Antibiotics:** Antibiotics are meant to kill pathogenic bacteria. Along the way, they can also kill off beneficial bacteria, allowing yeast and bad bacteria to predominate. Pretty much every woman is familiar with the frustrating cycle of treating a nongynecologic infection, such as a bladder infection or bronchitis, only to then deal with the inevitable vaginal infection.
- **Perimenopause and Menopause:** Anytime estrogen declines, vaginal pH rises. In fact, it is more useful for me to measure vaginal pH levels than to measure estrogen levels to determine the impact of hormonal fluctuations or decline. Vaginal atrophy is almost always associated with an elevation in pH. Vaginal pH may reach levels of 5.5 to 6.8 or higher in postmenopausal women.

An elevated pH is one indication that lactobacilli levels are low and "bad" bacteria are overpopulating the vagina. While some women with an alteration in the vaginal ecosystem have no symptoms, many have a funky odor and more discharge than usual. At its extreme, the result is bacterial vaginosis.

Bacterial Vaginosis

Bacterial vaginosis (BV), not yeast, is the most common cause of abnormal vaginal discharge, accounting for 40 to 50 percent of cases. While most women assume that any abnormal discharge is a yeast infection, it's usually not. A number of studies have shown that even if a woman has had a yeast infection before, she is correct in her subsequent self-diagnosis of a yeast infection only 35 percent of the time. The first thing most women do when they get that uncomfortable "something's happening down there that shouldn't be" feeling is to run off to the drugstore and buy one of the dozens of anti-yeast medications available over the counter. More times than not, these over-the-counter products do not work—not because they are not good products, but because BV, not yeast, is the culprit. So how do you recognize the difference between yeast and bacterial vaginosis before you spend a month's salary on the wrong medication?

Tampons

Since menstrual blood is known to increase pH, it makes sense that since tampons are *designed* to keep menstrual fluids in the vagina, they can further contribute to the problem, if there is a problem.

There's a Fungus Among Us: The Difference Between Yeast Infections and Bacterial Vaginosis

A vaginal yeast infection is caused by a fungus, usually by *Candida albicans*. This is a very common fungus, found on the skin or in the gastrointestinal tract. A small amount of the fungus can live in the vagina without causing a problem, but an overgrowth of yeast results in the all-too-familiar cottage-cheese-like discharge and extreme itching. Antibiotics that kill surrounding bacteria frequently allow yeast to flourish, which is why yeast infections often occur after treating another illness.

BV, unlike yeast, does not result from a predominance of a single abnormal fungus but is a result of an overall change in the vaginal environment that eliminates the lactobacilli and allows an overgrowth of many types of less desirable bacteria, the most common being *Gardnerella vaginalis*. These unwelcome bacteria produce enzymes, which in turn break down vaginal protein, causing an unpleasant discharge and odor.

Unlike yeast infections, which have a thick white appearance, the discharge associated with BV is thin, grayish, and watery. Yeast has no odor, or possibly a slightly yeasty odor. BV has a characteristic fishy odor that gets even more pungent after intercourse, since semen increases pH levels and therefore exacerbates the situation. Condoms minimize BV-related effects, so if you are prone to BV, you may want to use a condom.

Vaginal Discharge: The Perils of Self Diagnosis

For most women, the process of diagnosing BV goes like this:

Step 1: You notice a pungent smell, irritation, and a discharge that wasn't there before.

Step 2: You then make a midnight run to the corner pharmacy and after a humiliating conversation with the (male) pharmacist, you buy at least three products, usually spending your entire Starbucks budget for the month in the process.

Step 3: You get home and put disgusting cream into your vagina. You repeat for three nights, per directions. For the next few days you wear a panty shield in order to protect your underwear from the yucky medicine constantly coming out of your vagina, including the huge glop that plops out during the important presentation at work the next day. You make multiple excuses to your partner about why you don't want to have sex.

Step 4: You finally finish the round of medication only to discover that the disgusting odor and irritation haven't gone away.

Step 5: You call your gynecologist's office and beg for an appointment. You're told that the next available appointment is in two weeks.

Step 6: You send the receptionist flowers and beg for an earlier appointment, then get in on a cancellation, which happens to coincide with your weekly meeting with your boss. You tell your boss that you have an infection "down there" and you need to get to the doctor. Horrified, your boss asks for no further information.

Step 7: You take the afternoon off work to get to the doctor's office, sit in the waiting room, and then finally get in to see the doctor, who tells you that you don't have a yeast infection—you have BV, and you need to take an entirely different medication to make it go away.

Step 8: Relieved but frustrated, you go to the pharmacy, where you spend next month's Starbucks budget on a new medication. You get to choose between another disgusting vaginal cream that will plop out of your vagina or an oral medication that will require canceling all your social plans for the next week since you can't drink alcohol and you don't want everyone to think you're pregnant when you abstain. But finally, finally, in a few days you feel some relief.

What is the average time spent before getting a correct diagnosis of BV? At least two weeks. Average cost in time, money, and frustration? Way too high.

Vaginal Discharge: How Your Doc Checks It Out

As maddening as this process is, you really need to get an accurate diagnosis, especially if you have never had BV before. So how does your doctor make the diagnosis when you finally get your appointment?

He or she will put a speculum in, just like for a Pap test, and then use a swab to collect a sample of the discharge. If there is a suspicion of BV based on appearance and odor, some doctors simply check pH and look at the discharge under the microscope.

While this is not the most accurate way to make the diagnosis (other things can alter pH, and sometimes someone has more than one kind of infection), it is the least expensive and also generally the quickest way to figure out what is going on. Many doctors do not keep a microscope in the office and therefore rely on other tests that are more accurate but also more expensive. The most thorough way to determine if the culprit is indeed BV is to test the discharge for the presence of the DNA of *Gardnerella vaginalis*. While 95 percent accurate, (especially if combined with a measure of pH), these DNA probes are expensive and take anywhere from 12 to 72 hours to get a result.

Another approach your doctor may use is to test pH and the by-products of *Gardnerella* with one of the rapid-test office kits. These tests, while quick and less expensive, are not as accurate as the DNA tests—usually they have an 85 percent accuracy rate. If one of these tests comes back negative, you might want to go for another test if you are very concerned that you have BV.

What About Home Tests?

You can buy a kit (which is very expensive) at the drugstore that is supposed to determine if you have a yeast infection or a bacterial infection. This kit is nothing more than a pH test. They are most useful if your pH tests in the normal range, as this is a reasonable indication that your itching and discharge is the result of a yeast infection. An elevation in pH could mean BV, but it could also be atrophic vaginitis, the presence of menstrual blood, another infection like trichomonas, or semen. Save your money and go to your doctor instead.

Make It Go Away!

Once you have a diagnosis, the goal is to get rid of the discharge and odor ASAP.

In the United States, BV is treated with oral or vaginal metronidazole, clindamycin, or tinidazole. Each of these antibiotic products requires a prescription.

Being Proactive and Taking Care of Your Vaginal Health

The good news is that BV is treatable and pretty much any of the previously mentioned medications will make it go away. The bad news is that it comes back 30 to 50 percent of the time and most women who have had BV don't need a trip to the doctor to know they have it again. With such a high recurrence rate, it makes sense for women to be proactive and take steps (described below) to maintain a normal pH and let the lactobacilli do the work to prevent the overgrowth of bacteria instead of relying on recurrent courses of antibiotics to kill the offending bacteria once they have established residency.

Some women, in spite of doing everything right, still have a high recurrence rate. It's crucial to make sure there is nothing else going on. I had one patient who was treating her "BV" for months and finally at my insistence reluctantly came to the office to see what was causing her persistent vaginal odor and discharge. She was mortified when I pulled out a tampon she had forgotten from her last period—seven months earlier.

If you continue to have recurrent BV despite maintaining a normal pH and avoiding triggers, a more intense antibiotic regimen is in order, such as a prolonged course of oral metronidazole or tinidazole followed by twice-weekly applications of metronidazole gel for three to six months.

Not surprisingly, this long-term antibiotic approach can result in increased *yeast* infections. So unfair.

When women complain about a smell down there, I ask whether it smells like fish or smells like the zoo. If it smells like fish, more often than not it is bacterial vaginosis; if it smells like a zoo, the cause is usually a tampon that they forgot to remove.

Do You Even Need to Treat It?

Bacterial vaginosis will spontaneously resolve in up to one-third of women if the lactobacilli are able to charge in, take control, and give off lots of lactic acid so that the pH corrects itself. This is less likely to occur in a menopausal woman, however, because her baseline pH is well above the normal range.

The Consequences of BV Go Way Beyond a Smelly Discharge

It's not just about an irritating discharge. Women with BV are at risk for many more serious medical conditions, including preterm delivery, post-hysterectomy infection, and an increased tendency to acquire sexually transmitted infections such as gonorrhea and chlamydia. They also have an increased risk of pelvic inflammatory disease and subsequent infertility.

When BV-Like Symptoms Are Not BV

Occasionally a patient will complain of odor and irritating discharge but the tests for BV are negative. Sometimes the unpleasant smell and "discharge" are not even coming from the vagina. Incontinence (involuntary loss of urine) affects up to 30 percent of women. Urine on the outside of the vagina is extremely irritating. Urine on underwear is eventually going to smell. Sometimes it's hard to tell the difference.

In some cases the pH is "off" just enough to cause an odor without having full-blown BV. A course of Rephresh, an over-the-counter pH-regulating vaginal gel, often will correct the problem. In other situations, however, women are suffering from a more complicated condition known as atrophic vaginitis.

At first glance, atrophic vaginitis and BV seem to be the same thing. Both are associated with an elevation in pH. Both have an irritating discharge. The difference is that you can develop BV if you have normal estrogen levels. In fact, most BV is in young women, not menopausal women. Vaginal atrophy, on the other hand, is a direct result of low estrogen levels, which most typically is a result of the ovaries winding down during perimenopause or after menopause.

Atrophic vaginitis refers to a condition of low vaginal estrogen levels along with symptoms such as vaginal dryness, burning, itching, discharge, and bleeding. In addition, women with atrophic vaginitis have thin and inflamed vaginal tissue that not only bleeds easily but, yes, tears easily. Even a Pap test can cause bleeding and pain. It is no surprise, then, that intercourse for these women can truly be a nightmare. If that wasn't bad enough, women with vaginal atrophy are also at increased risk for recurrent urinary tract infections, urinary frequency and/or discomfort urinating even in the absence of an infection, yeast infections, and bacterial vaginosis. The treatment for atrophic vaginitis is vaginal estrogen (see chapter 13), which decreases the pH, thickens the vaginal tissues, and eliminates these symptoms. The vaginal moisturizer Replens is an option for women who prefer not to take estrogen.

Maintaining the Balance

Preventing recurring infections is always better than treating recurrent infections, and many women who suffer from recurrent BV infections find that their period or intercourse is the event that sets them in motion time after time. Some women ask how something as natural and normal as menstruation or intercourse can cause such a problem. Aren't women intended to have periods and sex? The answer is that, while most women's bodies can tolerate periods of pH elevation, in some women even a slight imbalance can tip the scales. In addition, women were never meant to have so many menstrual periods.

Biologically, women are supposed to be pregnant and/or nursing during their reproductive years. Today the average woman has two or three pregnancies, may start menstruating as young as eight or nine, and keeps on going until the early fifties. Modern women have on average 450 to 500 periods in a lifetime, as opposed to the

50 periods that our prehistoric ancestors experienced. No wonder our vaginas are exhausted! So no, I am not going to suggest that you stop having sex. I'm not going to suggest that menstruating women stop using tampons. (I consider tampons to be one of the top ten most important inventions of the twentieth century, right up there with sliced bread.) Luckily, there are a number of more practical strategies to maintain normal pH.

Don't Douche!

While douching is an incredibly tempting "quick fix," it will only freshen things up for about ten seconds and then inevitably make things worse. Not only does douching elevate the pH, it also dries out the tissues and washes away whatever lactobacilli you have. Scented douches can irritate things even more. In addition, douching is associated with an increase in pelvic inflammatory disease and subsequent infertility.

Consider Using Estrogen Therapy

In post-menopausal women, persistent odor and irritation, more often than not, is from vaginal atrophy, pH imbalance, or vaginal infections that will be corrected with systemic or local estrogen therapy. (See chapters 13 and 14 for more information.)

Avoid Menstruating

If, you are using hormonal contraception, such as a low-dose birth control pill, you can avoid the whole change in pH caused by menstrual blood by avoiding menstruation. That's right! Take your pill straight through the placebo days and skip having your period. And yes, this is safe. As discussed in chapter 9, skipping menstruation is a common treatment for endometriosis.

Vaginal Products for Normal pH

In addition to behavioral choices, there are a number of products available to restore and maintain normal pH.

- RePhresh is the over-the-counter vaginal gel that restores normal pH. It can be used every three or four days. In Europe it is actually approved to treat BV.
- RePlens is intended to be used as a long-acting vaginal moisturizer (see chapter 5), but like its sister product Rephresh, it also maintains a normal pH. Replens is a good alternative for women who are reluctant to use estrogen.
- A daily oral probiotic containing lactobacillus has been clinically shown to help maintain the normal amount of vaginal lactobacilli. Pro B, for example, contains two probiotic lactobacilli strains called *Lactobacillus rhamnosus GR-1* and *Lactobacillus reuteri RC-14*. These unique strains can naturally balance yeast and bacteria to maintain good vaginal health.

How Is Your Healthy pH Balance Relevant to Sex?

At the risk of stating the obvious, an imbalance in pH—whether it is due to vaginal atrophy, BV, or both—is pretty much going to sabotage your sex life. Here's why:

- Vaginal walls that are inflamed are not going to lubricate properly, making intercourse extremely uncomfortable.
- Unpleasant odor and discharge are not particularly conducive to feeling sexy or encouraging intimacy.
- Intercourse will generally result in even more discharge, inflammation, and odor.

Dr. Streicher's SexAbility Survey

When asked if they avoided receiving oral sex because they thought their vagina might smell or taste bad,

> 27.0 percent of women said yes
> 73.0 percent said no

Interestingly, nearly the same percentage of men avoided *giving* oral sex because of their partner's unpleasant vaginal odor or taste:

> 29.9 percent of men said yes
> 70.1 percent said no

The one thing that yeast infection, BV, and atrophic vaginitis all have in common is an alteration in the normal vaginal environment. Keep your pH normal and your vagina will thank you.

Myths

Myth: Wearing tight, wet bathing suits increases the risk of vaginal infections.
Truth: Wearing tight, wet bathing suits does not cause vaginal infections.

Myth: A probiotic intended for colon health also works for the vagina.
Truth: A probiotic *can* help keep healthy balance of good and bad bacteria in your vagina, but you need to take a vaginal, not a colon, probiotic such as Pro B.

Myth: Putting yogurt in your vagina is a good way to treat a yeast infection.
Truth: I happen to be a big fan of yogurt and eat it almost every day for breakfast. It is a great way to keep your weight in balance, but not your vagina. Eat it if you like it. Do not put it in your vagina.

Myth: Thong underwear increases vaginal infections.
Truth: Never!

Myth: BV and yeast infections are sexually transmitted infections.
Truth: While not sexually transmitted, they are sexually associated since intercourse can alter pH and increase susceptibility.

Myth: You can't have both BV and a yeast infection at the same time.
Truth: It's actually not uncommon to have both, since some of the same triggers that cause the lactobacilli to diminish also cause yeast to flourish. If you have both, you need to treat both.

part two

SEXABILITATORS:
ESSENTIALS TO FIX WHAT'S BROKEN

SLIP-SLIDING AWAY: LUBRICANTS AND MOISTURIZERS

The right product makes all the difference between sandpaper sex and slippery sex

Most drugstores have a dizzying selection of personal lubricants and moisturizers that promise everything from making things more slippery to increasing libido. There are shelves of vaginal lubricants that warm up, light up, and come with a theme song. Inexplicably, these products are generally located in the "family planning" section. That's right: the 65-year-old with vaginal dryness has to shop next to the 16-year-old surreptitiously buying a pregnancy test. As far as I'm concerned, the only family planning a 65-year-old with vaginal dryness should be thinking about is how to cut objectionable relatives out of the will.

When it comes to buying a lubricant, most women resort to one of two strategies. Either they grab the first product they see before they run into someone they know while stocking up on shampoo and deodorant to hide the fact that vaginal lubricant is the only thing on the list, or they grab a product that they have seen advertised. Women willing to linger often pick the brand that promises the most. Inevitably, the results are disappointing.

Here's the truth of the matter: Not all lubricants are created equal. In addition, lubricants and vaginal moisturizers are lumped together, even though they are intended to serve very different purposes. The only way to know what you are getting, and what you should use, is to understand what a lubricant is, what a moisturizer is, and what ingredients you need to look for to ensure that you are getting a product that does what you need it to do.

Lubricants: Slip-Sliding Away

A lubricant is to be used at the time of intercourse to reduce friction. Most lubricants are liquids, but there are some gel forms as well. They work immediately and are not absorbed.

A lubricant is recommended if your vagina is dry as a result of menopause, postpartum, cancer treatments, or a myriad of other conditions that will be discussed in the coming chapters. In any case, the key is to use a lube *before* attempting intercourse. Once you try and then experience the agony of sandpaper sex, it's pretty much "game over," since your vagina will go into protective mode to prevent another painful attempt. The pelvic muscles will spasm and tighten, the vaginal opening will be constricted, and the walls will become even drier than usual. Once that happens, you can pretty much forget it. A bathtub full of lube is not going to help. So slather the lubricant on you and your partner before you start. The worst that will happen is that it will be too slippery.

There are three basic categories of commercially available lubes: water-based, silicone-based, and oil-based. Hybrid lubes combine water and silicone.

Water-Based Lubricants

Water is interesting in that it can be really slippery (think slipping on a thin pool of it as you step out of the shower), but if there is a lot of friction, water can make things tacky or sticky. To combat this problem, most water-based lubes contain glycerin to keep things on the slippery side. Glycerin is similar to glucose, a sugar, and since yeast thrives on sugar, one of the problems with water-based lubricants is that they may promote vaginal yeast infections. Another ingredient often found in most, but not all, water-based lubes is a preservative known as propylene glycol, which many women find irritating.

The biggest issue with water-based lubes is that they tend to be gloppy and sticky and simply don't last very long. The major advantage to water-based lubes is price and availability.

Silicone-Based Lubricants

Silicone lubricants, on the other hand, are very slippery, long-lasting, and non-irritating. Like water-based lubes, they do not destroy latex and are condom-compatible. Since they don't break down in water, they are by far the best choice if you like having sex in the sauna, tub, or shower. (If you have never had sex in the shower, it's time that you did.)

The downside to a silicone lubricant is that they are generally more expensive, but remember: a little bit goes a long way. Another minor negative is that for those without a flesh-and-blood man on hand, silicone lubes should not be used with silicone vaginal toys or devices, since they will react with and roughen the surface (see chapter 20 for more on toys).

Also, alas, silicone lubes can stain the sheets, especially if they are satin. If that is a problem, you can always throw down a towel or a "sex sheet" over your regular sheet. If there is a stain, concentrated stain removers will usually remove it. Not to mention, it's not as if you are lying in a pool of the stuff. A lubricant generally stays where you put it . . . on his penis and in your vagina. The water-based lube manufacturers make a big deal out of the fact that their products don't stain, but I have yet to have a patient tell me that the silicone lubes are unacceptable because they ruin the sheets. Not to mention, it is far better to ruin the sheets than to ruin your sex life.

So where do you get silicone lubricants? Because of the higher price point, your local drugstore is unlikely to have much of a selection, and the silicone options, if they are even there, are often buried toward the bottom. Erotica shops, on the other hand, generally have a terrific assortment. The Internet is also a great way to find a selection of silicone lubes. Just be sure to specify silicone *vaginal* lubricant in your search or you are likely to come up with products meant for your carburetor.

Before a session of fantastic, slippery sex, you can even use a dab of silicone lubricant on your hair to make it smooth and shiny. Yes, the silicone product you put in your hair is essentially the same stuff that is manufactured to use as a vaginal lubricant. Just don't use an item intended for your hair in your vagina since the hair products have perfumes, which can be irritating.

And for the really thrifty shopper, there are a number of other uses for your silicone lube that have nothing to do with your genitals. Smear it all over your finger to get off that too-tight ring. Quiet a squeaky door. Polish your shoes. It's great for massages. It is also the perfect substitute for shaving cream when you have an "unexpected" sleepover guest. Not to mention, it allows for a close smooth shave anywhere on your body.

Oil-Based Lubricants

There are a handful of commercial lubricants that are oil-based rather than silicon- or water-based. Oil-based lubricants are not condom-compatible. They are also . . . oily. Some women like them because they are thinner and feel more like the real deal. While there are no studies that actually compare the various types of lubes, I have yet to have a patient tell me that an oil-based lube lasted as long or was as slippery as a silicone product.

Special Lubricants
Flavored Lubricants

Cookies and Cream, Sun-Ripened Strawberry, Chocolate-Raspberry, Passion Fruit, Cinnamon, Wild Cherry, Kiwi Strawberry, Lemon-Lime, Hot Strawberry, Orange-Mango, Watermelon (no seeds!), Bubble Gum, and Raspberry Kiss. Ben & Jerry, eat your hearts out.

There are three reasons why you might buy a flavored lubricant. One is that you have an unpleasant vaginal odor you are trying to cover up. If that's the case, find out *why* there is an odor and make it go away! The second reason to use a flavored lube is if the man in your life doesn't like the way a normal vagina tastes or smells. While that's his problem, his problem becomes your problem, and if that's the only way he will agree to oral sex, so be it. The third reason is that he loves the way you taste and smell, but you both think it would be "fun" to try a flavor. Some people even like to lick chocolate off each other's genitals. This goes in that category. And far be it from me to get in the way of fun.

Water-based flavored lubes are edible. Silicone-based flavored lubes are not considered edible, but if you swallow a little it won't cause any harm.

Warming Lubricants

The idea behind warming lubricants is that in addition to reducing friction they intensify and increase pleasurable sensations. An ingredient such as capsaicin, a component of chili peppers, causes the warming sensation. (I couldn't make this stuff up.) There are no scientific studies that have determined whether warming lubricants actually have a positive sexual effect. Anecdotally, and not surprisingly, many of my patients report a stinging or burning with these products. But if you put chili peppers in your vagina, maybe you should expect some burning to be involved.

Kosher Lubes?

There is only one lube that has gone to the trouble to pass the stringent requirements necessary to bear the "kosher" stamp that observant Jews require for any product used internally. Wet lubricants "kosherized" their production plant and passed rabbinical inspection to ensure that none of Wet's products contain ingredients derived from pigs or shellfish, and that any other animals used to create the lubes were treated humanely.

As Rabbi Shmuley Boteach, author of the bestselling book *Kosher Sex,* says, "It's nice to see that rabbis are not shying away from addressing sexual aids, which will facilitate great excitement in the bedroom," he said. "People misunderstand Orthodox Jews, in that they believe that they have sex through a sheet with a hole in the middle, that Orthodoxy is profoundly prudish. Orthodoxy is profoundly passionate. Orthodox couples have great sex lives."

And now, thanks to Wet, they are even better.

Oily Things

Good old petroleum jelly might seem like a good idea, but it's not. Not only is it just about impossible to wash off, but the jelly also traps bacteria and makes infection and irritation far more likely. In fact, a recent study showed that women who use Vaseline are more than twice as likely to develop bacterial vaginosis. In addition, petroleum products cause deterioration of latex, as in condoms, diaphragms, and cervical caps, which in turn increases the risk of pregnancy and sexually transmitted infections.

So use Vaseline on the lips on your face, not on the lips on your vagina. Or as one patient told me, the best sexual use of petroleum jelly is to slather it generously on the bedroom door to prevent the kids from coming in.

Baby oil is another popular lubricant, especially among women who are experiencing unexpected dryness postpartum. While readily available (postpartum, duh), it's not the best choice since, like petroleum jelly, baby oil can cause vaginal irritation and is associated with latex condom breakage. Oil-based products are also associated with a high rate of vaginal yeast infections.

Your Kitchen Pharmacy

Why not just slather on a little olive oil, butter, vegetable shortening, coconut oil, almond oil, or apricot oil? Here's the problem. Cooking oils, like petroleum jelly, dissolve latex and shouldn't be used with condoms. In addition, they don't rinse off easily and can trap bacteria. I also don't really see the allure of your vagina smelling like olive oil. In other words, these are great to use when making lunch, not when making love.

Already-There Lubricants (Bodily Fluids)

The human body produces lubricants that have the obvious advantage of being readily available and free, but they are not always enough to do the job. Saliva is a combination of mucous and water and is arguably the oldest sex lube. While not harmful, spit is primarily water, and it doesn't do much to decrease friction or make things slippery. In a pinch, it's better than nothing.

Pre-ejaculate is really slippery but low in volume, making it inadequate by itself. It's also not always available. And of course, the vaginal walls are supposed to provide lubrication, but if that were working for you, you wouldn't need a lubricant, would you?

Getting It Where It Needs to Go

So once you've selected the lubricant that will work for you, how do you use it? The easiest approach is to put a generous amount of lube on your (or his) fingers and apply it to the outside of your vagina. Coat his penis in it as well. (I guarantee he will like this part.) Let his penis be the delivery system to the inside of your vagina.

If you don't want to get it all over your hands, purchase a "lube shooter" or small cylinder with a plunger that is inserted in the vagina in order to squirt lube inside. This is also a strategy to use if for some reason you don't want him to know that your slippery moisture is not all "you" and you want to apply it in the bathroom before things get going.

Special Circumstances

Women who are trying to conceive are often faced with the conundrum of having to have intercourse on demand, even if they are not in the mood. "Honey, come home, I'm ovulating *right now!!!!*"

These women need extra lubrication, but most lubes affect sperm viability. Pre-Seed is currently the only lube on the market that has been tested and has demonstrated no impact on sperm motility or survival.

Then there are the "sensitive types" who get irritated no matter which lube they choose. If even silicone lubes are irritating to you, an iso-osmotic lube that is also glycerin-free, paraben-free, and preservative-free may not be the most slippery product, but is probably your best bet.

In general, most of my patients tell me that a good silicone lube makes all the difference in the world. So splurge. Trust me, if you spring for the good lubricant, your vagina, your partner, and even your hair will thank you.

> The power of the right lubricant is truly awe-inspiring. One patient told me that recommending it was the most valuable thing I had ever done for her. Apparently, even her three children that I'd delivered were of lesser importance.

A Moisturizer Is *Not* a Lubricant

All women of a "certain age" are well aware that the sure road to wrinkles is a dry face. Rare is the woman who doesn't apply some kind of lotion or cream on a regular basis to combat the lack of moisture.

The vagina also requires moisture to remain moist and supple, but the ravages of menopause, medications, postpartum, or chemotherapy can make plump, grapelike vaginal wall cells shrivel up like raisins.

Even the best lubricants do not thicken or alter the resulting dry, thin vaginal tissues; they just provide a slippery coating to reduce friction at the time of intercourse. A true long-acting vaginal moisturizer, on the other hand, is used regularly to increase the water content *inside* the cells that line the vagina, resulting in tissue that is more elastic, thicker, and better able to naturally produce lubrication. *It is used in anticipation of intercourse, not at the time of intercourse.*

Buyer, Beware!

In spite of claims from dozens of products that call themselves "long-acting moisturizers," most products labeled as "vaginal," "personal," or "feminine" moisturizers are actually vulvar moisturizers or lubricants. Only one product, Replens, has been proven in scientific studies to actually thicken vaginal walls, increase lubrication, and decrease painful intercourse.

That's right. Just because a product is labeled as a "vaginal moisturizer" doesn't mean that it alters or hydrates the vaginal walls. A gel, cream, or lotion that calls itself a "vaginal" or "personal" moisturizer may be something that goes in the vagina or something that goes outside the vagina; it may be a lubricant, or it may soften tissues at the entry of the vagina; it may actually reverse atrophic changes inside the vagina, or it may do nothing at all. The reality is that labels can be misleading. And there is a reason why.

Because moisturizers are classified as cosmetics, the companies that make them are under no obligation to back up their claims. Just as a face cream can promise to make you look ten years younger with regular use, a vaginal moisturizer can claim to make intercourse more comfortable. Unlike prescription medications, the companies that produce and market these products are under no obligation to the Food and Drug Administration to conduct scientific studies to prove that a product does what it claims to do. If a product is classified as a cosmetic, it only needs to demonstrate that it is not harmful when used as directed.

If you are confused, you're not alone. I was totally confused when I first started to research the world of vaginal moisturizers. Getting worthwhile information from product websites or directly from the various manufacturers was next to impossible. What I finally figured out was that a product labeled as a "personal," "feminine," or "vaginal" moisturizer generally falls into one of three categories:

Lubricants that call themselves moisturizers
External (vulvar) moisturizers/lubricants
Long-acting vaginal moisturizers

Lubricants That Call Themselves Moisturizers

Many lubricants that are intended to be used at the time of sexual activity are labeled as "moisturizers" because the manufacturer thinks that makes the product sound more appealing. Lela, the company that makes really lovely upscale vibrators, sells a companion "moisturizer" that is, by the company's own admission, a lubricant. Lela is just one of the many companies that focus on marketing over providing accurate information. Another popular product, K-Y Liquibeads Vaginal Moisturizer, is not a moisturizer but a lovely silicone vaginal lubricant. Period.

Purchasing a "feminine moisturizer" is a far easier sell for many women than buying a "lubricant" that is clearly intended for sexual purposes. The manufacturers are operating under the assumption that nice ladies buy moisturizers and wanton sluts buy lubes. It's misleading and confusing, and it works.

In addition, if a lubricant is labeled "for vaginal use," the FDA requires specific safety trials, including testing the product in animal vaginas to ensure that there are no harmful effects. While this is a boon for the rats that suffer from vaginal dryness, it adds an enormous expense to product development. It's cheaper and easier for manufacturers to just avoid the word "vagina" altogether on their labeling.

Vulvar Moisturizer/Lubricants

Many "personal" moisturizers instruct the user to apply the product to the outside of the vagina. If that is the case, the purpose is to soften and hydrate vulvar skin and the entry to the vagina, not to moisturize vaginal walls. Think of these products as vulvar hand creams. Use them if they make your vulva and vestibule feel more comfortable, but don't expect internal vaginal walls to become less thin or dry. Many also have lubricating ingredients, which is why instructions encourage not only daily use but use during intercourse.

Silk-E Vaginal Moisturizer is a good example of a product that markets itself as a vaginal moisturizer but is actually a vulvar moisturizer/water-based lubricant. According to the company, it provides "immediate comfort" for those who follow the recommendation to use it daily to moisturize "intimate areas" in addition to applying it during intercourse. The company also recommends, inexplicably, that it be applied to both the *inside* and outside of a condom. Is Silk-E also a penis moisturizer? Vitamin E (a lubricant) and aloe (a skin softener) are the active ingredients.

Long-Acting Vaginal Moisturizers

The only true *vaginal* moisturizer is a product that is meant to be inserted inside the vagina to increase the water content of cells so that the vaginal walls thicken and produce more natural lubrication. A true long-acting moisturizer is not intended to be used at the time of intercourse but on an ongoing basis. Any product that is applied to the *outside* of the vagina is *not* a vaginal moisturizer!

To be considered a long-acting vaginal moisturizer, the product ideally should offer the following:

A **"bio-adhesive"** *component to ensure that the product adheres to the walls of the vagina*

A **hydration** *component that sucks water into the vaginal cells to "plump them up"*

A **long-acting** *component to ensure that the lubricating results last for days, not minutes or hours—unlike a lubricant, which only needs to make things slippery during intercourse*

*A result that is **pain-free** or **pain-reducing,** since a true vaginal moisturizer helps to make sex hurt less.*

Two popular products that claim to be true vaginal moisturizers intended for internal use are Replens and Luvena.

Replens is a bio-adhesive gel that adheres to mucous membranes in the vagina and increases intracellular water by facilitating transfer into the cells. Studies show that cells treated with Replens carry up to sixty times their weight in water. The active ingredient is polycarbophil, which is the bio-adhesive that sticks to the walls of the vagina and sucks the water into the cells. Polycarbophil is also a weak acid that buffers vaginal tissues to lower the vaginal pH to between 3 and 4.5. These effects last for three days. Just as in a rich estrogen environment, the good lactobacilli can once again populate the neighborhood when the pH is lowered. When used as directed (twice weekly) vaginal tissue thickens, increases in elasticity, and shows a restoration of normal lubrication. The end result is that symptoms of dryness and discomfort are reduced.

Replens is the only long-acting moisturizer that has been approved by the FDA. It has gone through rigorous testing, including multiple clinical trials that have been published in the scientific literature. Replens is the only product that has been compared to topical estrogen in scientific studies in terms of delivering similar results.

Replens is the only over-the-counter product that actually meets the strict FDA criteria that have been set for estrogen products to get approval for use in treatment of vaginal atrophy. In other words, it not only increases lubrication and lowers pH but also decreases discomfort with intercourse. Many women who are not sexually active use Replens to reduce chronic vaginal irritation and infections.

Luvena is touted as both a long-acting moisturizer and a lubricant. It claims to restore a healthy vaginal pH and eliminate dryness, odor, and itching in addition to decreasing recurrent vaginal infections. It contains lactoperoxidase, lysozyme, and lactoferrin, which, according to the company, are "natural bio-active enzymes and proteins." Luvena is a "pre-biotic" that supposedly facilitates the growth of beneficial bacteria and is recommended to reduce vaginal infections and increase lubrication. While a few published studies have looked at some laboratory findings on this product, no published clinical trials have been conducted with actual women. Luvena may work, but the proof is pending. In June 2014 the FDA filed a complaint for permanent injunction stating that the manufacturer of Luvena is in violation of the Federal Food, Drug, and Cosmetic Act for illegally distributing a product that is "unapproved" and "misbranded." Stay tuned, but it doesn't look good for Luvena.

Vulvar Creams

And then there's V Magic. This amazing herbal product claims to "help take care of your sacred yoni" and "make the vagina a better place." The company promises to alleviate itching, burning, soreness, dryness, and tenderness. "Magic" would be the operative word, since no scientific studies have proven the claims made for this product. The only thing missing from V Magic's ad is a picture of Harry Potter.

Neogyn Vulvar Soothing Cream is in an entirely different category. It is not a moisturizer, nor is it a lubricant. It is a "human fibroblast lysate cream," intended for women to use on their vulva for a variety of reasons such as dryness, lichen sclerosus, or vulvodynia, all of which we'll discuss later. Essentially, this product is made up of skin cell proteins (taken from cultures of fetal fibroblasts) and growth factors, which have anti-inflammatory properties that promote collagen formation. Neogyn essentially "rejuvenates" and heals damage to the vulvar skin. A number of scientific studies have shown that this product *is* effective in wound healing and reduction of pain in a number of situations. Neogyn has a rich emollient base, which also has soothing properties. Recommended use is twice daily, and it has shown clinically significant results in six to eight weeks. Neogyn is not available in stores but can be ordered online.

How to Know What You Are Really Buying

Before you throw a lubricant or moisturizer into your shopping cart, check the ingredients and instructions to figure out if the product is a silicone lubricant, a water-based lubricant, a vulvar moisturizer, or a hybrid lubricant/vulvar moisturizer.

If all else fails, call the company and ask where the product goes, what it is supposed to do, and what the company's claims are based on. Good luck getting an answer.

The following guide to the ingredients commonly found in lubricants and moisturizers will help you figure out what you are buying and what it will do (or not do) for you. Some specific products to get you started are listed in the resources section.

M = Moisturizing properties
L = Lubricating properties

Aloe vera (M): *A plant that is purported to have soothing, healing, and skin moisturizing properties*
Benzoic acid: *A preservative that is also sometimes used as a topical antiseptic*
Calendula: *A plant that is used as an anti-inflammatory, to soothe irritated tissues, and for abdominal cramps and constipation*
Carbomer (M): *A chemical change to a molecule that is associated with water-absorbing compounds*
Cetyl alcohol: *Used as an emollient, emulsifier, or thickening agent in many skin creams and lotions*
Chorhexidine deglutinate: *A chemical antiseptic that is also commonly used in contact lens solutions and mouthwash*

Citric acid: *Decreases pH*

Diazolidinyl urea: *An antimicrobial preservative commonly used in cosmetics*

Dimethicone (L): *A nontoxic, inert, and nonflammable silicone substance that is used to make things slippery, is the main ingredient in silicone vagina lubricants, and is commonly used in hair products to make hair smooth, shiny, and more slippery*

Ginseng: *A plant that is a phytoestrogen and used for many medicinal purposes*

Glycerin (glycerol, glycerine) (L): *A colorless, odorless, slippery, thick liquid that is commonly used in vaginal lubricants, is a slightly sweet-tasting sugar alcohol, and may increase vaginal yeast infections with regular use*

Hyaluronic acid (M): *Stimulates a tissue's ability to retain water*

Hydroxyethyl cellulose: *A gelling and thickening agent derived from cellulose that is widely used in cosmetics, cleaning solutions, and other household products*

Methyl paraben: *An antimicrobial preservative that has sparked some concern that it has a weak estrogenic effect, though this has not been confirmed in studies and no link to breast cancer has been shown*

Mineral oil (L): *An oily substance from a nonvegetable source such as petroleum, this lubricant is commonly used in baby lotions and cosmetics and increases vaginal infections*

Paraffin (M): *The liquid form of paraffin, also known as mineral oil, that is used as a moisturizer in many cosmetics, such as Vaseline*

Pectin: *A polysaccharide from the walls of plants that is often used as a jelling or thickening agent in foods and is sometimes used to treat diarrhea*

Polycarbophil (M): *Absorbs water into vaginal cells and is used in many anti-diarrhea medications to absorb water in the gastrointestinal tract*

Polysorbate 60: *A sorbitol-based emulsifier*

Propylene glycol: *A colorless, odorless, viscous, clear liquid compound that not only is commonly found in vaginal lubricants and* *moisturizers but also has many industrial uses (and is an irritant for many women)*

Sodium benzoate: *An antimicrobial preservative*

Sorbic acid: *An antimicrobial preservative*

Sorbitol: *A sugar-free sweetener used both in sugar-free gum and other foods and as a laxative*

Vitamin E (Tocopherol acetate) (L): *A slippery, fat-soluble vitamin*

If intercourse is painful despite a bucketful of lube, then thin, dry tissue sometimes needs help beyond what an over-the-counter lubricant or moisturizer can provide. Keep reading. Chapter 13 will discuss specific prescription products to thicken vaginal wall tissue and alleviate sexual pain.

6

KEGELS WITH A KICK

A trip to the gym for your pelvic floor and the ergonomics of sex (who knew?)

I've heard it a million times. I will be talking to my patient about the steps she needs to take to fix her particular problem. As I bring up lubricants, moisturizers, medications, and doses, I can see her nodding. It's when I introduce the topic of pelvic physical therapy that I get reactions like:

> *"You're kidding, right?"*
> *"She's not going to put her hands in there!" (This is accompanied by a horrified look.)*
> *"Do I really need that? Can't you just give me a different medicine?"*

Well no, I'm not kidding. Yes, she is going to put her hands in there. Yes, you do need that, and no, I can't just give you a different medicine.

Consider if you broke your arm. Once the cast comes off, working with a physical therapist is a standard part of rehabilitation and restoration of normal function. After a break or serious injury, your muscles atrophy because they haven't been used for a period of time.

The same goes for the muscles that support your pelvic organs. If your vagina or pelvis has been traumatized by surgery, menopause, chronic pain, endometriosis, or painful sex, physical therapy is a key component to your recovery. You need a personal trainer for your pelvic floor, if you will.

Dr. Streicher's SexAbility Survey

Asked if they had ever heard of physical therapy for the vagina:

18.5 percent of women said, "Of course, everyone should have a personal trainer for her pelvis!"

81.5 percent of women said, "No, you're not serious are you?"

Your Pelvic Floor

The pelvic floor is made up of multiple muscle groups that support and surround all the good stuff—your clitoris, vagina, bladder, and bowels.

Pelvic Muscle Floor

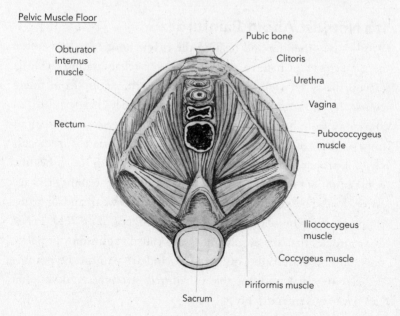

If you imagine a woman in a standing position, these muscle groups function as a strong trampoline that supports not only the bladder but also the uterus and rectum.

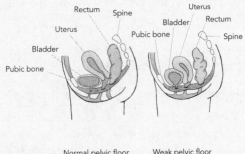

Normal pelvic floor   Weak pelvic floor

When all of the muscles work together, the "trampoline" is able to contract and relax in a coordinated fashion. If these muscles are not strong and healthy, they will not be able to function properly and may be a source of pain. In addition, if the muscles and connective tissue are damaged (think overstretched hammock), organs will sometimes prolapse, or drop down from their normal position.

It's Not Just About Painful Sex

While strengthening and healing the pelvic floor muscles is often necessary to eliminate pain, the benefits of rehabilitating this part of your body go well beyond eliminating the agony from intercourse. It is no coincidence that many women who have painful sex also suffer from urinary incontinence and constipation. Pelvic floor muscles that are able to contract and relax appropriately are necessary for proper bladder and bowel function. In addition, a healthy contraction of pelvic floor muscles contributes to the ability to have an orgasm! The general term used to describe weak and/or painful pelvic floor muscles is pelvic floor dysfunction, or PFD. Pelvic floor muscles that are hypertonic—also called vaginismus or pelvic floor tension—are tight, often spasm, and are painful. Hypotonic muscles are weak and not able to contract strongly. And yes, you can have an element of both.

> ## Benefits of a Healthy Pelvic Floor
>
> Bladder control
> Bowel function
> Proper placement of pelvic organs (bladder, uterus, rectum, bowel)
> Ability to orgasm
> Improved vaginal tone
> Pain-free intercourse

So as you work your way through the next few chapters and learn how to solve the vaginal dryness problem, lichen sclerosus, vestibulitis, endometriosis, or whatever condition created the initial pain, for many women there is one more step to take before reclaiming their sex life: pelvic physical therapy.

With the presence of these issues, vaginal tissues have been traumatized not only by the inflammation but also by the "pain memory" that lingers even after the initial problem has been eliminated. Both can create stubborn obstacles to intercourse. Your vagina—in fact, your entire pelvis—has been in protective "keep out mode" for so long that your pelvic muscles will continue to contract involuntarily in an attempt to keep out a penis, which could cause pain. Muscle memory does not know that vaginal tissues are now well lubricated and that whatever originally caused the pain has been eliminated. And that is where pelvic physical therapy comes in.

One patient came to see me after she'd had enough of "peeing everywhere but the toilet." In her midthirties, she had not been seeing a gynecologist because her husband, an internist, had been acting as her primary care physician. On further questioning, not only did I learn that she had stress incontinence, but she also admitted that she had experienced pain with intercourse for the past several years. She was frustrated, embarrassed, and close to feeling hopeless. When I recommended pelvic physical therapy and described what the therapist could do for her, she practically hugged me she was so relieved.

Pelvic physical therapists have done additional, very specialized training in the treatment of pelvic disorders, including gynecologic, urologic, muscular, and neurologic problems. Many women are skeptical when advised to seek the help of a physical therapist. These same women usually become the greatest advocates of the treatment. As a gynecologist, I can almost always fix the problem that initially caused the pain, but the PT is the only person who can erase the muscle memory, eliminate pelvic floor muscle tension, strengthen atrophied muscles, and restore normal, healthy functioning.

In my practice, I rely so much on my team of pelvic physical therapists that I refer to them as my "magicians."

Working with a Pelvic Physical Therapist

Since it is a mystery to most women what a pelvic physical therapist does, it helps to know what to expect when signing up. When you arrive at her office, she will first want to take a very detailed history, not only about your sexual issues but your general health. Since bowel and bladder issues often play into pelvic pain, she will ask questions about urinary and gastrointestinal symptoms as well.

After asking you these initial questions, you will be asked to undress for a physical exam. In the first part of the physical exam, the PT will evaluate things like your posture, abdominal strength, and general physical fitness. The pelvic exam is kind of like a gynecologic exam without the speculum; however, it's likely to include a number of elements that are unfamiliar to you. It starts with a thorough visual evaluation of the vulvar skin and vestibule (the mucosal tissue surrounding the opening of the vagina). The PT uses a cotton swab to touch each zone to see which areas are painful. She then gently introduces a gloved, lubricated finger into the vagina in order to systematically touch specific muscle groups that make up the pelvic floor. (Yes, you can say "Stop!" at any point if it becomes too painful.)

By gently applying pressure on various pelvic floor muscle

groups, the therapist determines whether the problem is due to tight muscles, known as a hypertonic pelvic floor. She feels for inappropriate knots, contractions, and inflammation of not only the muscles but the connective tissue as well. She may identify a specific, isolated tender spot, known as a trigger point, that when touched reproduces the pain felt during intercourse.

The physical therapist also evaluates your overall muscle strength and coordination by asking you to squeeze her finger using your pelvic muscles. This is similar to the maneuver you do when performing a Kegel exercise (see page 99).

The experienced pelvic physical therapist not only treats the problem but also plays an important role in helping your physician determine the source of the problem in the first place. In performing a thorough musculoskeletal evaluation of the pelvis, spine, and hips, she often finds pelvic asymmetry and muscle imbalances in women with pelvic and sexual pain. Often the location of the pain is not where the pelvic pain originates. For example, tight hip flexor muscles tilt the pelvis and cause tension in the pelvic floor muscles, which contributes, in turn, to pelvic pain and dysfunction. A pelvic PT often uses ultrasound to "see" what the muscles in this area are actually doing.

Once the source of the pain is identified, the therapist uses a number of modalities for treatment, including techniques such as myofascial (tissue) release and joint mobilization. Muscle spasms are eliminated using manual soft tissue work and trigger point release directly on the pelvic floor muscles through the vagina and occasionally the rectum. (This is definitely a hands-on treatment!) These techniques really work to eliminate pain, improve tissue integrity via increased circulation and tissue oxygenation, and restore normal resting muscle tone and length.

Your PT may also use biofeedback, which involves placing electrodes either externally or internally to register the electrical activity of the muscles. The information displayed on a monitor while your muscle activity is occurring shows you when your actions are causing muscles to tighten or relax. Since muscles that remain tense and contracted at all times cause pain, one of the major goals of biofeedback is to reteach the muscles to relax completely when they are not needed and learn to recruit the muscles in a coordinated fashion when they are. Ultimately you learn to control your muscles without the feedback.

In addition, sometimes electrical stimulation of the pelvic floor muscles is used to passively contract and relax the muscle as a way to strengthen it. (The e-stim does the work, not you!) While this may sound like a variation on a medieval torture, most women actually find it to be quite soothing.

If your case is severe, your physician or physical therapist may augment therapy with strategies to relax your tight muscles, such as diazepam suppositories (Valium for your vagina!), trigger point injections with local anesthetic, or Botox injections.

Ultimately, pelvic physical therapy allows a woman to improve function and also allows her to engage in intercourse without the vaginal and pelvic floor muscles painfully and inappropriately contracting. This therapy works, and in the coming chapters there will be many scenarios in which I will recommend PT as an adjunct to other therapies.

Conditions That Benefit from Pelvic Floor Physical Therapy

- Vulvar vestibulitis
- Vulvodynia
- Interstitial cystitis
- Vaginismus
- Dyspareunia (painful intercourse)
- Pelvic organ prolapse
- Dysmenorrhea (painful periods)
- Constipation and irritable bowel syndrome (IBS)
- Incontinence
- Inability to orgasm
- Pelvic pain

Finding a Pelvic Physical Therapist

Unlike dentists and hairdressers, you can't just ask a savvy girlfriend who her pelvic physical therapist is and go with her recommendation. If your gynecologist works with a PT, he or she will make a referral. Most major medical centers have a large PT department, including pelvic PT.

But beware: not every physical therapist does pelvic work, and you don't want to end up in the hands of someone who usually works with patients recovering from hip or knee replacement! When you call to make an appointment ask, "What percentage of your practice is devoted to pelvic physical therapy?" If the response is less than 50 percent, you may want to keep looking. A good starting point is to go to www.hermanwallace.com, a national website exclusively devoted to pelvic therapists. For a more extensive list, go to the American Physical Therapy Association website, www.womenshealthapta.org.

Some women do not have an experienced pelvic therapist in their area or do not have insurance that will cover the cost of the sessions. Fortunately, not everyone needs pelvic floor therapy, but the treatment of many conditions that will be discussed here does require, at a minimum, some of the techniques routinely used by pelvic physical therapists.

The following SexAbilitators will allow you to replicate on your own many of the techniques utilized by pelvic floor therapists.

SexAbilitators to Strengthen Your Pelvic Floor

The first thing every woman (somewhat defensively) says when I mention that something needs to be done to strengthen her pelvic floor muscles is, "I do my Kegels!" And I'm sure you do.

Kegel exercises are familiar to most women, as the solution commonly recommended to prevent or treat urinary incontinence. Theoretically, in addition to preventing incontinence, Kegel exercises should also help alleviate sexual issues such as pain or the inability to orgasm. But here's the problem. Studies show that the majority of women do not perform Kegels correctly.

And no wonder. When I went online and searched "how to perform a Kegel exercise," I was shocked at the number of credible websites that gave instructions like "tighten the buttocks," "stop the urine stream," and "tighten your abs."

The correct way to perform a Kegel is to tighten the pelvic floor muscles while *relaxing* the thighs, buttocks, and abdomen. It helps to insert two fingers in your vagina and feel the muscles contract, but that said, it is very difficult for most women to do Kegels correctly without the help of a therapist.

Moreover, it is the rare woman who is not disappointed in the results even when she is contracting and releasing her muscles correctly. Her muscles, like an overstretched rubber band, may simply be too weak to contract even if she Kegels perfectly.

So don't feel guilty if you abandoned your Kegels. You are far from alone, and it probably would have made no difference even if you faithfully did them.

Home Pelvic Floor Strengthening Devices

Given that Kegels are generally useless, creative entrepreneurs have come up with literally dozens of devices available to tone your pelvic floor. It wouldn't surprise me if in the future some upscale gym decided to devote a room to the pelvic floor, with vaginal cones, beads, balls, and barbells. The problem would be wearing the proper attire. Stay tuned for the Nike vagina line! In the meantime, you will have to purchase your own equipment to use in the privacy of your home.

The basic purpose of all these devices is to strengthen pelvic floor muscles by facilitating or reproducing Kegel contraction and relaxation exercises.

Apex

Apex is an inflatable silicone vaginal probe that uses battery-operated electrical muscle stimulation to "teach" the pelvic muscles to tighten and relax. This "automatic pelvic floor exerciser" is marketed as "a trip to the gym for the pelvic floor."

Apex essentially does the Kegel for you. Once the muscles get stronger, and because you experience a correct Kegel, over time you are able to reproduce a pelvic floor contraction without the device. Some pelvic physical therapists even use the device as an adjunct to PT. InControl, the company that makes Apex, also makes two other pelvic floor strengthening devices: Intone to treat incontinence, and Intensity to treat problems with achieving orgasm. I'll be discussing these two devices in later chapters.

Balls, Beads, Cones, etc.

If you can't afford to purchase an Apex (it retails for about $200 and requires a prescription), the other option is to purchase one of the dozens of balls, beads, cones, and other devices advertised online that claim to "strengthen your pelvic floor, improve sexuality, and give you explosive orgasms."

The problem is that, while the companies that make these devices make all kinds of promises and the ads feature enthusiastic testimonials of satisfied customers, there is no way to know if they do what they say they are going to do. On the other hand, the financial output is minimal, you get to peruse fun websites, and there is no harm in "experimenting." If you don't improve, it doesn't mean your situation is hopeless—it just means that you may need to bite the bullet and make an appointment with an actual human pelvic physical therapist.

Magic Banana

One of the most popular products is the Magic Banana, a resistance cord housed in smooth tubing in the shape of a long closed loop. The Magic Banana claims to not only strengthen muscles but also increase orgasms and help with bladder control. The Magic Banana is inserted into the vagina with the curve of the tubing loop facing up. Squeezing and releasing will cause the loop to contract and offer resistance to theoretically strengthen pelvic floor muscles.

The Ultimate in Multitasking

In addition to the Magic Banana, there are assorted varieties of weighted balls and cones designed to be inserted in the vagina and worn for hours (perhaps while you are making dinner or reading a book). As one manufacturer suggests, "Once you have the beads comfortably inserted, you can walk, run, swim, or clean the house." Some balls even vibrate to massage and exercise the pelvic floor muscles. The companies make all kinds of promises. "Better Orgasms!" "Less Pain!" "Eliminate Incontinence!" These promises, of course, have not been published in any scientific publication other than the *Journal of Wishful Thinking*. But why bother with expensive studies when websites can be loaded with testimonials from satisfied customers who evidently are having mind-blowing sexual experiences from vacuuming with vibrating balls in their vaginas. And yes, there is even a vaginal barbell. Try that, Arnold Schwarzenegger!

I need to stress that *nothing* takes the place of working with an expert pelvic physical therapist. However, if you live in an area where you don't have access to someone with this kind of specialized training or you cannot afford this type of health care, give one of these devices a try.

Vaginal Dilators

Another tool that pelvic physical therapists and physicians use is the graduated vaginal dilator. This instrument has two purposes. One is to get the vagina used to having something inside of it. Even if the size of your vagina is normal, painful sex for any reason initiates a cycle of pain–fear–muscle spasm–more pain that results in the vagina constricting at any attempt to have intercourse. Dilators are often needed after the cause of the pain has been eliminated to decondition the vagina and pelvic floor from going into protective mode. By starting small and then increasing gradually to whatever penis size is in your life, the vaginal tissues "learn" to accommodate having something inside without a pain response being triggered. That way, when you have sex with an actual penis, your pelvis won't panic.

A vaginal dilator is also a way to gently and gradually stretch tissues that are tight and have lost their elasticity, which is often the case if a woman has vaginal atrophy from hormonal changes or skin conditions or her vagina has been shortened by radiation or surgery. Scarring and shrinkage of the vaginal opening is almost always reversible! The other important advantage to using a dilator is that you will know when you are ready for intercourse.

Situations or Conditions That Often Require a Vaginal Dilator

Vaginismus
Vaginal atrophy
Postsurgery
Postradiation
Interstitial cystitis
Lichen sclerosus
Vulvodynia
Vestibulodynia
Painful intercourse
Hypertonic pelvic floor

Graduated dilators can be purchased individually, but generally come in sets of five to eight, ranging from ½ inch to 1⅝ inches in diameter. I know what you are thinking. Just what is the diameter of an "average" erect penis? The average diameter of an erect penis is 1.5 inches (3.8 centimeters), so if you can get the 1⅝-inch dilator in comfortably, you are good to go. If you want to know the diameter of your partner's penis, use a piece of string or ribbon to take a measurement. (I will leave you to come up with the creative response as to why you are putting a ribbon around his erect penis.) Tell him his result in centimeters, not inches, since that always sounds much bigger. No matter what the measurement, look impressed. *Never* use the word "average" when announcing a man's penis diameter.

Where Do You Get a Dilator?

Medical dilators in graduated sizes can be ordered through your physician but are expensive and not always readily available. If you order them through a pharmacy with a prescription, your insurance may cover the cost. The easiest option is to visit an erotic shop or website. (Check the resources section at the end of the book.)

"Alternative" Dilators

Since dildos and vibrators come in different sizes, you can simply buy the one or two sizes you need instead of a whole set. Remember, unless you have a short vagina, diameter is more important than length.

While it's tempting to use phallic-shaped items from your kitchen (celery, zucchini, banana, cucumber) or candles (birthday, Hanukkah, tapers, pillars), I don't recommend it. Ask any ER doc who has removed one of those objects from a mortified patient. If you must, put a condom over it in case of breakage!

Once you own a dilator, what do you do with it? For now, put it away. Unlike the new shoes that you can't wait to wear, you need to be patient. A dilator is rarely the first step in eliminating sexual pain.

How to Use Your Graduated Dilator

Once you get the go-ahead, here's what to do:

Step 1: *Start with a warm bath (to relax you and your pelvic floor muscles) and make sure you have at least 15 minutes of privacy. Putting a dildo in your vagina if your teenage son is about to burst into your room is not going to work.*

Step 2: *Lie in bed on your back with your knees bent and slightly apart. This is not yoga class. Be comfortable! Use pillows to support your head and back.*

Step 3: *Apply a generous amount of lubrication to the opening of your vagina and to the tip of the smallest dilator. If your dilator is silicone, be sure to use a water-based lubricant.*

Step 4: *Bear down slightly and gently slide the dilator in as far as it will go.*

Step 5: *If there is no pain or resistance, continue to insert larger dilators. The dilator that should be used to initiate your therapy is the dilator that does not cause pain with insertion but does create some resistance or slight discomfort when you insert it. Don't push it. This is not the gym, and you don't need to use the heaviest weight. You will get there eventually.*

Step 6: *Leave the dilator in place for 5 to 15 minutes. Concentrate on letting your vaginal tissues relax around it. Your buttocks and thighs should be relaxed as well. Don't forget to breathe. A little Mozart is not a bad idea.*

Step 7: *Repeat steps 1 through 6 on a daily basis, if possible. Don't panic, however, if you miss a day.*

Step 8: *When you are at the point where the dilator you're using slides in without resistance or discomfort, it is time to go up to the next size. This usually takes 3 to 4 weeks.*

Step 9: *When you are ready to go up to the next size, use the smaller dilator to start your session for at least a few days before you insert the next size.*

Always wash your dilators with antibacterial soap and water and dry them well before you put them away. Store them in a box labeled 2012 TAX RETURNS so your teenage daughter will not find them when she is raiding your drawers to borrow some tights.

When first using a dilator, a little spotting is not unusual, but you should *never* experience severe pain or heavy bleeding. If you do, or if you are unable to comfortably insert a dilator, see your doctor before proceeding.

Sometimes it is necessary to coat the dilator with local anesthetic jelly (you will need a prescription for this). In other cases, a muscle relaxant is useful. (Valium for your vagina!) Once you can comfortably put something in your vagina that is slightly larger than your partner's penis, you are ready for the real thing.

In subsequent chapters, I will discuss a number of medical situations for which I will recommend using vaginal dilators. Now that you are familiar with what they are, you can refer back to these instructions if you need a refresher on how to insert them.

Sexual Ergonomics

I would be surprised if this is a phrase you are familiar with, because until a very short time ago I had never even heard of it myself. Like most doctors, I go to a lot of medical conferences, which are great opportunities to meet with colleagues and learn about the latest research. But of all the conferences I attend, none even come close to being as fun and informative as ISSWSH—the International Society for the Study of Women's Sexual Health. At a recent ISSWSH conference, I was introduced to the concept of sexual ergonomics by Dr. Heather Howard, who has a PhD in sexology. (Who knew!)

Ergonomics refers to human factor engineering—in other words, ergonomics helps adapt the human body to function optimally in physical situations. You may have heard of ergonomic desk chairs that support your back while you sit at a desk, or keyboard hand rests to help you avoid carpal tunnel syndrome. There's ergonomics for riding a bike without injury, and there's ergonomics for having sexual pleasure even in the face of physical challenges.

Think about it. A woman with severe arthritis can't open a pickle jar, and she also can't give her partner a hand job or self-stimulate holding a vibrator. A woman with limited strength from chronic illness not only can't climb two flights of stairs but also can't support herself in a female superior position to have intercourse. There is no end to the physical limitations that can sabotage the ability to receive or give sexual pleasure. Given that roughly 50 percent of the middle-aged and older population suffer from some sort of chronic illness or disability, there are millions of adults who struggle with the mechanics of having sex and, more often than not, just give it up. Well now, thanks to the innovative work of Dr. Howard, who has spearheaded this innovative field, nothing is impossible.

For the woman who desires penis-vagina penetrative sex but cannot part her legs (think hip replacement or pelvic fracture), Dr. Howard proposes a variety of intercourse positions that keep her legs together, such as "spooning."

The woman who desires sexual stimulation but has urinary or fecal incontinence and avoids sexual activity because she doesn't want to change the sheets afterward (think pregnancy, stroke, diabetes, spinal cord injury, cancer) can protect her bed with an elegant and machine-washable "waterproof throw blanket." This is also useful for those who ejaculate during sexual stimulation or experience incontinence during sleep.

Acknowledging that vaginal-penile sex is not always possible or desired, Dr. Howard also explores alternatives. You name it, Dr. Howard has thought of safe, comfortable, and inventive ways to maximize pleasure when you are experiencing physical obstacles or challenges that limit your sexual experience.

There are many SexAbilitators that will be useful to women who are challenged by a physical disability, muscle fatigue as a byproduct of cancer, or one of the medical issues discussed in chapter 15. Check out the resources section for further information.

The Power of the Right Pillow

Pillows and bolsters optimize comfortable positions not only for intercourse but also for cunnilingus, anal play, and self-stimulation. The right pillow needs to be the correct shape, size, and firmness. It also needs to be in the right place. While you can certainly use any pillows you have around the house, there are pillows specifically designed to facilitate comfortable sex. Ergoerotics.com probably has the largest assortment of sexual support pillows, along with suggestions for placement depending on the issue and the desired sexual activity. If style is important, the Liberator foam wedge is designed for maximum support during sex and comes in a variety of fabrics to match any decor! Only you will know that it is not something your designer chose.

Easy Rider

Pillows are not the only way to facilitate support if you don't have sufficient muscle strength to hold a position. The Body Bouncer (not to be confused with a bouncy baby seat!) is a rubber saddle mounted on a steal frame that allows the "rider" to bounce on the penis with zero effort. The very helpful (and graphic) website illustrates 27 different positions to facilitate sexual activity, including "The Bliss Box," "The Cat Cage," "The Flow Job," and "The Arch Angel." All promise "pleasure without strain, neck cramps or burning arms."

No Partner, No Problem: Choosing the Right Toys to Make Pleasure Possible

Once you have read chapter 20 (no skipping ahead!), you will doubtless want to invest in an assortment of toys. Physical challenges can have an impact both on the sort of toy you can hold and on your ability to get the toy to touch yourself (or a partner, or partners) where you want it to. No matter what the medical issue, finding the right sex toy and then figuring out how to successfully use it can be daunting.

First consider what you want to do with the toy. Are you interested in clitoral stimulation? Penetration? If you want to use a vibrator, can you hold it, reach the right area, and keep it in place for a prolonged period of time?

The woman who desires self-stimulation but cannot reach her genitals or hold a vibrator (think arthritis, cerebral palsy, amputation) can position herself over a "hands-free vibrating cone." A surprising number of vibrators and dildos have suction cups so you can affix them to a chair or dresser and lean up against it. (After writing this book, nothing surprises me.) A harness designed to hold a dildo or vibrator does not necessarily have to be fixed to a person; it can also be fixed to an object, such as a bed.

If a traditional vibrator is too heavy to hold, consider a wand vibrator with a broad surface area. You can put it between your legs and prop it up with pillows so you don't need to hold it.

The Handy Harness Glove is the perfect solution for anyone who fatigues easily or has grip issues. If you are handy and want to make your own version, take a little bullet vibrator and drop it in the finger of a glove, put on the glove, and you're good to go.

Grasping and holding may not be an issue, but flexibility may be. If so, toys such as Flex-A-Pleasure, with long flexible shafts, help you reach all the right places.

Some vibrators can be worn. You may want to check out the Remote Butterfly and the Ruby Remote 3-Speed, which can be worn on the body; neither one needs to be held in place. Some vibrators go around the waist or are placed in a panty with a pocket to sit in front of the clitoris. There are also vibrators that can be worn on a finger and are very light.

Sex as Sport

The Sports Sheet is an innovative accessory intended for couples who like bondage. But guess what? A sheet with Velcro arm and leg cuffs also offers the perfect solution to keeping body parts in place for maximum function and comfort. While you are on the website (http://www.sportsheets.com), check out the five-piece vibrating position pillowcase. Maybe treat yourself to a body tickler.

7

SAY YES TO DRUGS

Sometimes a prescription doesn't just make sex better, it makes it possible

On the one hand, women are saying, "Where's my Viagra?"

On the other hand, they're saying, "I only want to use something that's natural."

So what is best? Take drugs? Avoid drugs? I say, in many cases, *Say yes to drugs*. But sadly, you won't be saying yes to the female equivalent of Viagra anytime soon.

If you ever wondered why that's the case, you're not alone. It's true that there are relatively few prescription drugs specifically for women's sexual health. It's not that no one is doing research or that there is no interest. Sexual health research is alive and well in many of the major universities and sexual health clinics across the country.

In addition, the pharmaceutical companies that often fund research are profit-motivated and well aware that with increased life expectancy come a greater number of women living after menopause. Clearly, this points to a lot of money that could be made in addressing vaginal dryness and lost libido in women. But since product development is expensive, excruciatingly slow, and dependent on Food and Drug Administration approval—another necessary and frustrating roadblock to the timely release of new drugs—this kind of drug will be slow getting to market. Even if someone does discover the perfect pill to keep women lubricated, interested, and highly orgasmic, the chance that the FDA will approve that pill before our daughters are grandmothers is extremely small.

The average time it takes for a drug to get to your pharmacy is *15 to 25 years.* Here's why. Once a brilliant scientist has an idea for a drug that will give women incredible orgasms, she (the scientist) needs to go through the following steps. First she has to sell a major pharmaceutical company or major investor on the idea. Then:

Lab research takes two to ten years
Preclinical testing takes three to six years
Clinical trials take six to seven years
FDA review takes one to two years

Millions of dollars are needed for research, development, and trials, and it is more than likely that the drugs will never make it to your pharmacy anyway. It's the FDA's job to establish that a drug works and that its benefits outweigh its risks, and because of this arduous process we enjoy one of the safest pharmaceutical systems in the entire world. But it can be really frustrating to not have access to drugs that are sometimes available in other parts of the world and may benefit women.

While all of this is true for any new drug, it has proven particularly challenging for a woman's sexual health drug to get FDA approval. Contrast the process just described to the ease with which drugs get approved for men's sexual health:

There are 15 drugs that are FDA-approved to treat various sexual issues in men
There are only 6 drugs that are FDA-approved to treat vaginal dryness
There are 0 drugs that are FDA-approved to treat lack of libido in women

It's hard to make an argument that the FDA is just being careful when only 3,000 men were in the trial to get Viagra approved, but libido drugs such as flibanserin and testosterone were rejected despite the fact that 11,000 women were in the trial for flibanserin and 10,000 women were in trials for testosterone, both with strong safety and efficacy data.

"Off Label" Doesn't Mean "Off Limits"

However, getting around the FDA is sometimes okay. In some cases a drug is prescribed for a condition even if it was approved for a different purpose or for a different population. Prescribing drugs that are not FDA-approved for the use they were originally intended for is known as "off-label" prescribing, and it's something every doctor does. When a drug is prescribed off-label, it doesn't mean that the drug is illegal, or that it won't work, but simply that it is being used to treat something other than what it was developed and originally intended for. Hundreds of drugs are prescribed off-label. In gynecology, the medications most commonly prescribed for off-label uses are birth control pills. Every birth control pill has been FDA-approved to prevent pregnancy. But 30 percent of birth control prescriptions are legitimately prescribed for reducing menstrual cramps, treating endometriosis, or decreasing heavy bleeding, all "off-label" reasons.

Testosterone is a good example of a sexual health drug that I recommend off-label. The testosterone products on the market are intended for—and FDA-approved for—men who have low testosterone. While many scientific studies show that women with low libido benefit from small doses of testosterone, the FDA has not approved testosterone products intended for women, even though it is safe and testosterone for women is approved in Europe. So when I prescribe testosterone to enhance a woman's libido, it's not illegal and it's not malpractice; it's just not approved by the FDA.

"Custom" Drugs from Compounding Pharmacies

Another approach is to use compounding pharmacies, which are not under the umbrella of the FDA. Historically, all pharmacists "compounded." In the 1800s, a doctor would give his patient a prescription to take to the local pharmacist, who would then mix the drug up per the doctor's specifications. As large commercial pharmaceutical companies came on the scene in the 1950s, compounding became the exception, not the rule, and was used only for products that were not commercially available.

Then compounding pharmacies took on an entirely different role when they began marketing and distributing so-called bio-identical hormones. In fact, "bio-identical" is not a scientific term. It is a term originally made up by savvy market research gurus to describe hormones distributed by compounding pharmacies.

The use of the word "bio-identical" was brilliant. It was catchy, it sounded "natural," and it also sounded like something different than the duplicate FDA-approved plant-derived hormone products produced and distributed by commercial pharmacies. And it worked. A $1 billion industry was launched by an actress and supported by women who distrusted the pharmaceutical industry and were desperate to feel better.

Compounding pharmacies promote the idea that their bio-identical hormones are customized for an individual based on hormone levels in saliva and blood, even though it has been scientifically proven that salivary levels are affected by diet and other variables and that serum levels do not correspond to efficacy. In addition, the compounded hormones are now almost never customized. In fact, many compounding pharmacies mass-produce hormone preparations that are almost exact copies of those produced commercially. So why not get your hormones from a compounding pharmacy?

Issue 1: If It Sounds Too Good to Be True, It Probably Is Too Good to Be True

Since the FDA does not regulate compounding pharmacies, they can make whatever claims they want. So they tell women what women want to hear—namely, that compounded bio-identical hormones have fewer risks and fewer side effects and are more effective than identically structured, commercially produced hormones, even though there is no scientific evidence to prove that claim. Some promoters of compounded hormones claim that their products reverse aging, enhance sex, and prevent cancer.

While women generally distrust the pharmaceutical industry—which is legally obligated to back up its claims, do testing, and report all safety risks and negative findings—the general population seems to have little problem trusting companies that have no such efficacy or safety standards. This, combined with aggressive advertising and misleading marketing, has resulted in women believing that compounded products are safer than commercial products.

Another way to understand the issue is to think of the estrogen in hormone therapy as the sugar in a cookie. A cookie with the same amount of sugar can be sold either by Nabisco—where it is commercially prepared and packaged with a specific list of ingredients and a calorie count on the package to let you know that if you eat a lot of cookies you will get fat—or by the corner bakery, which puts no listing of ingredients on the package and is free to say that its cookies will not make you fat.

Transdermal progestogens from a compounding pharmacy *are* potentially dangerous, since there is no evidence that they prevent the lining of the uterus from developing precancerous or cancerous cells. Only oral progestogens have been proven to offer that protection.

In 2005 the American College of Obstetrics and Gynecology released a committee opinion stating that there is no scientific evidence to support claims of increased efficacy or safety for individualized hormone therapy regimens prepared by compounding pharmacies.

Issue 2: Quality Control

Lack of FDA oversight also means that quality is not ensured in drugs from compounding pharmacies. The public became acutely aware of this in 2012 when 749 people became ill and 63 of them died of meningitis after a compounding pharmacy in Massachusetts manufactured and distributed contaminated steroids. In 2013 the FDA conducted 31 unannounced inspections in 18 states of other compounding pharmacies and found rust and mold in "clean" areas along with tears in workers' gloves. Unsterile and potentially risky conditions were found in all but one of the inspected compounding manufacturing plants.

Compounding pharmacies don't manufacture hormones—they just mix them. The problem is that, according to the evidence, they don't generally mix them very accurately.

In 2013 investigative reporter Cathryn Ramin, on behalf of *More* magazine, commissioned lab tests of hormones distributed by 12 popular compounding pharmacies and found that, despite identical prescriptions for estrogen and progesterone, there was no uniformity in what was compounded. Virtually every sample was either significantly lower than what was prescribed or significantly higher. There was even variation in capsules from the same pharmacy. A woman who has been prescribed 50 milligrams of estradiol might actually be taking 25 milligrams one day and 100 milligrams the next.

The bottom line when it comes to compounded "customized" hormones is that there is no benefit and there is also, despite the illusion of safety, potential risk.

"Natural" Drugs

Consumers tend to feel relieved when a medication is labeled "natural." Indeed, when it comes to hormones, pretty much every one of my patients requests a "natural" medication. But know this: "natural" does not equal "safer." We can all name many things that are natural but also unsafe. Arsenic, anthrax, and strychnine come to mind.

In addition, natural products do not always work better than synthetic products. Once again, it all comes down to marketing. The term "natural" is appealing to consumers and implies an advantage over "synthesized" pharmaceutical products. No one wants Premarin, a common hormone drug prescribed by many doctors. Premarin is derived from PREgnant MARes' urINe. Get it? Instead, patients request the "natural product." When it comes to hormone therapy, the only thing that is truly natural is to eat the plant that contains the hormone or drink the horse urine. In reality, both forms of estrogen require synthesis to put them in a usable form.

Even plant-derived hormone preparations, whether they come from a compounding pharmacy or a large commercial pharmacy, require a chemical process to synthesize the final product into a powder that can then be put into a cream, a spray, a patch, or a pill. And face it . . . what's more natural than *horse urine?* Premarin is pretty natural stuff. Horses are actually much closer to humans than plants. I rarely prescribe estrogen synthesized from horse urine, however, not because I prefer something "more natural," but because other products have scientifically been proven to be better and safer.

Most menopause and sexual health experts in this country prescribe and recommend FDA-approved "bio-mimetic" plant-derived estrogen, produced and distributed by companies that have quality control and are obligated to tell you not only the benefits but the potential risks as well. An added bonus to these commercial products is that your insurance company is likely to cover their cost. The non–FDA–approved compounded versions will require you to open up not only your ability to trust but also your checkbook.

While it is important to understand the limitations of a compounding pharmacy, it is also important to understand when they are useful. Do I use a compounding pharmacy? You bet. I use a compounding pharmacy whenever I need a preparation for my patient that is not commercially produced. However, even though I work with pharmacies I know, I make a point of disclosing to my patient that the drug I am prescribing is a non-FDA-regulated product.

Specific Drugs

Throughout the book I will recommend specific drugs, or categories of drugs, that require a prescription. Keep in mind that some categories of drugs are used in multiple scenarios but may only be described fully in a section that does not pertain to you. For example, the prescription options for treating vaginal dryness are discussed fully in the chapter on menopause since that is the most common reason to prescribe vaginal estrogens. However, some women who are years away from menopause also suffer from vaginal dryness, perhaps because of postpartum issues or as a side effect from cancer treatment. So, if I direct you to a section that doesn't seem relevant to your specific problem, understand that while the cause of the problem may not be the same, the solution is.

The Economics of Midlife Sex

I would be remiss if I did not acknowledge that all of these prescription and nonprescription medications, lubes, moisturizers, and products that I recommend are not free. I was reminded of this when I was sitting across from Jill, a long-term patient of mine who was in for her annual exam. The year before we had spent a lot of time talking about strategies to deal with the painful intercourse that had left her pretty much in avoidance mode. She had left my office with a prescription for a local vaginal estrogen product along with a number of over-the-counter recommendations.

"So how are things going sexually?" I asked. She gave a dismissive wave of her hand and said, "We gave up on that."

"What about all the things we discussed last year?" I asked.

"Frankly," she said, "between my husband's issues and my issues, we added it up and realized we couldn't afford it. It's okay."

Couldn't afford sex? Sex is one of the few pleasures in life that's free! That's like saying you can't afford to go for a walk, or can't afford to give your partner a nice massage. And for some people, that's true. But shame on me, I had never really considered the cost of the products that, for some people, don't just make intercourse pleasurable but make it possible. Even though some insurance plans cover part of the cost of prescription products, many Americans are uninsured, underinsured, or have a prohibitively high deductible. And over-the-counter products are rarely covered.

So I added it up myself, and I was shocked at the average annual cost for a typical couple who have sex twice a week and require help to keep things going. Here's what I found:

Silicone lubricant (four bottles/year at $16 each)	$64
Local vaginal estrogen ($40–80/month)	$720
Long-acting vaginal moisturizer ($20/month)	$240
Erectile dysfunction medication ($35/pill)	$3,360
Doctor's visits to get prescriptions	$300
Annual total:	**$4,684**

Not everyone requires all these products, but depending on what your needs are, it may be dramatically cheaper to go to the movies once a week than to make love. And that's not including the cost of some new lingerie, candles, a vibrator, and maybe the occasional bottle of champagne. I wondered how many of my patients had given up their sex lives not just because it was difficult or painful, but also because, given a choice between buying groceries and buying Viagra, eating trumped pleasure.

The solution? You can get some breaks by checking out the coupons on the pharmaceutical websites. Ask your doctor for samples, and also whether half a Viagra, or vaginal estrogen once a week rather than twice a week, would do the trick. Beware the mail-order stuff (it's almost always fake!), and tell your husband that next Mother's Day he can skip the flowers and give you some lube.

part three

SEXABILITY SABOTEURS

IT HURTS!

Turn vaginal agony into vaginal ecstasy

You've been there . . . a beautiful romantic evening . . . passion and expectation leading to kissing, touching, arousal, and an attempt at intercourse . . . only to find that despite a really great guy and a bucketful of lubricant, the realization that *nothing,* no how, no way, is going in there . . . or even worse, he enters, but instead of cries of delight there are cries of "Ow, *ow, OW, OMG . . . please stop!"*

Burning, knifelike, searing, pinching . . . these are the words I have heard my patients use when trying to describe their experience.

For some the agony ends when he withdraws, but other women are in pain for hours, days, or weeks after an attempt at intercourse.

No wonder women decide to go into avoidance mode.

Finding out what is causing pain with intercourse may well be one of the most frustrating things that women must contend with. It's not unusual for a patient to come to me after seeing three or four other doctors who have said either, "I don't know why you are having pain," or worse, "Everything *looks fine,* just relax!"

Every woman with sexual pain has a story, and I want to hear it. When I ask the following questions, I can begin to understand both the nature of the pain a woman is experiencing and what the cause, or causes, might be.

When did the pain start?

Do you ever have pain-free sex?

What medications are you taking?

Is the pain primarily on the vulva, in the entry of the vagina, or inside the vagina?

Does it hurt immediately on entry or only once he's inside? Or both?

Does it feel dry?

Does it hurt when you use tampons? When you sit on a bike?

Is there a discharge? Itching? Burning? A rash?

Are there other associated problems, such as incontinence?

Is there pain with bowel movements?

By the time a woman has answered these questions, I generally have a pretty good idea what is going on, but until I take a look and do some testing, nothing is certain.

Dyspareunia: The Name for Pain with Intercourse

The medical word for painful intercourse is "dyspareunia," which is categorized in two general ways. "Superficial dyspareunia" refers to pain that is limited to the entry and walls of the vagina when there is an attempt at intercourse. In general, superficial dyspareunia is caused by one of the vulvar or vaginal conditions covered in this chapter. "Deep dyspareunia" is the term for when the penis or toy negotiates getting into the vagina just fine, but any thrusting movement causes pain that ranges from achy to sharp to intolerable. The cause may be a gynecologic condition such as endometriosis, a medical condition such as ulcerative colitis, or a side effect of cancer treatment. There are actually more than fifty conditions that may be responsible for deep pelvic pain. Many women experience both kinds of pain: it hurts for him to get in, and then it hurts deep in the pelvis during thrusting.

It's also not unusual to start with just one kind of pelvic pain—either superficial dyspareunia or deep dyspareunia—but in time end up with both. The reason is simple. If you initially have only superficial dyspareunia, your vagina is not stupid: it is going to try to protect itself from further agony by tightening your pelvic floor muscles to keep the penis out. If you start with deep dyspareunia, the best way for your pelvis to prevent a penis from entering is by not lubricating. In other words, the dryness may not be the initial problem but becomes a protective mechanism to prevent intercourse from occurring. One triggers the other. This is exactly how you get into a vicious cycle of pain.

The body's protective response to this cycle is often called vaginismus, which refers to the general physical reactions that make intercourse out of the question. The vagina spasms closed, and the slightest touch on the vestibule is excruciating.

An international committee of scientists who met in 2002 defined vaginismus as the "persistent difficulties to allow vaginal entry of a penis/finger/object, despite the woman's expressed wish to do so. There is a variable involuntary pelvic floor muscle contraction avoidance and anticipation/fear/experience of pain."

Keep in mind that the anticipation of pain is just as harmful as actual pain, which is why many women are still unable to have intercourse even after the initial physical problem has been eliminated. In other words, vaginismus is not a disease . . . it is a defense mechanism.

Many women respond to this physiological cycle by losing hope. They say to themselves (and sometimes to me), "I will never get better or have pleasurable sex again." Often they experience persistent anxiety even when they just think about being sexual. A total loss of libido is pretty much inevitable. The only way to break the cycle is to find the cause of the pain, eliminate it, and, if present, treat the vaginismus. This sounds pretty obvious. But in many cases the cause may seem elusive.

Physical Conditions That Can Cause Superficial Dyspareunia

Estrogen deficiency
Vulvovestibulodynias
Lichen sclerosus
Lichen planus
Female genital mutilation
Radiation therapy
Chemotherapy
Graft-versus-host reaction
Congenital malformations
Hypertonic pelvic floor
Dermatologic conditions
Vulvar cancer

Physical Conditions That Can Cause Deep Dyspareunia

Endometriosis
Adhesions
Constipation
Irritable bowel syndrome
Ovarian cysts
Uterine infection
Pelvic organ prolapse
Adenomyosis
Fibroids
Interstitial cystitis
Bladder cancer
Diverticular disease
Fibromyositis
Pelvic infections
Hypertonic pelvic floor

The Exam

The pelvic exam for someone who is having sexual pain goes way beyond the standard annual exam of looking at the vulva, putting in the speculum, and feeling the uterus and ovaries.

First, I do a visual inspection of the skin covering the entire vulva and the vestibule mucosa to check for redness, ulcers, scarring, change in pigmentation, sores, rashes, or dryness.

I then use a cotton swab to touch every part of the vulva and vestibule to detect which parts are painful. Certain conditions affect very specific parts of the vulva and vestibule. Most important is determining whether the pain is inside or outside the Hart's Line, which is located just inside the labia minora.

Cotton Swab Testing

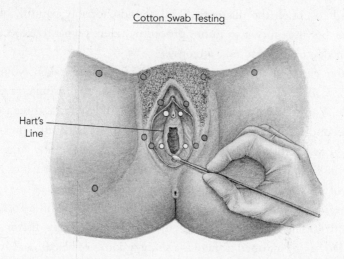

Hart's
Line

Yes, I need to put a speculum in, but if a patient is having severe pain, I use the very smallest speculum possible. In severe cases, I can also use an anesthetic jelly to numb the vaginal opening before inserting the speculum. I then take a careful look at the vaginal tissue to check for any atrophic changes, evidence of infection, or inflammation. Often I check the vaginal pH. If there is an abnormal discharge, I take a sample of the fluid to check for infection.

The speculum exam is followed by the standard bimanual exam (one hand on your belly, with one or two fingers in your vagina) to check your uterus and ovaries for any abnormalities or pain. In addition, I gently push on the bladder to see if there is specific bladder pain consistent with interstitial cystitis. (See chapter 9 regarding pain in the pelvis.) This is followed by a thorough digital exam (applying pressure with a finger inside the vagina) of the pelvic floor to determine which muscle groups are painful or tight. It's important to differentiate pain from pressure. Sometimes there is a specific trigger point that causes intense pain, as discussed in chapter 6.

"You're Going to Take a Biopsy from Where?"

In some cases, a sample of tissue from the vulva or vestibule is needed to clinch the diagnosis. This sounds horribly painful, of course, but in reality it's a minor procedure. Here's what to expect if your doctor needs to take a biopsy.

After cleaning the area where the biopsy will be taken, your doctor will inject a small amount of local anesthesia, using a tiny needle. You will feel a stick and a burn that will last about three to five seconds. You will feel nothing further other than a little pressure. Your doctor will obtain a tiny sample of tissue (slightly larger than the tip of a match) and then use either a dissolvable stitch or a drop of medication to stop any bleeding.

After the local anesthesia wears off, you may be a little sore. Usually 400 milligrams of ibuprofen will take care of any discomfort. Do not be alarmed if there is a slight amount of bleeding. You can apply pressure using a pad or tissue. In the rare case of bleeding that is heavy or continuous, you should call your doctor. If the biopsy site burns when you urinate, either gently pat-dry or rinse with warm water. Do not rub the area. Using a blow dryer on a warm setting is soothing if you are sore. Biopsy results generally take three to five days but may take a little longer if the sample is sent to a specialist in interpreting vulvar tissue.

Conditions That Cause Superficial Dyspareunia and Their Fixes

The causes of sexual pain are often complex to diagnose and complex to treat. As much as I wish you could fix anything that's causing your pain simply by reading this book, that's not realistic. *This is not a cookbook, and my approach is not the only approach.* More likely than not, if you suspect that you have one of the following conditions, you will need to see a doctor, not only to get appropriate prescriptions but to confirm the diagnosis. What follows are explanations of the conditions that cause superficial dyspareunia, a general approach to how they are treated, and suggestions on how to facilitate the healing process. Being informed will not only help you when you get to your doctor's office but calm your fears, I hope, before you get there.

Superficial dyspareunia is generally caused by one of three D's:

1. Dynias
2. Dystrophies
3. Dryness

The Dynias: Vestibulodynia, Vulvodynia, and Vulvovestibulodynia

When Charlotte on *Sex in the City* was diagnosed with vulvodynia (aka "the burning vagina syndrome"), awareness of this problem, which affects as many as 15 percent of women, exploded. *Dynia* is the Greek root for "pain." Even though the term "vulvodynia" is often used to describe all external genital pain, many women actually have vestibulodynia, also known as vestibulitis. Vestibulodynia is pain confined to the vestibule. This is where pain "mapping" with a cotton swab is important and Hart's Line (just inside the labia minora) becomes an important landmark. Women with vestibulodynia do not have pain outside Hart's Line. Vulvovestibulodynia (sometimes called generalized vulvodynia) can affect the entire vulva, including the vestibule. The terminology is confusing, particularly because the same condition may go by various names. I've tried to include the most common names to go with the descriptions.

Women with vestibulodynia, no matter what the cause, have severe pain on entry if intercourse is attempted. For some women, the pain and burning associated with vestibulodynia (and vulvo-dynia) is so severe that it interferes with activities such as riding a bike, wearing jeans, inserting a tampon, or simply sitting and doing nothing. The vestibule may look completely normal, or there may be redness.

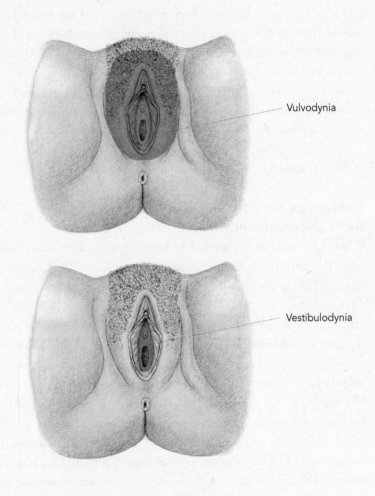

Vulvodynia

Vestibulodynia

Strictly speaking, vestibulodynia is not actually a diagnosis; it is a symptom, essentially "pain in the vestibule." And just as a pain in the stomach might be gas, it also might be appendicitis. In every case, the burning and pain are due to the proliferation and hypersensitivity of the nerve endings located just outside the vagina. One way to think of it is that women with vestibulodynia have "too many nerve endings." The result is pain with any physical contact or pressure.

Acquired Vestibulodynia, Inflammatory Vestibulodynia, and Provoked Vestibulodynia

This is the classic "burning vagina" syndrome that women describe as "burning, raw, cutting" pain. Sometimes this condition is a result of chronic inflammation from infections, allergies, or irritants, such as antifungal creams that are used for a presumed infection. There is no end to the possibilities that can cause inflammation to the vestibule—everything from a scented panty liner to that recurrent yeast infection. Any chronic vaginal discharge can cause itching and burning of the vestibule. Allergic reactions also fall into this category. Anything from latex to semen may be the culprit. In many cases there is no identifiable cause.

The Fix

Identify and treat any abnormal vaginal discharge.

Bacterial vaginosis, yeast, desquamative inflammatory vaginitis (see page 142), or even a nasty cervical infection can be the culprit. This is a situation in which you do not want to self-treat a presumed yeast infection.

Eliminate irritants and allergens.

It's amazing how many everyday products, even those intended for genital use, are loaded with potential irritants. Think of how many products touch your vulva or are applied to your genitals every day—your soap, lubricant, lotion, even your towels if they have been washed in detergent and dried using a fabric softener. Anything with a chemical can be a problem. Take a look at the labels of everyday products and you will be shocked at the number of ingredients you can't even pronounce, much less would want to intentionally apply to your vulva.

Potential Vaginal Irritants and Allergens

Perfumes
Dyes (as in toilet paper)
Scented soaps
Liquid soaps
Preservatives used in lotions, lubes, and creams
Toilet paper
Sanitary pads
Laundry detergent
Fabric softener
Vaginal lubricants
Antifungal medications
Feminine sprays
Spermicides
Vagisil Feminine Cream

Use medication to "quiet" the nerve endings.

Once irritants are eliminated, the goal of treatment is to desensitize the nerve endings. It can be a frustrating process since a medication that works for one woman may not work for another. Keep the faith. A solution is there, but it might take a little trial and error to figure it out.

Neurologic drugs that "calm nerves" (including vulvar nerve endings!), such as gabapentin and pregabalin (Lyrica), have been successfully used for treatment. If you are prescribed an antidepressant, it is not because your doctor thinks depression is causing your symptoms (even though you may be depressed about them), but because antidepressants that decrease norepinephrine are known to alleviate symptoms. The dosages of the antidepressants prescribed for this purpose are significantly less than those used for depression.

In some cases, an injection of local anesthesia into the painful area or a nerve block injection will "down-regulate" (turn off) sensitized nerves. Capsaicin, an extract from red chili peppers, is an interesting treatment. Initial application causes burning (hardly shocking), but continuous use actually decreases pain since the neurotransmitter that causes the burning sensation gets depleted over time. Don't expect relief for weeks, but this strategy can work.

Topical Cromolym spray is usually used to treat allergic rhinitis (a runny nose) but can also be sprayed on the vulva. A compounded Cromolym cream is also sometimes prescribed. Antihistamines such as Allegra or Singulair calm the inflammatory response too.

When all else fails, surgical removal of the tender vestibular tissue, a procedure known as vestibulectomy, often solves the problem. It is appropriate as a last resort after every other treatment has been tried, and it is critical that the procedure be performed by a doctor who is very experienced to ensure that you get the best result and also to avoid complications that might make the problem worse.

Congenital Vestibulodynia

About 5 percent of women with vestibulodynia were born with it. So teens who have congenital vestibulodynia don't use tampons—not because they love wearing pads, but because inserting a tampon is so painful that it's out of the question. Usually these young women find their way to a gynecologist when they attempt intercourse and experience excruciating pain. Congenital vestibulodynia is one of the most common causes of unconsummated marriages.

The pain associated with this condition is a result of a developmental abnormality that occurs before birth and results not only in vestibular hypersensitivity but also, in 60 percent of cases, umbilical hypersensitivity. So if you are one of those people who hates, *hates* to have anyone touch inside your belly button, and you also have painful sex, you may have been born with this problem.

The Fix

The same strategies for acquired vestibulodynia are usually the first step in treating the congenital kind. Many experts believe that the *only* thing that is going to eliminate the pain from congenital vestibulodynia is a vestibulectomy. It sounds radical, but women who have *never* had pain-free intercourse rarely need to be talked into it.

Atrophic Vestibulodynia, aka Atrophic Vestibulitis or Hormonally Mediated Vestibulodynia

Atrophic vestibulodynia is not the same as vaginal atrophy. With vaginal atrophy, it is specifically the walls of the vagina that are thin and dry. In atrophic vestibulodynia, it is specifically the vestibule, and sometimes the vulva, that is painful from lack of estrogen. In addition to the tissue appearing dry and sometimes thin, there are often bright red patches at the opening of the vagina with this condition. Most women describe the pain on entry during sex as being knifelike. A lack of estrogen is not the only cause of this condition. There are androgen receptors as well as estrogen receptors throughout the vestibule, and these require testosterone, so a lack of testosterone can affect this area as well.

Menopause is the number-one cause of atrophic vestibular issues, which can occur with or without vaginal atrophy. It can also occur in any other condition associated with low estrogen, such as breast-feeding, and with the use of medications that block estrogen pathways, such as certain chemotherapy drugs, tamoxifen, and aromatase inhibitors. Atrophic vestibulodynia is also the number-one cause of sexual pain in young women and is almost always traced back to using a low-dose birth control pill (see chapter 12).

The Fix

Local estrogen treatments, as discussed in the upcoming chapter on menopause, will alleviate the pain, but in addition to a vaginal ring, cream, or tablet, estrogen cream should be applied directly to the vestibule.

A young woman with vestibulodynia who is on hormonal contraception must stop taking the pill and apply estrogen creams to the area. In addition, a topical testosterone cream may also help.

Don't expect to see any significant improvement for six weeks, since hormone receptors need to be reactivated. It can take up to six months to be 100 percent better.

Posterior Vestibulodynia

The symptom of posterior vestibulodynia is pain that is limited to just the bottom half of the vestibule and does not include the tissue around the urethra. This condition specifically arises from pelvic floor muscles being tight and tender. It really doesn't make sense that tight, painful muscles would cause pain in the tissue just outside the vagina, but it does. One theory is that since the pelvic floor muscles come together behind the vestibule, there is decreased blood flow and buildup in lactic acid from persistent muscle contraction and chronic inflammation. This can cause not only deep dyspareunia but also vestibular pain and burning as well.

This is why the skin and mucosa look entirely normal with this condition, but the patient experiences excruciating pain at the slightest touch with a cotton swab or finger.

The Fix

As any pelvic physical therapist will tell you, once the pelvic floor muscles are healed (see chapter 6 on pelvic physical therapy), the pain in the vestibular tissue disappears as well. It's a leap of faith to try pelvic physical therapy, but go with it.

Generalized Vulvodynia

Vulvodynia is, again, not a diagnosis but a description of *where the pain is*. Many women who are told they have vulvodynia actually have vestibulodynia. Sometimes the condition is referred to as "generalized vulvodynia" to cover all the possible locations for pain—labia, vestibule, clitoris, perineum. In other words, generalized vulvodynia refers to any pain *outside* the vestibule.

Vulvar pain may be caused by any of the conditions listed earlier that cause vestibulodynia, or it may be caused by one of the following dermatologic, allergic, hormonal, or neurologic conditions. In addition, pelvic floor dysfunction (see deep dyspareunia, page 124) can also result in vulvar pain.

The Fix

The key to dealing with any kind of vulvar pain is getting the correct diagnosis and treating the specific condition. You may need one drug, a combination of drugs, and/or pelvic physical therapy. Your doctor may be able to help you, but you may need a consultation with a specialist.

Should Your Vulva Be on a Diet?

A 1991 study suggested that foods high in oxalate (such as peanuts, pecans, and tofu) could cause vulvar burning and pain. While popular for a time, recent studies have shown that a low-oxalate diet is not only almost impossible to maintain but probably doesn't help with this issue. Some women do find that eliminating certain foods can make a difference. I have one patient whose symptoms disappeared after she eliminated the little red cinnamon candies (sky high in oxalate!) that she was addicted to.

Pudendal Neuralgia

This neurologic syndrome is caused by an inflammation of the pudendal nerve. The pudendal nerve carries sensation from your genitals. The problem occurs if the nerve becomes damaged or entrapped following a coccyx (tailbone) injury or pelvic surgery. Some experts even propose that it can occur from bicycle riding. It is usually one-sided, and the pain extends outside the vestibule to involve the entire vulva and sometimes the clitoris. It is generally at its worst when sitting, but sex is excruciating. Any perineal pressure can cause discomfort, burning, and aching, which is why it is sometimes confused with a vulvodynia. The pain is usually relieved if lying on your stomach or standing.

The Fix
This condition must be treated by a specialist. The pudendal nerve is injected with a local anesthetic, and a medication such as gabapentin or Lyrica is prescribed to desensitize the nerve. Sometimes surgery is required to release an entrapped nerve. Pelvic floor physical therapy is an essential component of treatment.

The Dystrophies

The dystrophies are dermatologic (skin) conditions that are unique to the vulva and vestibule. The majority of women with vulvar dystrophies are peri- or postmenopausal. In the case of dystrophies, the skin does not look normal. There may be discoloration, bleeding, bumps, fissures (splits in the skin), or a rash.

Nearly every one of these conditions can result in chronic itching, discomfort, and scarring if untreated. Scar tissue can even form over the clitoris—and yes, that is painful—and over time the vaginal opening can shrink. This creates a major barrier to entry. While each of these skin conditions has its own characteristic appearance, a biopsy is generally needed to clinch the diagnosis, particularly because constant scratching can make the tissue really inflamed and the condition unrecognizable to the naked eye. A biopsy will also determine whether there is a condition such as eczema, psoriasis, or a vulvar cancer or precancer.

Lichen Sclerosus

There is nothing to like about lichen sclerosus (LS). Just about every woman has experienced at least one itchy crotch episode that was so unbearable it culminated in an emergency midnight trip to the drugstore. Over-the-counter remedies will generally do the job if a yeast infection is the culprit, but in the case of lichen sclerosus, no amount of antifungal medication will give relief.

Lichen sclerosus is not an infection or a sexually transmitted disease, but a chronic inflammation of the skin that causes an itching so severe that some women literally scratch until they bleed. One of my patients hadn't had a decent night's sleep for months—every time she would drift off she would awaken to find herself scratching furiously. Another patient even confessed to using her hairbrush in a desperate attempt to get some relief.

While LS most commonly affects peri- or postmenopausal women, I have seen it in every age group, including the occasional teen. It's not clear how or why women get LS, but it is relatively common and affects about one in 70 women. There does seem to be a genetic predisposition, and in many cases it is associated with an immunologic problem such as thyroid disease.

Lichen sclerosus usually occurs on the skin around the clitoris and/or labia, which appears white, thin, and slightly wrinkled. In addition to intense itching, there can be cracks in the skin, bleeding, and pain. Scarring due to this inflammation can cause the labia minora to essentially disappear, and in severe cases the clitoris completely scars over, a condition known as clitoral phimosis.

LS sticks to the vulva and never affects the vagina. However, women with lichen sclerosus have a 4 to 6 percent risk of developing vulvar carcinoma. Lichen sclerosus has been found in more than 60 percent of cases of squamous carcinoma of the vulva. Therefore, treating LS is *not* optional. A biopsy should be performed, and close follow-up is essential.

Most women know something is amiss because of the itching, the presence of vulvar pain, or the inability to have intercourse. Up to 79 percent of women with lichen sclerosus report chronic vulvar pain. Other women have no symptoms, which is why it is never a good idea to skip your annual gynecologic exam. Someone (other than your sexual partner) should look at your vulva annually even if you don't need a Pap test!

The Fix

Once the diagnosis is made, relief can be found in the form of Clobetasol, a prescription-strength, high-potency steroid ointment. Clobetasol works best if you take a warm bath first and then massage the cream into the affected area for two to three minutes. A mirror is helpful to ensure that all areas are treated. A follow-up appointment two or three months after initial treatment is important to ensure that all areas have healed. Any areas that have not responded to treatment must be biopsied to ensure that there are no precancerous or cancerous changes to cells.

Once-daily treatment is recommended for the first few weeks, but then is tapered down to once a week. This condition has a high rate of recurrence, so it is important to keep using your medication until cleared by your doctor. While some women are able to eventually stop using the cream and apply it only if symptoms come back, most need to apply the medication on a weekly basis indefinitely to prevent recurrence.

Steroids tend to make the skin thin, so many treatment protocols also require adding a topical estrogen or estrogen/testosterone cream to make the tissue thicker and more elastic. It's a balancing act: the right combination of steroid and hormone cream does the trick for the majority of women. The hormone cream needs to be applied frequently at first, and then, like the steroid cream, is tapered down to a maintenance dose.

Occasionally a minor surgical procedure may be needed to remove scar tissue, as in the case of a clitoral phimosis.

The most important thing to know is that this is a manageable problem. Virtually every patient with LS is able to restore her sex life and her sanity. So if these symptoms sound familiar, put the hairbrush away and go see your gynecologist.

Lichen Simplex Chronicus, aka Pruritus Vulvae or Hyperplastic Dystrophy

Lichen simplex chronicus is the result of the itch that just doesn't go away. Basically, some irritant causes an itch. The itch causes scratching, and the scratching causes inflammation and thickening of the skin (known as lichenification) along with the release of histamine. This causes more itching. Sometimes the itching is so bad that the skin starts to bleed or gets infected.

This itch-scratch-itch cycle can be set off by any number of allergens or irritants. In addition, discharge from a vaginal infection may be the root cause of the irritation.

The Fix

Since it is generally impossible to figure out what started the problem, every irritant or allergen must be eliminated to find a root cause. That means no soap, no detergent, and no scented panty liners. Any vulvar or vaginal infection should be treated with oral, not topical, medication if possible. A topical steroid cream such as Clobetasol is then applied once daily. Nighttime scratching can be prevented with a bedtime vulvar ice pack and a low dose of amitriptyline, a tricyclic antidepressant. Unlike other vulvar dystrophies, once treated, lichen simplex chronicus does not return, unless a new irritant is introduced.

Can You Be Allergic to Sex?

It's pretty obvious that the best way to cope with the average allergy is to simply steer clear of whatever it is you are allergic to. So, while sometimes inconvenient, it is certainly doable to avoid penicillin, shellfish, peanuts, or cats. But what if you are allergic to sex? Yes, there are women who literally break out whenever they have intercourse . . . and abstinence is clearly not a positive solution. Women who are allergic to sex don't get a rash all over their bodies. Typically, their vestibule gets red and swollen after intercourse. There is no pain, discharge, itching, or odor.

And unlike most infections, the reaction occurs within minutes after intercourse, as opposed to days later. In most cases, the symptoms spontaneously disappear within a few hours, but on occasion hives and/or trouble breathing can occur.

So what is it exactly that causes the allergic reaction? The problem is actually not the penis or the sperm, but the semen, or more specifically, the proteins that are present in seminal fluid. Before you replace your partner, be aware that once you are allergic to semen, you often react to the proteins in any semen, not just a specific man's semen. Sometimes, though, the allergens are in certain medications, food, or even cola ingested by the man and then transmitted through the seminal fluid, thus causing an allergic reaction in his partner.

A true semen allergy is a difficult predicament. Using a condom is the simplest way to eliminate the problem. If condoms are not an option, the use of an antihistamine or vaginal cromolym sodium (an allergy medication) will often help, especially if you have a mild case. It's important to first have your gynecologist make sure that no infection is present. An evaluation by an allergist is the next step to confirm that what you are experiencing is indeed an allergic reaction. In addition to making the diagnosis and prescribing an appropriate medication, allergists can actually "desensitize" a woman to semen using injections similar to allergy shots.

If the problem occurs only after having sex with a condom, keep in mind that a latex allergy is another cause of post-intercourse redness and swelling and can be acquired even after years of successful condom use. In that case, the remedy is to use a lambskin or polyurethane condom. Also, nonlatex condoms break more often than latex condoms, so a spermicide backup is a good idea. The nonlatex female condom (FC2) is also an option. As an aside, if you have a latex allergy, it's important to inform your gynecologist so that he or she will know to use nonlatex gloves during your examination.

If it's not his semen and not latex condoms, it could be your vaginal lubricant or spermicide that is eliciting the allergic reaction. So before you give up sex altogether, it's probably a good idea to try eliminating that strawberry-flavored lube your boyfriend gave you last Valentine's Day.

Lichen Planus

Lichen planus (LP) is a less common inflammatory autoimmune disease that affects the vulvar skin. It is most commonly found in the soft tissue of the mouth and gums. Approximately 25 percent of women who have oral lichen planus also have genital lesions. Whereas lichen sclerosus is white and looks a little like cigarette paper, lichen planus has bright red shiny patches with lacy borders. Like other vulvar skin conditions, women with lichen planus experience itching, burning, pain, and soreness. Unlike lichen sclerosus, the lesions of lichen planus can also be found on vaginal tissue and can even obliterate the vagina if there is severe scarring.

The Fix

Lichen planus is more challenging to treat than lichen sclerosus. A steroid cream such as Clobetasol, along with a calcineurin inhibitor (a cream usually used to treat psoriasis), is usually successful. Vaginal dilators are usually recommended not only to prevent vaginal adhesions but also to apply steroid cream to the vaginal walls.

Desquamative Inflammatory Vaginitis

Desquamative inflammatory vaginitis (DIV) is a vaginitis that has gotten so out of hand that excessive discharge loaded with white blood cells pours out of the vagina and leaks onto the vulva. Women often describe yellow, sticky, gluelike discharge with this condition. DIV can be initiated by a vaginal infection or by severe inflammation from vaginal atrophy. Women with DIV are the ones who don't dare go out without a panty liner to protect their underwear. Usually the vaginal pH is elevated with DIV, since the good lactobacilli have vacated the neighborhood.

The Fix

A vaginal antibiotic such as metronidazole or clindamycin, along with a vaginal estrogen, will usually alleviate this problem. Sometimes a vaginal hydrocortisone is used as well. DIV usually clears up quickly (in a week or two) once it is properly treated.

Superficial Dyspareunia and Dryness

Vulvovaginal atrophy—or more simply, dryness—is also a common cause of superficial dyspareunia. As discussed throughout the book, while lack of estrogen from menopause is the most common cause of vaginal dryness, it is not the only cause. Circumstances that reduce natural lubrication in younger woman include:

Postpartum
Hormonal contraception
Chemotherapy or radiation treatment

Stress is also known to have an impact on dryness. I don't mean stress about being dry, but rather life stress that affects the vagina's natural ability to lubricate. Add medications such as antihistamines, decongestants, anticholinergics, and tamoxifen to the list, along with cigarette smoking and infrequent intercourse—all of these things can create dryness issues.

No matter the cause of vaginal atrophy, the fixes are available and covered in chapter 13. If the dryness is a reaction to pain from another source, the pain must be eliminated.

Further Tips on Healing

No matter what the condition, your vulva, vagina, and pelvic floor have been traumatized and need to heal. In addition to the specific treatments recommended by your physician, the following tips will help the healing process. Many have already been mentioned but bear repeating:

Avoid Irritants

Avoiding irritants and allergens is critical. Make sure your lubricant is free of preservatives (see chapter 5). Many doctors prescribe an antifungal cream assuming that the pain is from a chronic yeast infection. If yeast has not been diagnosed, chances are that you don't need this medication and it will be a huge irritant. Find a soap and a detergent that are not loaded with chemicals, or better yet, just wash your body (and your underwear) in warm water.

Keep in mind that urine, because it is acidic, is also an irritant.

No, I'm not going to suggest that you stop urinating, but separate your labia to ensure the urine stream goes straight into the toilet instead of splashing all over your vulva. Toilet paper is also a problem. If you are lucky enough to have a bidet, use it! If not, a bottle with a squirt top is ideal to use in washing the area with warm water before patting it dry with a cotton cloth. Some women also apply zinc oxide ointment or Aquaphor to protect the skin.

Numb the Area

Whether you are attempting intercourse or inserting a dilator, it sometimes helps to numb things up. Keep Cool Water Cone dilators (coolwatercones.com) in the fridge and place in your vagina both pre- and post-intercourse to relieve the burning and pain. Benzocaine, which is the anesthetic in Vagicaine and Vagisil, is often irritating and a common cause of allergic contact dermatitis and should be avoided. Your doctor can give you a prescription for lidocaine gel or ointment to both alleviate pain and short-circuit the nerve impulses. When you first apply the gel, it may be irritating, but if you give it a minute, numbness will set in. Some women apply it right before intercourse and find that it makes an enormous difference. Partner alert: let him know his parts may get a little numb as well.

Neogyn

As previously discussed, Neogyn is marketed as a "vulvar soothing cream." Although it may well win the prize for worst advertising campaign ever ("Do you suffer from chronic feminine discomfort . . . DOWN THERE?"), it happens to be an excellent product that facilitates healing of any vulvar condition when applied twice daily. The active ingredient is a cutaneous fibroblast lysate with human cytokines. In English, these are proteins that aid in wound healing.

It has been shown to be effective for pretty much any of the conditions discussed in this chapter to promote healing and decrease pain. In some studies, it is used *instead* of prescription medications for the treatment of vulvar dystrophies and vulvovestibulodynia. While I wouldn't recommend that (it's too early to know if it is effective enough), it is an excellent adjunct to prescribed treatment. Do not expect results for at least six weeks. It can be purchased without a prescription but currently is only available directly from the manufacturer's website (www.neogyn.us).

When dealing with any kind of pain associated with intercourse, sometimes you are better off avoiding an actual penis until the problem has been solved. Since in severe cases superficial dyspareunia will cause your pelvis to panic and your vagina to contract as a protective mechanism, pelvic physical therapy and/or vaginal dilators may be needed to teach your vagina that putting something in it will not be painful.

Nothing Is Working

I've just discussed the most common causes of sexual pain that arise from vulvar and vestibular conditions, but there are other, less common conditions that can be culprits as well. When it comes to pinning down one of these sometimes elusive diagnoses, or if you've been treated for one of the conditions I've discussed here and it is not getting better, a visit to a vulvar vaginal center (see the resources section) is in order, even if it means getting on an airplane to do so. As one woman I met when I was visiting Dr. Andrew Goldstein's clinic, the Center for Vulvar Vaginal Disorders in New York, said, "This trip is costing double what my trip to Florida last winter cost, but when I got home from Florida, I still had painful sex. I figure this is a much better use of my money."

More information about vulvovestibuldynia can be obtained

by going to the National Vulvodynia Association website, www
.nva.org.

The Small Vagina Issue

Before I close the chapter on superficial dyspareunia, I want to address those women who have a vaginal opening that has become
too small and inelastic for the penis in their life. Normal vaginas are
able to stretch enough to accommodate a baby's head and should
therefore be able to accommodate a penis of pretty much any size.
Sometimes a vaginal opening has shrunk, however, and is no longer
elastic owing to scarring, poor blood supply, radiation treatments,
lack of estrogen, surgery, or a vulvar dystrophy. There is also such a
thing as a vagina that is too tight following reconstructive surgery.
Obviously, during a surgical repair of a gaping or scarred vagina,
the surgeon has to make a judgment call as to the appropriate size
to make the opening. Fortunately, vaginal tissues are elastic and
will accommodate pretty much any size penis. Sometimes, though,
even with lubrication, intercourse after repair is impossible since
the vaginal opening may be too small and has lost elasticity.

All of these scenarios are fixable, but there is no getting around
the need for dilators and in some cases additional surgery.

Partners

While sexual pain sometimes comes when a dildo or vibrator is
used, most painful entry disorders include a male partner. I would
be remiss to not at least address the fact that, unless you are entirely
self-sexual, some of what may be causing you pain is the other
person involved.

Indeed, studies show that many women, despite severe pain,
continue to have sex to please their partner. They do this primarily because they fear the loss of the relationship. I have had more
than one woman tell me, "I really feel sorry for him, so I grit my
teeth and do my best to get through it." The guys are generally well
aware that the pain is occurring, and sometimes, in a well-meaning

way, they make it much worse by saying things like, "This pain is terrible. I'm worried you are never going to get better!" A 2013 study in *the Journal of Sexual Medicine* showed that this kind of "support" actually makes sexual pain worse.

It's also not unusual to "protect your pelvis" by intentionally or unintentionally sabotaging your relationship so that he doesn't even attempt intercourse. In any case, be aware of the profound effect that painful sex has on your relationship, communicate what is going on, and consider couples therapy to fix the emotional and relationship damage that your broken vagina may have caused.

9

A REAL PAIN IN THE PELVIS

Some sexual pain can be an indicator of a deeper problem

My new patient Valerie was beyond frustrated.

"You're the fourth doctor I have seen about this. Every other doctor I talk to about painful sex just keeps telling me to use more lube. If I use any more lube, my husband and I are going to both slide off the bed!"

She went on to tell me that she never felt dry, even without the bucketful of slippery stuff she had been advised to use. Her problem was that the slightest little thrust caused excruciating pain. The first doctor Valerie had consulted informed her that her exam was "normal" and told her that she should keep at it. The second ordered an ultrasound and CT of her pelvis. Also normal. The third sent her and her husband for couples therapy. At that point getting a concussion from sliding off an overlubed bed and banging her head seemed infinitely more likely than getting any relief from her pelvic pain.

Distinct from superficial dyspareunia (which you read about in chapter 8), deep dyspareunia can be gynecologic in nature, but it can also be due to gastrointestinal, bladder, musculoskeletal, psychological, or neurologic problems. Fibromyalgia and other pelvic floor muscle disorders have also been identified as culprits.

The cause of deep pelvic pain related to sexual activity is often challenging to diagnose. Your gynecologist may not be thinking about irritable bowel syndrome, your internist may not be thinking about endometriosis, and nobody may be thinking about interstitial cystitis. To make things more complicated, most of these problems are not detectable through blood work, ultrasound, or X-rays. What is required is a high level of suspicion and thinking "outside the box." It is not unusual for a woman to visit two (or three or four) doctors to get the right diagnosis. In many cases the correct diagnosis isn't made without a surgical exploration. The purpose of 20 percent of the laparoscopies conducted today is to evaluate chronic or persistent pelvic pain.

Sometimes no identifiable cause for the pain can be found. When this happens, a woman is often told, "It's all in your head." This may be true for a very rare few (those suffering from psychiatric conditions, for instance, or from post-traumatic stress due to a history of sexual abuse), but it is not common.

If you are not getting answers to why you experience persistent pelvic pain, it is worth finding one of the gynecologists who specifically deal with chronic and deep pelvic pain. Only when the cause of the pain has been determined can treatment be instituted. What follows is a brief discussion of the conditions that can be responsible for deep dyspareunia. This is not intended to be a complete list, but rather an introduction to the more common conditions to point you in the right direction. More details, including a comprehensive discussion of treatment options, can be found in my book *The Essential Guide to Hysterectomy.*

Endometriosis

While there are many problems that can cause pelvic discomfort, there is no question that endometriosis is the culprit for the vast majority of women who suffer from the chronic pelvic pain associated with deep dyspareunia. Basically, endometriosis is a condition in which the glandular tissue that normally lines the uterine cavity appears in other places, such as the lining of the pelvis, the fallopian tubes, the ovaries, the bowel, or the bladder, and even in unusual places like the lung. Each month during menstruation, this tissue responds to hormonal changes, just like the tissue that lines the uterine cavity. Since the tissue is not where it's supposed to be, various problems can ensue, such as inflammation, ovarian cysts, painful intercourse, infertility, adhesions, and excruciatingly painful periods that get worse with time. The degree of pain is not necessarily related to the visible severity of the endometriosis. Women who appear to have minimal endometriosis sometimes suffer the most.

Who Gets Endometriosis?

Any menstruating woman can have endometriosis, but it is most commonly found in women who have no children and who are between the ages of 25 and 40. It is estimated that 7 to 10 percent of premenopausal women have endometriosis. Historically, teenage girls just weren't supposed to have endometriosis. The monthly pain that would make an otherwise healthy 16-year-old eat ibuprofen like candy, miss school, and crawl into bed on a Saturday was just "bad cramps." We now know that is not the case. In fact, one study showed that 52 percent of teenage girls with severe chronic pelvic pain had surgically proven endometriosis.

There can also be a genetic predisposition for endometriosis. Women with an affected first-degree relative, such as a mother or sister, are at higher risk than women with no family history of this disorder. Women with shorter intervals between periods and women who bleed eight days or longer are also at increased risk.

How Do You Get Endometriosis?

There are lots of theories for how the endometrial glands get outside the uterus, but no single one explains the disease in everyone.

Most researchers in the field feel that there is no one explanation for endometriosis but that many mechanisms are responsible for it. Everyone agrees that it is not infectious or sexually transmitted.

How Do You Know if You Have It?

Endometriosis doesn't show up on ultrasound or X-rays. Often, it is suspected on the basis of symptoms such as painful periods, pain during intercourse, and infertility. A pelvic exam is sometimes suggestive, but the only way to know definitively if someone has endometriosis is to surgically look inside. Obviously, it's not appropriate for every woman with severe cramps to have surgery to determine if endometriosis is the cause, but if things are no better despite treatment, a laparoscopy is in order. Many cases of endometriosis are discovered when women have surgery for other issues.

The Fix for Endometriosis

Most conservative treatments for endometriosis do not require definitive diagnosis. If a woman has horrible periods and painful intercourse and endometriosis is suspected, it is perfectly reasonable to seek improvement of symptoms by trying different medical treatments.

It is also reasonable to do nothing in a known case of endometriosis if a woman has minimal or no symptoms, is not interested in conceiving, or is very close to menopause.

Treatment is divided into two categories: medical and surgical. Sometimes medical and surgical treatments are combined. The choice of treatment depends on the age of the patient, the desire for pregnancy, and the severity of the symptoms.

Medical Treatments for Endometriosis

Nonsteroidal Anti-inflammatory Drugs

Nonsteroidal anti–inflammatory drugs (NSAIDs) such as ibuprofen have always been useful to treat the pain associated with endometriosis, but they are usually not adequate for women with severe cases. It helps if the medication is started as soon as there is any pain, or even better, before there is pain. If women who have predictable periods start medication before bleeding starts, they can usually get much better relief than if the pain is well established.

No Period—No Problem

The easiest way to suppress mild to moderate endometriosis is to suppress menstruation, and the best way to do that over the long term is by taking continuous hormonal contraceptives. Some women are uncomfortable with the idea of eliminating their period and worry that there will be a buildup of tissue or some other side effect. In reality, women on the pill have thin uterine linings that do not require monthly shedding, and it is in no way detrimental to long-term health or fertility to not get a period.

There is actually no medical reason for a woman to take a week off and get her period if she is taking hormonal contraceptives. The scientists who developed the pill provided a pill-free week in which a "period" occurs only so that women would be more comfortable taking it. There is also documentation that the early developers of the pill naively thought that the Catholic Church would accept the pill as "natural birth control" and permit its use if it maintained normal menstrual cycles. Some even believe that misguided (male) scientists thought that women taking the pill would still want to get their period—to make them feel young and womanly!

Not only is it okay to fool Mother Nature, but for many women there is a significant medical benefit in not having a period. Menstrual cramps, hormonal migraines, heavy bleeding, and pain from endometriosis are all reduced or eliminated by taking an active pill every day. In truth, estrogen/progestin pills should be known by a name other than "birth control pills" since many women take them solely for the noncontraceptive benefits.

Some women are concerned that it is not "natural" to eliminate a period. That's true. But it also is not natural to be on the pill.

What is natural is to be pregnant or nursing all the time. And then you die.

Traditionally, since insurance companies covered only 12 packs of pills a year, no matter how many polite letters (using small words) they were sent explaining the medical logic, taking continuous pills has been a logistical nightmare. Fortunately, though, many companies are now manufacturing extended-cycle regimens, which make this an easier approach. The development of the birth-control patch and the vaginal ring has also expanded options for the woman who finds it difficult to take a pill every day.

For some women, menstrual suppression is not an option. While most women feel well on hormonal contraception, some women simply don't tolerate it and despite multiple attempts with multiple varieties continue to have problems with breakthrough bleeding, headaches, depression, or other side effects. Some women can't take estrogen, such as those with a history of blood clots, smokers older than 35, or women with breast cancer. And of course, there are the women for whom hormonal contraception causes a loss of libido or vaginal/vestibular pain (see chapters 8 and 11). Progestin-only contraception, such as a Mirena IUD, has also been shown to suppress endometriosis and can be used even by women who cannot take estrogen.

GnRH Analogue Injections

Gonadotropin-releasing hormones (GnRH) analogue injections temporarily shut off estrogen production and suppress menses, causing endometrial implants, inflammation, and cysts to become inactive and to regress. GnRH is not recommended for more than six months, since low estrogen levels over a long period of time may result in bone loss. Once GnRH is stopped, endometriosis recurs.

One use of GnRH is to test a woman to determine the source of pain. If it's not clear whether chronic pelvic pain is from endometriosis or some other cause, a course of GnRH will clarify the diagnosis. Pain from a urologic or gastrointestinal problem will not improve with GnRH. Sometimes a short-term course of GnRH is followed by long-term menstrual suppression with hormonal contraception.

Surgery—Conservative

In conservative surgery, the effects of endometriosis are removed but the uterus and ovaries are preserved.

One of the limitations of conservative surgery is that doctors can only remove what they see. Some endometriotic glands are always present microscopically within tissue, invisible to the naked eye, and therefore go untreated. If pregnancy does not follow surgery, suppression with continuous hormonal contraceptives is usually recommended to delay or prevent recurrence.

Surgery—Definitive

Definitive surgery is hysterectomy and removal of the ovaries. The decision to choose conservative or definitive surgery for endometriosis is made based on the severity of symptoms, age, the desire for pregnancy, and personal preference.

Hysterectomy is appropriate if pregnancy is not desired and if debilitating symptoms persist despite medical treatment. Removal of the ovaries in young women is, of course, controversial. Since endometriotic implants occur outside the uterus and respond to hormones released from the ovaries, removal of the uterus alone will not prevent endometriosis from persisting in the ovaries, pelvic lining, bladder, and other organs if the ovaries remain and continue to cycle. Traditionally, the recommendation for women with severe endometriosis has been to remove the ovaries in order to ensure that no residual endometriotic implants can be stimulated. Post-hysterectomy estrogen therapy is appropriate and has not been shown to cause recurrence of endometriosis symptoms.

Many women, in spite of severe endometriosis, do not want to go into menopause and choose to preserve their ovaries. While removal of the uterus alone will definitely lead to improvement of symptoms, issues related to endometriosis may still occur until the onset of natural menopause. If a woman is made aware of that, preservation of ovaries is an option. The only real "cure" for endometriosis is menopause, either natural or surgically induced.

Adenomyosis

It's beyond maddening to contend with monthly heavy bleeding, incapacitating cramps, and pain during intercourse, only to be told that it's not due to fibroids, endometriosis, hormonal problems, or any other identifiable gynecological issue. One diagnosis that is overlooked far too often is adenomyosis, a condition in which the glands that usually line the cavity of the uterus infiltrate deep into the wall of the uterus, resulting in bleeding and pain beyond even the worst of menstrual periods.

Adenomyosis is essentially a cousin to endometriosis. Whereas in endometriosis the glands that line the uterus get *outside* the uterus, in adenomyosis the uterine glands that usually line the cavity of the uterus burrow *into* the muscle (the myometrium) of the uterine wall. This condition results in an enlarged, softer than usual, and quite tender uterus. Painful periods and abnormally heavy bleeding are common in women with adenomyosis, but many women feel no symptoms at all and the disorder is discovered only when the uterus is removed for another reason.

Deep dyspareunia is often present with adenomyosis and is triggered when the penis hits the swollen, inflamed uterus. The diagnosis of adenomyosis is rarely made with certainty, since the only way to be certain is to look microscopically at a uterus that has already been removed. Women with adenomyosis often also have a painful hypertonic pelvic floor as a result of chronic pain.

Like endometriosis, adenomyosis doesn't show up on an ultrasound or X-ray. Since the glands are buried in the wall of the uterus, they can't be seen during laparoscopy, which inspects only the outside of the uterus, or hysteroscopy, which surgically visualizes the interior cavity of the uterus. An MRI can sometimes be useful in getting to a diagnosis but is not routinely done owing to its high expense.

The Fix

Treatment options for adenomyosis are essentially the same as for endometriosis. A trial of continuous oral contraceptives, or GnRH, may be beneficial. If medical therapy doesn't result in adequate relief, the definitive therapy continues to be hysterectomy. Unlike endometriosis, removal of the ovaries is not beneficial or necessary with this issue, since the problem only occurs inside the uterus. Symptoms resolve with the onset of menopause, so waiting it out is always an option, though not a very pleasant one.

Adhesions

Adhesions are commonly thought of as "scar tissue" but are not the same thing as scar tissue at all. Scar tissue refers to changes that occur as part of the normal healing process. Adhesions, on the other hand, refer to an abnormal tissue reaction that causes internal organs or structures, such as the small intestines, to adhere or stick to other structures. Adhesions can occur as a result of surgery, infection, endometriosis, or inflammation, or for no apparent reason whatsoever. Prior surgery is generally the biggest culprit, but some types of surgery are more likely to result in adhesion formation than others. In general, laparoscopic or robotic-assisted surgery, as opposed to traditional surgery performed through a large abdominal incision, tends to minimize the likelihood of adhesion formation.

Most women with adhesions have no symptoms and are unaware of their presence. But adhesions can be responsible for a myriad of problems, including bowel obstruction, infertility, and, in some cases, pelvic pain.

For example, structures such as ovaries, tubes, or loops of bowel can adhere to the back of the vagina and be responsible for deep dyspareunia. The pain when the penis hits the ovary is much like the pain a guy experiences when he gets kicked in the testicles.

Interestingly, the way a skin incision heals is not a reflection of the way things heal on the inside. Many women with invisible abdominal scars have terrible intra-abdominal adhesions, yet someone with a thick, raised scar may be perfect inside.

The Fix

Not infrequently, the tissues soften up and the pain dissipates over time and with continued sexual activity (if you are able). Pelvic physical therapists are often able to work with tender trigger points from trapped nerves or adhesions to manipulate tissue and decrease inflammation.

On occasion, however, a surgical procedure is needed. One memorable patient started to have excruciating deep dyspareunia following a very straightforward laparoscopic removal of an ovarian cyst. After months of pain, I did a follow-up laparoscopy and found that a single band of tissue had caused her ovary to attach to the back of her vagina. One snip to cut the adhesion freed the ovary and resulted in pain-free intercourse.

Interstitial Cystitis

The only thing more distressing than having chronic pelvic pain, a constant urge to urinate, *and* dyspareunia is to have a doctor who has no idea what might be causing this. For women who suffer from interstitial cystitis (IC), also known as bladder pain syndrome, that is all too frequently the case. Recently, however, there has been an increased awareness of this debilitating condition that affects anywhere from 700,000 to 7 million women (depending on whose statistics you believe). Unfortunately, it is still an average of five years from the onset of symptoms until diagnosis and treatment for this condition. One of the reasons diagnosis is so complicated is that IC symptoms are not limited to the bladder. Pain frequently radiates to the back, thighs, or lower abdomen, and yes, this condition can also occur in men.

Usually when doctors talk about *cystitis,* they are referring to a bacterial bladder infection. IC is *not* an infection, but an inflammation of the wall of the bladder. Urine cultures are always negative for bacteria, and antibiotics don't help. Most researchers feel that IC is caused by damage to the inner lining of the bladder, resulting in an elevated pain response to the normal components of urine. Since there is always at least a little urine in the bladder, there is essentially always some degree of pain. Women with mild IC have occasional flares triggered by food, sex, or stress; women with severe IC have chronic, debilitating pelvic pain, urinate as often as 60 times a day (and night!), are unable to have intercourse, and are pretty much nonfunctional.

Diagnosis of IC has always been a challenge, which is why identification of this condition is often delayed. Women who have urinary frequency or urgency should first have a urine culture to make sure there is no infection. A visit to your gynecologist is also in order to eliminate other pelvic problems. Often a urologist is the one to make the IC diagnosis. A few years ago, a questionnaire was developed to help women recognize if they might have IC. The PUF (Pelvic Pain and Urgency/Frequency) patient symptom scale is an eight-question test that measures the presence and severity of IC symptoms and identifies those women who are likely to have IC as opposed to another bladder condition.

Since Antibiotics Don't Work, What Will?

In the past, the only advice doctors could give patients for dealing with IC was to tell them to avoid foods that were known to irritate the bladder, such as caffeine, alcohol, fruit juices, vinegar, and spicy foods. In 2011 the American Urology Association released guidelines to assist in the diagnosis and treatment of interstitial cystitis.

First-line treatments include diet modification, over-the-counter products, and avoidance of activities that trigger pain, such as exercise or certain positions during sexual activity. Second-line treatments include pelvic floor physical therapy and various prescription drugs such as Pentosan polysulfate (Elmiron), an FDA-approved oral medication specifically for the treatment of IC. A number of other treatments are available for the most severe cases, but they are best administered by experts in the IC world.

Additional information about interstitial cystitis, including the details of bladder-friendly foods and available treatments, can be found at www.ic-network.org.

Ovarian Cysts

Ovarian cysts are common. Pain from ovarian cysts, including pain during intercourse, is not. Having said that, very large cysts can sometimes hurt, which is why it's not unreasonable for a patient with deep pain during intercourse to be sent for an ultrasound in order to eliminate the possibility of a problematic ovarian cyst.

Frequently a tiny one- to two-centimeter cyst is detected and is cited as the cause of the pain. Small cysts do not cause pain, however, and the surgery that some women end up having to remove them is unnecessary.

I had one patient who had a very well-endowed new partner. She experienced deep pelvic pain whenever she had intercourse, and lo and behold she was found to have a large ovarian cyst that turned out to be an early-stage ovarian cancer. We joked about how her new boyfriend's penis saved her life.

If you are found to have a cyst on ultrasound, keep in mind that only 7 percent of persistent cysts in women under the age of 50 are cancerous. After age 50, up to 30 percent of cysts are cancerous. Size and other characteristics help determine the likelihood of a potential cancer, the likelihood that the cyst is responsible for your pain, and most important, the appropriateness of surgical removal.

Fibroids

Like cysts, fibroids are common, but do not commonly cause severe pelvic pain.

If a woman has sexual pain and is found to have fibroids, it is far more likely that she also has endometriosis or adenomyosis that is causing the problem and that the fibroids are just a red herring.

The official nomenclature for a fibroid tumor is uterine leiomyoma. Also referred to as myomas, fibroids are benign (noncancerous) tumors that arise from the smooth muscle cells of the uterus. They are solid, as opposed to cystic (fluid-filled), and vary widely in size. Often they are microscopic, but they can also grow to the size of a beach ball.

In most cases, fibroids are too small to create symptoms and, if found, can be ignored. It's not just the size but the position of the fibroid that predicts who is going to have an issue, and what kind of issue. As any good real estate agent knows, it's all about location, location, location. When it comes to heavy bleeding from fibroids, there's no worse location than fibroids that grow into the cavity of the uterus. Even small fibroids can cause the "change the tampon every hour" heavy periods that not only are miserable to deal with but also can result in anemia. While heavy bleeding can cause wicked menstrual cramps, small fibroids in the cavity of the uterus do not cause dyspareunia.

The truth is that most fibroids do not cause pain, but there are always exceptions to the rule. Degeneration results if a portion of a large fibroid outgrows its blood supply and dies. The result is pain and a tender uterus. This is more common during pregnancy, when fibroids grow very quickly, but can also happen just because the fibroid is large.

Women with large fibroids that exert pressure on other pelvic structures (known as "bulk symptoms") are the ones who generally experience discomfort during intercourse. If the fibroid is located on the front of the uterus, the woman knows every bathroom within a five-mile radius of her home and work. There is a constant pressure "down there," resulting in the feeling of needing to urinate even when her bladder is empty. And when the bladder starts to fill . . . well, there's not a whole lot of room to spare.

If the fibroid is on the back of the uterus, constipation and rectal pressure may become problematic. Women who have had a baby know that incredible feeling of pressure on the rectum as the baby's head moves down the vagina right before delivery. Women with large fibroids sitting on their rectum experience that sensation on a regular basis. And really large fibroids can make even the slimmest of women look pregnant. Unlike pregnancy, however, the belly bulge doesn't disappear after nine months with fibroids, and there is no cute little baby to make you forget all the discomfort. It goes without saying that looking like you are about to deliver, when you're not, doesn't do a lot for body image or that sexy feeling.

Any woman can get fibroids, but some women are more likely candidates than others. Fibroids most commonly appear during the years in which women produce estrogen and progesterone—in other words, the reproductive years. Most women develop symptoms from fibroids during their thirties and forties, but some women continue to have problems even after menopause. Many women assume (and bank on the assumption that) their fibroids will disappear after their periods stop. They generally don't, but they do usually stop growing and eventually shrink over time postmenopause.

As with ovarian cysts, the presence of a fibroid doesn't always mean the fibroid is causing the problem. Twenty-five percent of women in the reproductive years have fibroids that they are aware of, either because they've had symptoms or the fibroids were discovered during a routine gynecologic examination. Small, asymptomatic tumors exist in the uteruses of up to 80 percent of women, most of whom are totally oblivious to their presence until the fibroids are identified serendipitously on an ultrasound done for another reason.

The Fix

We've come a long way since your grandmother's time when the only option for dealing with fibroids was hysterectomy requiring a big abdominal incision and a long recovery. If a hysterectomy is required or desired to treat your symptoms, it can almost always be performed laparoscopically or robotically as an outpatient procedure. But sometimes your uterus doesn't need to be sacrificed to deal with symptomatic fibroids.

Myomectomy is an alternative to hysterectomy that surgically removes fibroids and leaves the uterus behind. Most women who undergo myomectomy still end up with an abdominal incision and require a six-week recovery even though if the fibroids are in the uterine wall or project outside the uterus, laparoscopic or robotic-assisted removal is often an option.

Hysteroscopic myomectomy is another underutilized minimally invasive uterus-sparing technique that removes problematic fibroids inside the uterine cavity without an incision. This procedure is performed on an outpatient basis, takes less than an hour, and requires essentially no recovery.

Here's how it works: Most women are familiar with dilatation and curettage (D&C), a procedure in which the cervical opening is made slightly larger in order to put an instrument into the uterine cavity to scrape away the lining of the uterus. It would be nice if a simple D&C could eliminate fibroids, but scraping the lining of the uterus to remove a fibroid is like raking leaves and expecting to remove the boulder in the ground. D&Cs are useful for *evaluating* bleeding, but are not really meant to *treat* the bleeding.

When I perform a D&C, it is always accompanied by a hysteroscopy in which I slide a slender scope with a camera and light attached to it through the cervix in order to see what's going on inside the uterus. If a fibroid is present, I insert a small instrument through the hysteroscope to cut the fibroid into small pieces, a process known as fibroid resection, or morcellation. The small pieces of fibroid then are easily removed. The patient goes home that day, fibroid-free.

Uterine artery embolization is another minimally invasive approach to treat fibroids and involves an interventional radiologist injecting beads (using an MRI for guidance) to reduce the blood supply to the uterus and shrink fibroids.

The details of these and other treatments are covered in *The Essential Guide to Hysterectomy.*

Dr. Streicher's SexAbility Survey

From my survey of over 2,000 women about why they decided to ultimately have a hysterectomy:

> My uterus was the size of a small loaf of bread because of the fibroid tumors. The bleeding had me soaking through a super-size tampon and extra-heavy pad in an hour. My periods lasted two weeks. It detracted greatly from my quality of life.

> I bled 27 days out of 30 and was exhausted for well over two years. I just had enough! I'd tried everything the doctors wanted to try and finally just said, "Enough! I want this nightmare to end. Do the surgery—please!"

> Possibly due to the birth of 10-pound baby, years later my uterus severely prolapsed so it was very awkward physically and for sex. Also during exercise/sneezing urine came out. At the time I was going through a divorce. Pre-op appt. the doctor asked if I would be having sex later in life. I'm not really sure what that question had to do with the surgery but my sex life is great.

> I was finished having children was one of the main factors and I was just tired of the pain that I was having. Intercourse was awful to the point I would make up excuses not to do it.

> My husband and I made the decision due to the fact that I was experiencing extremely painful intercourse. My doctor stated it was because my uterus was prolapsed and so was my bladder after multiple pregnancies. Also to reduce my risk of uterine cancer as my mother had uterine cancer.

> *My story is about making excuses. I made every excuse to not go to the doctor. Until I was able to feel the fibroid tumors in my belly, I put off making the appointments. I had every symptom and still put it off, making excuses about why my period was so heavy. For two years, I told myself it's just my body changing. It was stupid and I ended up without a choice. For me, it worked out, but it was very scary for me and for my husband. It could have been cancer, it could have ended badly. Take-away here. Go to the doctor for your annual exam. If I had, I would still have my uterus.*

Uterine Prolapse

Uterine prolapse is just what it sounds like: the uterus drops down into the vagina, and in severe cases outside the vagina. Weakened pelvic floor connective tissues (as in muscles, ligaments, and fascia) that should support the uterus don't, gravity wins out, and the uterus descends from its usual position.

Women who have uterine prolapse frequently have other displaced organs due to weak pelvic tissues. A cystocele results when a prolapsed bladder bulges through the front of the vagina; a rectocele occurs when the rectum bulges through the vaginal floor, or back wall of the vagina. The general term used to describe these conditions is POP, as in Pelvic Organ Prolapse, not as in "Yikes, my uterus has popped out."

Uterine and Pelvic Organ Prolapse Are Associated with Sexual Problems

If the cervix is outside the vaginal opening, there may be bleeding, discharge, and vulvar pain. Let's not forget the effect of your uterus or bladder hanging outside your vagina on your body image. The urinary or fecal incontinence associated with prolapse is a significant sexual sabotage. (I cover this in greater detail in chapter 15.)

What causes the pelvic pain associated with prolapse is a very weak, dysfunctional pelvic floor (remember chapter 6?). In other words, the weak pelvic floor that contributed to the prolapse also causes pain.

Who Gets a Prolapsed Uterus?

A vaginal delivery, particularly if the labor is long and the baby large, is the greatest risk factor for a uterus that has gone south. It's not the only risk factor, since most women who deliver vaginally don't end up with POP, but 75 percent of prolapse can be attributed to pregnancy. Family history is also a major factor. Tissue prone to damage is an inherited tendency, and it's not unusual for a woman with uterine prolapse to mention that her mother and grandmother had the same problem. Take a genetic predisposition, add a nine-pound baby and three hours of pushing . . . something is going to give. Once the tissue is damaged, it never completely regains its strength and elasticity; the effects of gravity and age then compound the problem.

Obesity is also a significant risk factor. Women with a body mass index over 25 are two times more likely to have prolapse than normal-weight women. Smoking is another culprit. Even though the pelvis is a long way from the lungs, the effects of smoking on tissue are seen throughout the body. It doesn't help that smokers are often frequent coughers. Chronic constipation is also a risk factor. Pushing is pushing and whether it is a huge baby or repetitive efforts at getting out a bowel movement, tissue will weaken as a result.

While this distressing condition spares no age group, the likelihood of prolapse increases with age, and since women are now living longer, increasing numbers of women are destined to suffer from uterine prolapse.

My new patient was 92 years old and had a uterus that was completely hanging out. I asked her how long that had been the case, and she said, "Oh, I've had this since I was 75." When I asked her why she had never had it taken care of, she replied, "I didn't think I would get my money's worth—if I knew then what I know now, I would have had the surgery years ago!"

How Do You Know if You Have a Prolapse?

Symptoms are generally related to the degree of the prolapse—in other words, how far the uterus has dropped. In a first-degree prolapse, the uterus is only slightly lower than its normal position, and most women are totally unaware that something has shifted unless their gynecologist points it out. A further drop creates a second-degree prolapse, which is the point at which some women become aware that something is not quite right. Still, many women with a second-degree prolapse have no symptoms. By the time the uterus drops low enough for the vagina to be completely filled and the cervix reaches the opening of the vagina (third-degree prolapse), most women are definitely aware there is a problem. Even the most oblivious woman notices when her uterus drops outside her vagina (a fourth-degree prolapse), prompting an emergency visit. One woman actually called from her bathtub, appropriately upset, crying, "Something is floating out of my vagina . . . and I think it's my uterus!"

The most common symptom is the feeling that "something is falling down," which is not surprising since that is exactly what has happened. Nine times out of ten, a woman correctly diagnoses her own prolapse before any doctor lays eyes on her. Many women, in addition to constant pressure, actually feel a mass or bulge at the vaginal opening. A quick look in the mirror (a hand mirror with a long handle works well) and you can see something pink bulging out. In severe cases, women may be unable to have a bowel movement or urinate.

The Fix

Once the damage is done, what options are available to treat uterine prolapse? Surgery, almost always a hysterectomy, is the ultimate treatment. The first hysterectomy in history, as a matter of fact, in AD 200, was done vaginally for a completely prolapsed uterus. Today vaginal or laparoscopic hysterectomy is the standard treatment for symptomatic uterine prolapse. If surgery is not desired or medically appropriate, a doctor may recommend the placement of a pessary, a device that is placed in the vagina to support the uterus. This will sometimes give relief. Pelvic floor physical therapy is instrumental, with or without surgery.

Sex Post-Hysterectomy

If someone has a hysterectomy to *solve* a gynecologic problem, a common fear is that the surgery will create a sexual problem. Fortunately, that is rarely the case. Over 500,000 women in the United States undergo hysterectomy each year. One-third of women will lose their uterus by age 60. Virtually every one of those women will have worried about how hysterectomy will affect her sexual function, desire, and desirability. Unfortunately, studies have shown that only half of gynecologists initiate a discussion of sex during pre- or post-op appointments, and few patients (about 13 percent) are willing to bring it up themselves. That means a lot of women who worry about their post-operative sexuality do just that—*worry*.

Fortunately, studies show that unless ovaries are also removed along with the uterus, inducing menopause, the majority of women do not report adverse effects of hysterectomy on sexual function.

A patient of mine had a severe uterine prolapse and was in the pre-op area waiting to have a hysterectomy. The male medical student was eagerly asking her questions about her condition. She finally turned to him and said, "You just have no idea what it's like to have something hanging between your legs all the time!" Just as she realized what she had said, we rolled her off and mercifully put her to sleep.

A 1999 study published in *the New England Journal of Medicine* tracked over 1,000 women during the two years after their surgeries and, unlike many earlier studies, evaluated sexual function both before and after hysterectomy. The results of the study were reassuring and validated what most gynecologists (but not most pre-op patients) knew all along.

Seventy-seven percent of the women in the post-operative group were sexually active one year after surgery, in contrast to only 71 percent of the group the year before. This finding is not surprising given that the study also demonstrated that the number of women who experienced pain during sex decreased from 19 percent to 4 percent. The quality and number of orgasms increased, as did overall libido post-op. The bottom line is that frequency of sexual activity consistently increased and sexual dysfunction decreased after hysterectomy.

Even though there was a negative impact on sexual function in about 15 percent of women who took this survey, the improvement in general health evidently trumped the impact on their sex lives.

Women who become menopausal as a result of surgery have an additional set of issues to deal with. If estrogen supplementation is not initiated, it is likely that mood disturbance, vaginal dryness, and a much higher risk of sexual dysfunction overall will ensue. There is no question that estrogen and androgen supplementation will absolutely increase libido, lubrication, and sexual response. Some women are fine without it, but for many women the loss of hormones is a major blow to sexuality. These issues are further explored in chapters 12 and 13.

Dr. Streicher's SexAbility Survey

My own survey of over 2,000 women post-hysterectomy asked: "Is your sex life better or worse after hysterectomy?"

- 85 percent said that their sex life was better or unchanged
- 85 percent said that their orgasms were better or unchanged
- 92 percent said that they were glad they had the hysterectomy

Pain Post-Hysterectomy

While the overwhelming majority of women have no problems, some may experience postsurgical sexual issues.

Once you have had your final post-hysterectomy checkup, most doctors give the go-ahead to resume sexual activity. One big hurdle to overcome is fear. Many women are understandably nervous about having intercourse, thinking that it might create a problem or that they will experience pain. Partners are also sometimes leery, which hardly makes for a wild sexual experience. If your doctor has given you the okay, it really will be fine, but you won't believe that until you try.

Nevertheless, in spite of waiting the proper amount of time, using appropriate lubrication, and drinking a glass (or two) of chardonnay, things don't always go well.

New-onset superficial dyspareunia after hysterectomy is usually only an issue if things are dry. If your ovaries were not removed or you were already postmenopause prior to surgery, this should not be the case. If at the time of hysterectomy there were other procedures, like a bladder lift, your first attempt at intercourse may be uncomfortable due to vaginal stitches and healing vaginal or perineal tissue. Use plenty of lube and take it slow, but if things hurt, healing may be incomplete and you may just need a little more time. Once healing is complete, the opening to the vagina occasionally becomes too small or tight. In that case, dilators and local vaginal estrogen may be needed to restore functional anatomy.

Deep internal pelvic pain during intercourse after hysterectomy is generally not due to vaginal dryness.

> ### Dr. Streicher's SexAbility Survey
>
> 3.7 percent of women surveyed had sex two weeks post-op
> 11.7 percent had sex four weeks post-op
> 34.9 percent had sex six weeks post-op
> 32.5 percent had sex eight weeks post-op
> 7.2 percent never resumed having intercourse

Generally, the pain is caused by the penis hitting something at the back of the vagina, or behind the vagina. There are a number of things that could create this problem, all generally solvable.

Infection at the back of the vagina or behind the vagina occurs rarely after hysterectomy, but if it does it can be a cause of discomfort. Usually, a combination of antibiotics, time, and sometimes drainage of a pocket of pus (if there is an abscess) will solve the problem.

Pelvic adhesions are always a possibility, but occasionally there is an adhesion in the vagina where a band of tissue has formed during the healing process. You would have no way of knowing it's there until a finger or penis pushes on it, creating pain. The pain is usually sharp and occurs without warning. Your gynecologist can easily identify this condition by doing a speculum exam and can easily remedy it, usually in his or her office.

Persistent Pain

It's not unusual to treat the endometriosis, IC, or adenomyosis, yet still have pain with intercourse. No matter what the initial cause of deep dyspareunia and chronic pelvic pain, there is inevitably some degree of hypertonic pelvic floor dysfunction or a lingering vaginismus, even after the initial cause of the pain has been treated. Your vagina isn't stupid: it has spent years developing the same kind of protective mechanisms that women with superficial dyspareunia do.

Even if no gynecologic or medical cause of pelvic pain has been identified, in most cases your issues are caused by a pelvic floor dysfunction. *I can't emphasize enough* the importance of working with an experienced pelvic floor physical therapist to determine if that is the case. If so, that therapy can change your life.

> If deep penetration hurts, one strategy is to make penetration less deep. A Comeclose collision ring (http://www.comeclose.co.uk) placed around the base of your partner's penis will not detract from his pleasure, but may increase yours since the ring serves as a cushioned "spacer."

10

LOST MY MOJO

Want to find your mojo? Here's how.

Of all the conditions that get in the way of sexual health, libido is the most common, and also the most complex. In nature, the desire to have sex is driven by the need to reproduce. Once that is no longer an option or is biologically undesirable, there are a number of mechanisms in place that decrease libido. Evidently, whoever was in charge forgot to consider that sex is not *just* about making babies.

Consider the "cycle of sex" throughout our lives. In your twenties, it's all about sex, all the time. Then we get into the baby-making years, where sex has a purpose. And then, before we know it, the bedroom is a place where all we want to do is get a decent night's sleep after a long day.

The years go by, and suddenly it occurs to you that you're not having sex anymore. When you start trying to make it a priority again, your brain and your body don't even remember what it was like to have great sex.

Things get even more complex during the perimenopause and menopause years, when, in addition to plummeting hormones, factors such as illness, medications, problematic relationships, divorce, and stress can get in the way. It's hard to be in the mood when you just lost your job, your husband is having an affair, your kid just came home with another piercing, and you are dealing with a 20-pound weight gain. On top of that, as has been mentioned, once estrogen has plummeted, roughly half of couples find that if they do actually give it a go, it hurts. As a result, what's left of your libido completely evaporates and you simply get out of the habit of wanting it, or even thinking about it. Avoidance mode becomes the norm, and 10 PM seems like the perfect time to clean out the refrigerator to circumvent the discomfort of slipping into bed and trying to make yourself invisible—or worse, come up with yet another excuse why you don't want to have sex.

It's not just midlifers who have libido issues. Even if you are 30 and single, even if intercourse is pleasurable and orgasms are happening, even if your ovaries are still pumping out estrogen and menopause is years away, too many women find they simply don't think about sex and have zero interest in initiating it.

These are the patients who tell me they feel like something has been stolen from them, and they want it back.

When Lust Disappears

The medical term for lack of lust is hypoactive sexual desire disorder (HSDD), which is defined as an absence of sexual thoughts, fantasies, or desire for sexual activity that *causes distress or interpersonal difficulties*. The "causes distress" part is important. Many women acknowledge that they have no libido, but when I inquire as to whether they would like to address it, some of them will say very clearly, "No, it's fine. I don't care." In other words, their loss of libido doesn't seem to matter to them.

Another part of the definition is also key: "interpersonal difficulties." Some women come to my office saying that they have no interest in sex and are not particularly motivated to give things a boost, but their lack of interest is getting in the way of their relationship with their spouse or partner. The realization that their lack of libido is having a negative effect on the relationship is what causes distress, and ultimately it is also what gives them the motivation to do whatever it takes to get it back.

I, like many sexual health experts, have a problem with the "distress" requirement for an HSDD diagnosis. Women don't generally use the word "distress" when they have sexual problems. They tend to use the word "frustrated." In addition, it makes no sense to require someone to be distressed (or frustrated) by a lack of libido and seeking treatment to meet the criteria of HSDD. If a woman has a pain in the head, it is still called a headache even if she chooses not to take an aspirin.

So how many women have HSDD? Depending on the study, age group, and other criteria, rates range from 15 to 30 percent of premenopausal women. Well over 50 percent of women who are postmenopausal report diminished libido, but since only a fraction of them are "distressed" to the point of seeking treatment, the number of them who would be diagnosed with HSDD is much lower. In reality, however, if the women in my practice are any indication, the rates are dramatically higher.

In my experience, it is the rare woman who says that she never, at any time in her life, had an interest in sex. In other words, loss of libido is almost always an acquired condition—it isn't something you're born with. This also means it can be reversed, or at the very least addressed.

According to Dr. Jan Shifren's landmark study, 40 percent of women have sexual dysfunction, but only 12 percent care enough to do something about it. Many women stop caring that they have sexual problems simply because they have lost the urge to have sex. If you love to run marathons and then have to stop because of a knee injury, over time you'll have no incentive to have surgery to fix the injury if you no longer have a desire to run marathons.

The Causes of HSDD

An intact libido depends not only on sociocultural, psychological, and interpersonal influences but on intact biology as well. Anything that tips the balance in these areas is a potential problem. The list of ingredients in the biological libido cocktail includes the physical ability to have a healthy response, neurotransmitters firing correctly, and the right amount of hormones.

Physical Response

A functioning, intact libido is dependent on a physiological response that not only results in the ability to have intercourse but results in pleasure. No one wants to do something that doesn't feel good. Women who have sexual pain invariably lose libido and often become dysfunctional in arousal and orgasm as well. No one wants to do something that hurts, and it is hopeless to address libido issues without first eliminating the source of pain.

Neurotransmitters

While many women are aware that hormones such as estrogen and testosterone are needed for an intact libido, neurotransmitters are just as important. Neurotransmitters are released from the brain and control the pathways that determine how often we think about, and desire, sex. While there are many neurotransmitters that make a contribution, the essential ones are dopamine and serotonin.

Dopamine is all about desire. It's dopamine that creates that feeling of "I want sex, I need sex, I can't stop thinking about sex."

Serotonin is all about keeping desire under control so you can stop making love long enough to go to work and do the laundry. Serotonin is nature's way of ensuring that we don't have sex 24/7.

If there is too much serotonin, or too little dopamine, cleaning out the closet becomes infinitely more interesting than a sexual encounter. So it's all about balance—we need enough dopamine to want sex, and enough serotonin so we don't want it all the time.

And don't assume it's just older women who have trouble with their libidos. In Dr. Streicher's Sexability Survey (see box) almost 40 percent of women ages 30 to 40 answered *50/50!*

Hormones

While there are a number of hormones that contribute to libido, androgens and estrogen are the big players. Anything that interferes with normal hormone levels potentially interferes with desire. (Some researchers believe that loss of libido is less about hormones and more about the monotony of monogamy. More on this later!)

Menopause is the most obvious situation in which estrogen levels are pretty much nonexistent, but women who are postpartum or taking various medications can have low estrogen as well (see chapter 12).

Androgens are commonly thought of as male hormones, since men make androgens in large amounts and have minimal amounts of estrogen. In fact, all women make androgens as an integral part of the female hormonal milieu. The levels are lower than in men, but they are definitely there, and definitely female. The ovary produces two types of androgens: testosterone and androstenedione.

The majority of testosterone is bound to sex-hormone binding globulin (SHBG), a protein that circulates in the blood. For testosterone to be active, it must be unbound, or free. Anything that increases SHBG decreases the amount of unbound, or active, testosterone. SHBG levels are inversely related to body mass index. The more someone weighs, the lower the SHBG. Pregnancy, hormonal contraception, and oral estrogen therapy all increase SHBG, therefore decreasing the levels of testosterone that are free to actually do something, often resulting in lowered libido.

Androgens, in combination with estrogen, are responsible for increased sensitivity to sexual stimulation, sexual fantasies, arousal, enhanced capacity for orgasm, sexual energy, and a general sense of well-being. In short, androgens are what make women want sex and experience great sex. In menstruating women, there is even is a midcycle surge in testosterone around the time of ovulation— nature's way of encouraging sex for reproduction during this time.

Fortunately, for the thousands of women who have no ovaries or have nonfunctional ovaries, there is an androgen backup. Most women are relieved to know that the ovary is not the only source of androgens in the body; they are also produced in significant amounts by the adrenal glands, which sit on each kidney. There is a god.

How much estrogen and androgen are needed for a healthy libido and a great sex life? That is probably one of the most complex questions in the whole libido dilemma. It would be nice if there were precise amounts of each hormone required for a perfect sexual response, but it doesn't appear that that is the case.

Women with very low testosterone levels often have healthy libidos and amazing sex lives, while women with high levels may have no interest at all. A few years ago, I got a call from the husband of a patient: "My wife has absolutely no interest in sex. Can you check her testosterone level when she comes in for her annual exam?"

When his wife arrived, I mentioned her husband's concern, and she readily agreed to a testosterone blood-level check. I called her the next week and announced, "Well, I think I have found the problem. Your testosterone level is essentially zero!"

There was a long pause before she finally said, "That's really interesting—because, guess what? I am having *amazing* sex with my personal trainer twice a day."

So much for testosterone levels being a clear indicator. And that is precisely the problem. There is a wide range of "normal," and a number of other things beyond hormones (evidently a hot personal trainer is one of them) contribute to libido.

Prolactin, produced by the pituitary gland, which is located in the brain, is the hormone that can inhibit desire. Prolactin is normally elevated during breast-feeding. Biologically, a woman who is nursing is not ready to have another baby, so it makes sense for the hormone that stimulates lactation to also inhibit sexual desire.

So, does it make sense to measure hormone levels when trying to solve the libido puzzle?

I get this question a lot, and it's not unusual for women to come to a first consultation holding pages of hormone lab results from other doctors. During the perimenopause or premenopause phase, it is generally not useful to measure hormone levels, not only because they fluctuate wildly, but also because there are no specific levels that correlate with an intact libido. Postmenopause there is no reason to obtain an estrogen level because it is hardly informative or shocking that a 55-year-old woman who hasn't had a period in three years has low estrogen. It's kind of like getting a pregnancy test for someone who is about to deliver and being surprised that it is positive.

> If you regularly fantasize about having sex with men other than your partner, you don't need to check your hormone levels.

The Big Libido Saboteurs
Pain
Nobody wants to do something that hurts. I can pretty much guarantee that anyone who has one of the issues discussed in chapters 8 and 11 is going to have a limited libido at best.

Menopause
Menopause and pain often go hand in hand. Forty to 50 percent of women experience genital dryness and painful intercourse as a

result of lack of estrogen (see chapter 13). But genital dryness and pain are not the only effects of waning or absent estrogen. Hot flashes, mood swings, irritability, and insomnia from lack of estrogen also have a negative impact on sexual interest. But remember, estrogen is only part of the story. While estrogen alone is needed for normal lubrication and vaginal health, both estrogen and androgens are required for arousal and libido.

The postmenopausal ovary continues to make testosterone even after estrogen production ceases, but over time ovarian testosterone levels eventually decrease. Ovary removal results in an immediate 50 percent reduction in circulating testosterone.

Clearly, for some (but not all) women, the loss of estrogen and testosterone after the onset of menopause can have a profound effect on libido, and for many women hormonal supplementation may be all that's needed to not only alleviate menopausal symptoms but also get their mojo back.

Vaginal atrophy correlates strongly with sexual activity. In the CLOSER Study (CLarifying vaginal atrophy's impact On SEx and Relationships) of over 4,000 women, 65 percent of women with atrophy issues reported low libidos. Two-thirds rarely engaged in sex. And in fact, multiple studies prove that eliminating vaginal dryness, particularly in menopausal women, is often the variable that is most likely to wake up libido.

Hormonal Contraceptives

Some women who take hormonal contraception experience a dramatic decline in libido, despite the high levels of estrogen the pills deliver. The problem lies with the impact of the pill on SHBG and correlating testosterone levels. In part four ("Hormone Havoc"), we will go into deep detail about the effect of hormonal contraception on libido.

Selective Serotonin Reuptake Inhibitors

The most commonly prescribed antidepressants, selective serotonin reuptake inhibitors (SSRIs), are associated not only with HSDD but also with the inability to have an orgasm. This is too unfair for words. The reason why SSRIs, such as Celexa, Lexapro, Prozac, Paxil, and Zoloft, lower libido is the same reason why they alleviate depression. It all comes down to serotonin, one of the key neurotransmitters. Low serotonin is associated with depression. High serotonin levels can inhibit sexual activity and libido. SSRIs increase the amount of circulating serotonin, which does a great job to alleviate depression but in some cases kills the libido.

Studies report a wide variation in exactly how many women have sexual problems as a result of SSRIs. Some studies place it as high as 75 percent. Others put the number much lower, at 0 to 30 percent, especially if the women in the study group had libido issues prior to taking the SSRI. Since 70 percent of depressed women have sexual issues even if they are not taking SSRIs, it can be difficult to determine what is truly causing the loss of libido. Is it the depression, the drug to treat the depression, or both?

It's fair to say, however, that depressed women with an intact libido who lose that lusty feeling once they start an SSRI can probably blame the drug. Midlife women are particularly at risk for depression and are therefore the group that is most likely to be taking an SSRI. This is also the group that is most likely to have sexual problems from other causes. Does the loss of libido in a 55-year-old woman stem from her SSRI, her thyroid problem, her breast cancer diagnosis, or the mood swings, insomnia, and hot flashes she's enduring because of lack of estrogen?

In addition, SSRIs are not just used to treat depression. They are often prescribed off-label to menopausal women for relief of hot flashes. So losing the flashes may also mean losing your love life. Brisdelle, an SSRI that was recently approved by the FDA specifically for relief of hot flashes, is much lower-dose than SSRIs

Depression and Libido: The Catch-22

No longer having a libido is depressing. Losing your libido because of treating your depression is *really* depressing.

prescribed for depression and fortunately does not have the same effect on libido.

SSRIs are not the only class of antidepressants that kill libido, but they are the most commonly studied since their use is so high. Monoamine oxidase inhibitors (MAOIs) such as Marplan, Nardil, Emsam, and Parnate, along with serotonin and norepinephrine reuptake inhibitors (SNRIs) such as venlafaxine (Effexor) and duloxetine (Cymbalta), have also been associated with sexual side effects.

Medical Illness

Any medical illness will have an impact on libido. Biologically, someone who is sick is not someone who should reproduce. (See chapter 15 on the myriad of medical conditions that can affect your sex life.) For most women, illness brings a quadruple whammy:

1. Chronic diseases such as hypertension, diabetes, obesity, and cancer can inhibit the ability to have sex. For example, diabetics often have atherosclerosis, which results in decreased sensation, decreased lubrication, and decreased arousal.

2. The psychological stress caused by having a serious medical problem can inhibit desire. If you are concerned that you might lose your life, losing your libido is pretty much a given.

3. More likely than not, it is the older person who also has waning hormones who is the most likely to be sick.

4. People who are sick tend to take medications that in and of themselves may cause a decline in libido.

Libido-Killing Drugs

That's right, hormonal contraception and SSRIs are far from the only drugs that affect libido. Many other drugs used to treat medical illness are known to decrease libido, independent of other factors.

The drugs that can decrease libido fall into these categories:

Antihypertension medication
Antipsychotic medications
Tricyclic antidepressants
Monoamine oxidase inhibitors (MAOIs)
Serotonin and norepinephrine reuptake inhibitors (SNRIs)
Sedatives
Selective serotonin reuptake inhibitors (SSRIs)
Anticoagulants
Medications to control cholesterol
Chemotherapy
Hormonal contraceptives

Aging

It can sometimes be tricky to determine whether a loss of libido is part of the normal aging process as opposed to loss of hormones, medical problems, or simply the fact that older women tend to have been in relationships longer.

Age vs. Hormones

A 2006 study looked at the rate of HSDD by age and found that in the 20- to 49-year-old age group, HSDD had a prevalence of 15 percent in women with normal estrogen levels. Members of that same age group who had gone through menopause had a 25 percent incidence of HSDD. The 50- to 70-year-old group, regardless of estrogen levels, had a 10 to 15 percent incidence of HSDD. Therefore, it appears that both age and hormones are factors.

Age vs. Health

Some 70-year-olds are in perfect health. Other 70-year-olds have diabetes, heart disease, and arthritis. It's pretty much a guarantee that the healthy 70-year-old is more likely to have a terrific sex life than the sick 70-year-old. A 2007 study published in the *New England Journal of Medicine* addressed the issue of age and sexual function and confirmed that, while a loss of interest in sex is part of the normal aging process, an individual's general health is a much bigger factor in determining sexual health.

Age vs. Length of Relationship

If you have had the same partner for 45 years, chances are good that you are at least 70 years old. So, have you lost interest in having sex because you are 70 or because you've had the same guy in your bed for as long as you can remember? Having said that, while many couples maintain a sexual relationship into their eighties or even nineties, particularly if they are in good health, it is far more typical for interest to wane with age.

Other Things That Can Decrease Libido
Bad Habits: Smoking and Drinking

Add loss of libido to the ever-growing list of why you should stop smoking. A 2008 study found a 30 percent decrease in genital responses in women who were exposed to erotic films after chewing nicotine gum.

And then there's alcohol. Perhaps one of the few Shakespeare lines you might recall from your high school English class is "it provokes the desire, but it takes away the performance." In other words, a little alcohol will help your libido, but if you drink too much it was all for nothing. One study conducted by the University of Florence in 2009 reported that women who drank one to two glasses of red wine (not white) had increased libido, increased lubrication, and better overall sexual functioning. I suspect they didn't have a lot of trouble recruiting for that trial. I think it also helps to be Italian.

Most studies show that both male and female alcoholics have impaired sexual function. Granted, these studies are often difficult to interpret because heavy users of tobacco and alcohol often have poor mental and physical health, dysfunctional relationships, and unstable finances, all of which also have negative impacts on sexual function.

Relationship/Partner Issues

Relationships are one of the biggest variables in libido, obviously. Is it that you don't want sex, or is it that you don't want to have sex with him? Emotional intimacy, a feeling of commitment and trust, particularly in women, is often a greater motivator for physical intimacy than biology. This is particularly the case in midlife and older women. I am reminded of a patient who came to me to discuss her lack of libido. She had waited months to get an appointment and driven six hours from rural Illinois for her consultation. I was in the midst of taking a detailed medical and sexual history when she interrupted and said, "Doctor, I hate to interrupt you, but I realized something midway between southern Illinois and Chicago. I hate my husband, and the only thing I hate more than my husband is living in southern Illinois. I don't think I need you. I need to get a new life."

We both agreed it was a very successful appointment.

While she came to that conclusion on her own, many women benefit from individual or couples therapy to figure out if the relationship, not a lack of estrogen, is the ultimate cause of a lack of libido.

> ### HRT?
>
> Partner issues seem to correlate with sexual activity more than hormone levels, which is why some women would benefit more from Husband Replacement Therapy than Hormone Replacement Therapy.

Body Image

There is a reason why actors and actresses in the movies are constantly naked and constantly having sex. Wouldn't you take your clothes off at every opportunity if you had a perfect body? While some women seem to have no problem baring it all, many midlife women are self-conscious about their saggy boobs and muffin top and are less than eager to strip and have someone fondle their imperfections. Studies confirm that, while there are exceptions, gaining weight and feeling self-conscious about bodily imperfections (real or perceived) *at any age* impacts sexual desire.

Too Stressed for Sex

It may seem intuitive that stress in our lives poisons our libidos, but I do believe it's worth pointing out that if you're extremely stressed—whether it's because of financial issues, relationship issues, medical issues, or life issues—your libido is going to suffer. While for many men sex appears to be a stress reliever, for most women the expectation that they are supposed to want sex and be having sex often is just something else to add to their already sky-high stress level.

Insomnia

According to a 2007 National Sleep Foundation survey, 48 percent of women ages 55 to 64 report sleep issues from a variety of causes, including hot flashes, stress, restless leg syndrome, the snorer in the bed, and the need to get up several times a night to pee. Peri- and postmenopausal women are twice as likely to use a sleep aid as premenopausal women. Adults require six hours of sleep at a minimum, but ideally eight hours, and very few are getting what they need. Poor sleep is associated with irritability, weight gain, fatigue (duh), inability to concentrate, mood disorders, and . . . guess what? Lack of libido! Given a choice between getting some sleep and getting some sex, there is really no contest—women, hands down, will choose sleep.

The Monotony of Monogamy

Remember that feeling the first time you kissed a new boyfriend? The rush of incredible excitement the first time you practically ripped each other's clothes off and had heart-racing sex? Remember the newness and *excitement* of it all? Fast-forward 20 years. It is an irrefutable fact that familiarity and lack of novelty breed boredom in the bedroom. Women especially seem sensitive to the connection between familiarity and a fading libido. Having sex with your husband of 5, 10, 20 years, no matter how interesting, charming, and handsome he is, gets boring. It's just a fact.

Actually, forget 20 years. Hot sex evidently lasts on average about 18 months if a relationship is new, regardless of whether you're 40 or 70. If partners aren't living together, it takes a little longer. Studies have shown that the *length* of a relationship is actually a much bigger factor in determining libido than the *age* of the people in the relationship. This is the case not just in the heterosexual world, as pointed out by University of Washington sociologist Pepper Schwartz, who coined the term "lesbian bed death." These stats help explain why the roughly 20 percent of women who have sex outside of marriage find that sex to be far more exciting than sex with their husbands. It's new. It's different. It's taboo. And all of that translates into better sex.

Many scientists believe that more than any other factor, long-term monogamy most accurately explains the loss of libido. A new sexual partner overrides both a lack of estrogen and the day-to-day stress that life inevitably brings. While increasing life expectancy is an excellent thing, sex with the same partner for 50 years presents problems.

Same Old Same Old

My 60-year-old patient told me that she rarely had sex with her husband of 30 years in spite of the fact that she loved him very much. She just had very little urge. Two years after he died, she sheepishly confessed to me that she and her new boyfriend "were going at it like rabbits all day long."

The Fixes

As you can see, libido is complex and affected not only by hormonal and neurotransmitter status but also by psychological, physical, and relationship factors. Add the fear of pain during intercourse and you have a no-win situation. It doesn't help that a decline in libido means that this part of your brain has shut down as well. You need to stimulate your mind as well as your body. You need to wake up the part of your brain that has been hibernating, and it's not going to happen automatically.

Women who have issues with libido need to consciously decide that they want to make things better and are willing to put the time and effort into doing so.

It's never just one thing: the causes of a loss of libido are multifactorial, and the first step is to identify which libido killers discussed in this chapter are issues for you. Then you must make a conscious effort to change as many of them as possible. Let's look at how to get your mojo back, step by step.

Eliminate Pain

Humans generally don't desire things that hurt. So it's hardly a mystery why women who experience painful intercourse don't have the urge. It is futile to attempt to increase libido before eliminating pain associated with sex.

Just because you can't have intercourse doesn't mean you can't be sexual. Intercourse should not be the expected goal of touching, fondling, or kissing. Many couples avoid physical intimacy because they think their partner won't be satisfied unless it ends with the grand finale of intercourse. Wrong! There are lots of ways to have intimacy, orgasms, and sexual satisfaction even if intercourse is off the table. For many couples, acknowledging that they enjoy physical intimacy with no expectation of intercourse is a huge relief.

Menopause Matters

If your ovaries have gone out of business, you may need to fill your empty estrogen and testosterone tank. Keep in mind that if you had low libido long before menopause hit, a hormone cocktail is unlikely to help. The woman who says, "Everything was great until I went into menopause, and then it was as if someone just turned off the switch," is the one whose libido is most likely to benefit from hormone therapy. It is important to emphasize that many studies, interestingly enough, have not shown systemic estrogen to have a directly beneficial effect on libido. Many scientists believe that the effect is indirect—having your hot flashes eliminated and getting a good night's sleep are the factors that increase your interest in having sex.

Keep in mind that the local vaginal estrogen you use to treat your vaginal dryness and pain will not increase your blood estrogen levels. If you have been treated for your genital dryness and intercourse is no longer painful but you still have zero interest, you may want to consider systemic hormone therapy to add the needed spark.

Transdermal estrogen, absorbed through the skin as a transdermal patch, spray, or gel, appears to have a more favorable impact on libido than oral estrogen since it does not increase SHBG and maximizes the amount of available active testosterone.

Choose Your Drugs Wisely

If you have identified a drug on the libido killer list as one you're taking, such as an antihypertensive drug or birth control pill, don't assume that your doctor knows that your medication has destroyed your sex life. Not only may your doctor not be aware that reduced libido is a possible side effect, but he or she will also not be aware that you have been experiencing this negative side effect unless you bring it up. You would be surprised how often there are other options or medications to treat your medical problem. Your doctor won't know to offer alternatives unless you ask. (Specific strategies to deal with hormonal contraception are discussed in detail in chapter 12.)

If you are taking an SSRI, it is imperative that you not alter your dosage or stop taking this drug without the help of your doctor. Changing depression medications is not a do-it-yourself project.

However, you may be in the rather common position of not being able to change your SSRI; if that's the case, another approach would be to take an additional medication to counteract your SSRI's negative sexual side effects. Drugs like Viagra and Cialis have been shown in some reports to improve orgasms, but not necessarily libido. There is conflicting data, based mainly on anecdotal reports, about whether adding bupropion or buspirone (Wellbutrin) is helpful. Talk to your doctor to see what your options might be.

Dealing with Stress

Despite the proclamations of every woman's magazine, simply signing up for yoga is not going to improve your sex life. But studies have shown that real stress reduction does have an impact. It may be as simple as getting some help around the house. On *The Doctor Oz Show,* I recommended a vacuum cleaner (to be used by your husband) as the ultimate aphrodisiac. Nothing makes a woman hotter than to come home and find that the man in her life has vacuumed the house.

Therapy, either individual or couples, is really important—not just to improve a relationship that may be problematic but for stress and anxiety management as well.

I know you have heard this one before, but putting sex on your schedule really makes a difference. Too often, even with the best of intentions, life and exhaustion get in the way and sex just doesn't happen. Figure out a code phrase ("Dinner with the Spielenbergers"), add it to your mutual calendar ("Thursday, 8:00 PM"), and *don't cancel*. Make the Spielenbergers your new best friends and have dinner with them at least twice a week.

There are two reasons for scheduling sex. The first is that you don't have to be in the mood for sex to enjoy it once you have it. By reminding your body and your brain of the pleasure, you will start to desire sex more often. This goes under the heading of "use it or lose it." The more sex you have—assuming it is pain-free and pleasurable—the more you will want to have it.

The other benefit to scheduling sex is that you get to anticipate "dinner with the Spielenbergers," and the anticipation of sex gets your brain going. It also decreases stress to know that you have a special time for sex and don't need to try to work it in.

Repair Your Relationship

It goes without saying that disdain and anger are not aphrodisiacs. Fixing your relationship is beyond the scope of this book. But I can acknowledge that your libido is not going to improve unless you actually like the person you are supposed to have sex with.

If sex is unpleasant, many women consciously, or subconsciously, sabotage a relationship as a way of avoiding sex. If you are really mean to him, he won't even try to have sex with you. This is where couples therapy is key.

Your Body Image Matters

Childbirth and time are not kind to one's thighs or stomach, and virtually every woman expresses some insecurity about the appearance of her body. It's true that intimacy does involve nakedness and the extra pounds don't make one feel particularly sexy.

I always remind my patients that their partner is likely to be the same age or even a few years older, and that he's not likely to have kept either his 20-year-old eyesight or his 20-year-old body. His six-pack has usually morphed into a not so attractive one-pack. Savvy women can rely heavily on candlelight to create the right ambiance for a romantic interlude. Everyone will look more attractive.

Having said that, decreased libido is more common in overweight and obese women, and in a perfect world you would lose the weight. I am always reminded, however, that some of my larger patients are also the most sexual and their bodies don't seem to get in the way of a fabulous sex life one bit. Since sex-hormone binding globulin is reduced with obesity, large women generally have adequate testosterone. It is body image and other health issues that create problems for overweight women. If you feel sexy, you will be sexy. So do your best to lose the weight, but also indulge in some beautiful lingerie that makes you feel gorgeous no matter what size you are. Nothing says, "I'm not interested," like a pair of white cotton underpants that come up to your belly button. Burn them.

Sleep, Perchance to Dream . . .

You have to get some sleep. If hot flashes are keeping you up, give some serious consideration to systemic estrogen therapy or an alternative therapy. You would be surprised at the number of women who take estrogen in order to get a good night's sleep. If lack of estrogen isn't an issue for you, get yourself to a sleep specialist and/or a sleep clinic. Every major university hospital has specialists in this area. Call.

Do not underestimate the impact of insomnia on your quality of life. Fix the sleep issue and you will lose weight, move more, reduce stress, think more clearly, and function better. Fix the sleep issue and you will improve not only your sex life but your whole life.

Manage Your Medical Illness

Knowing there is a direct correlation between your high blood pressure, diabetes, or incontinence and lack of libido should motivate you to do everything you can to work with your doctor and get in the best shape possible. Finally, kicking the cigarette habit and cutting down on alcohol are always good ideas.

Eliminate the Monotony of Monogamy

If the boredom of having the same partner is the great libido killer, then the obvious fix is to either have an affair or leave your partner altogether. Just kidding. Unless, that is, you dislike your partner and had planned on making a change anyway. But if you love your partner and in every other way want to maintain the relationship, then the fix is to make it seem new. Switch it up. You don't need to put on a wig and pretend you are someone else, but a little imagination goes a long way.

My patients don't come in and say, "Sex is boring." They do come in and say, "I'm just not that interested anymore."

Some Tips to Spice It Up

If there are cornflakes on the table for breakfast every day, after about ten years you won't ever want to see another cornflake. If one morning you find chocolate chip pancakes on your plate, you might suddenly have a terrific appetite.

A combination of anticipation and creativity will eliminate the "same old same old" of 20-plus years of marriage. There are lots of books out there to help put a kick-start in a marriage (see the resources section), but here are a few ideas to get you started:

- If the only thing you own that vibrates is your cell phone, *it's time to go shopping.* A lot of couples think of a sex toy as something the woman uses alone while the guy goes out for a ham sandwich. Not true! See chapter 20 for more information.
- While you have your credit card out, buy some books, lingerie, candles, and an erotic movie.
- Add a blindfold to make sex play mysterious and to focus on physical sensation.
- At the risk of sounding like I lifted this from *Fifty Shades of Grey,* even the standard missionary position is a whole new experience when you are enveloped in darkness.
- Get out of bed. Stand up while he presses you against the wall. Wear a skirt and surprise him with no panties.

- Take it outside. Feeling the breeze on your breasts is very sexy—not to mention the eroticism of potentially "getting caught." If you are not that brave, you can always put a fan by the bed.
- Wear a wig. I said you didn't *have to* wear a wig. I didn't say you *couldn't* wear a wig. Have your honey "pick you up" in a hotel bar before heading upstairs.
- Wax away. A couples bikini wax may seem silly, but it will add a whole new dimension to the "69" position.
- Take him to the shower. A lap dance is perfect for the shower if you have a sturdy seat or bench for him to sit on before you "dance." A hand-held shower only adds to the fun. Silicone lube is a must, but be careful . . . it's really slippery on a shower floor. Good luck explaining that one to the paramedics.
- Eat! The idea of food as an aphrodisiac is hardly new. The list is long: hot peppers, (to make you "hot"), oysters, garlic, and even watermelon. Let's start with oysters. Casanova reportedly ate 50 dopamine-laden oysters for breakfast to prep for a day of lovemaking. Buddhist monks are advised to avoid garlic lest it stimulate their sexuality, a major monk no-no. And then there is watermelon. I was once asked to discuss the libido-boosting effects of watermelon on *Dr. Oz*. After a lot of digging, I learned that the watermelon rind contains citruline, which in turn releases arginine. Arginine is an enzyme that theoretically increases blood flow to the genitals . . . a Viagra-like effect. So while there is no proof that watermelon actually enhances arousal, the possibility has a group of Texan scientists very busy breeding special sex watermelons with lots of citruline. Chocolate, with its serotonin-like effect, is not on the aphrodisiac list, although you'll probably feel a flood of love for whoever was thoughtful enough to give it to you.

Drugs to Fix HSDD

I know what you're thinking. These suggestions aren't practical, possible, or helpful. Yes, it's important to eliminate stress, lose the extra weight, and address general health concerns, but some women need more than lifestyle changes to turn on what has turned off.

The guys get to just take a pill to help their problem. Where's our pill? The answer, of course, is that it is nonexistent. Despite the claims of several Internet ads touting products promising to revitalize a woman's lackluster sex life, a female equivalent to Viagra has proven elusive. Currently there are no FDA-approved medications to treat sexual problems in women other than vaginal dryness and pain with intercourse. As of now, the only available options to boost a woman's lagging libido are non–FDA-approved preparations from compounding pharmacies, over-the-counter neutraceuticals (dietary supplements, herbs, etc.), or prescription testosterone products intended for men.

Here's what's out there.

Testosterone Supplementation: FDA-Approved for Men but Not for Women

Since physicians and many women now recognize that androgens are part of the normal hormonal milieu, androgen supplementation has become an important component of hormone therapy for women. And yet, in spite of a great deal of scientific data demonstrating that many women benefit from testosterone supplementation, the FDA has approved testosterone only for men.

The exception is an oral combination of estrogen and methyltestosterone (formerly known as Estratest) that is intended for women but is actually only FDA-approved for the treatment of hot flashes. In general, it is rarely prescribed, since a transdermal testosterone is preferable. Oral testosterone can increase lipid levels and elevate the risk of liver function problems.

Intrinsia was the first testosterone product intended to increase libido in women, but the patch never got FDA clearance. Libigel, a testosterone gel intended for women, was in clinical trials for years and demonstrated an excellent safety profile, yet in 2011, after millions of dollars, 11,000 patients, and years of clinical trials, it too did not get the FDA nod. Essentially, the FDA was not convinced that it worked beyond the placebo effect since in the clinical trials "satisfying sexual experiences" increased by only two to four per month. Many experts think that "satisfying sexual experiences" was not the correct endpoint to use to determine efficacy and that the outcomes would have been different if the FDA had considered endpoints such as desire, arousal, pleasure, and decline in personal distress. Interestingly, most women in the trials indicated that they would like to continue to use the product. At this time, no company has taken up the challenge, and an FDA-approved female testosterone product is unlikely to appear anytime soon.

Despite what the FDA says, most sexual health experts (and women) feel that there is value in supplementing testosterone. The effect isn't immediate, and you need to stick with it for at least four months to know if it is doing anything for you.

Since there are no FDA-approved products for women, a lot of testosterone intended for men is prescribed off-label. As discussed in chapter 7, off-label does not mean illegal. Based on physician survey data, every year over 4 million testosterone prescriptions are written off-label for women. It is important to use supplemental testosterone only under the guidance of a physician who is familiar with dosing for women; otherwise, you may need to borrow your husband's razor or your teenager's acne cream.

The major downside to prescribing off-label is that insurance doesn't always cover it. Also, the manufacturer doesn't provide instructions or dosages that are appropriate for the alternative use. Many physicians prescribe testosterone on a regular basis for women and are very familiar with dosing for women. Most testosterone is in the form of a gel, but it is also available in patch or pellet form. Testosterone is also available from compounding pharmacies.

DHEA

Many women are familiar with DHEA as a supplement to facilitate libido. Essentially, DHEA is the hormonal precursor to estrogen and testosterone. In other words, your body requires DHEA to make estrogen. Women have their own supply of DHEA, thoughtfully provided by the adrenal glands. But with age comes a significant decline in adrenal DHEA.

As with other hormones, there is a wide range of normal when it comes to DHEA levels, and there is also a great deal of controversy regarding the correlation of the blood level of DHEA with libido. In addition, it is very controversial whether supplementing DHEA improves libido. In spite of the lack of evidence, women hoping to boost their libido "naturally" spend countless dollars every year buying DHEA supplements.

The only scientific study that looked at DHEA for libido did not find an effect beyond the placebo effect, but stay tuned. An exception may be women with adrenal insufficiency, whose libidos have shown some improvement when they take DHEA.

Known Dopamine Agonists

Since dopamine is the neurotransmitter of lust, it would seem that medications known to boost dopamine would also give a boost to libido. The most studied of these medications, bupropion (Wellbutrin, Zyban), an antidepressant, does in fact give a boost to libido in many women. Other women experience just the opposite.

Increased sexual urges can be a side effect with a number of other dopamine-type medications. This is not the reason, however, why I am not recommending that you use them. There just is not enough data yet to know if the libido benefits outweigh potential side effects. Some of these drugs are:

Cabergoline—used to lower elevated prolactin levels
Pramipexole—used to treat restless leg syndrome
Ropinirole—used to treat Parkinson's disease

What About Viagra?

Phosphodiasterase (PDE5) inhibitors such as Viagra and Cialis obviously work wonders for the guys. And you would think that anything that so effectively increases blood flow to the penis would also increase pelvic blood flow to the clitoris and vagina. These drugs have a physical effect on women, but alas, they don't affect desire.

Up and Coming

It's a funny thing about writing a book about sexual health. Things that never sounded sexual before suddenly take on a whole new meaning. "Up and coming" is a perfect example. But I digress.

Pharmaceutical companies, being the profit-motivated entities that they are, recognize that there is a lot of money to be made in female sexual problems. More important, a tremendous amount of research and development in this area is being conducted, and new drugs to increase libido may be available in the not-too-distant future. Among the drugs currently in clinical trials, the most promising are Flibanserin, Bremelanotide, Lybrido, and Lybridos.

Flibanserin

Flibanserin is designed to increase libido by working on the brain, not on blood flow to the genitals. This oral medication decreases serotonin, increases dopamine, and increases adrenaline. Essentially, it makes you have sexy thoughts. Boehringer Ingelheim poured millions of dollars into research and development of this drug, only to be denied approval by the FDA despite impressive safety and efficacy data. Several large trials for premenopausal women with HSDD found significant improvement in sexual desire and satisfying sexual events with this drug. The FDA felt that while results showed a statistically significant improvement in sexual satisfaction, the results were not impressive enough. The Flibanserin torch was picked up by Sprout Pharmaceuticals, and the product is now being reviewed again.

Lybrido

The idea behind Lybrido is to impact both the brain and genital blood flow to create both lust and response. Basically the premise is to put testosterone and a PDE5 inhibitor together to provide both the motivator (testosterone) and the physiological sexual response.

Lybridos

The same company that is working on Lybrido is also developing Lybridos. Like Lybrido, this pill has a testosterone component. Instead of a PDE5 inhibitor, the other ingredient in this medication is buspirone, an anti-anxiety medication that is used to elevate serotonin. Of course, the last thing you want is elevated serotonin (since serotonin decreases libido), but here's the interesting part. If you take buspirone every day, it does elevate serotonin, but if you take it on demand no more than every two days, there is a short-term reduction of serotonin. The beauty of this medication is that, like Viagra, you only take it when you need it. Spring break with the kids? Forget it. Romantic weekend in the Riviera? Don't leave home without it.

Both Lybrido and Lybridos have a peppermint-flavored testosterone coating that melts in your mouth (but not in your hand!). Bonus: you will have minty fresh breath for kissing. This company truly thought of everything. Preliminary data for both drugs is promising.

Bremelanotide

Bremelanotide has primarily been studied for its effects on libido and erectile dysfunction in men, but now it's being looked at for female libido as well. Data from the second phase of the clinical trial demonstrated increased sexual arousal, sexual desire, and number of sexually satisfying events.

> It is estimated that 20 percent of testosterone prescriptions written for men to use for their sexual issues are also used by their wives!

Herbs, Spices, and Wishful Thinking

Lots of neutraceuticals, or natural supplements, boost libido. Just ask the expert at Whole Foods. Keep in mind that the companies that produce these products are just as profit-motivated as pharmaceutical companies. They actually end up making more money since they are not required to spend massive amounts of money on research, development, and clinical trials to get FDA approval. As a result, a multimillion-dollar industry has evolved to promote "natural" products to a vulnerable population of women who are seeking effective products to boost their libido. While many people generally distrust the pharmaceutical industry, they seem to have little problem placing their trust in information and promotional ads placed by companies that have no efficacy or safety standards to meet. Just because something is "natural" doesn't mean it is safe. Just because the health food store clerk seems very knowledgeable doesn't mean he is.

Many women question why more studies haven't been done on herbal preparations. Some studies are in progress, but they are extremely expensive and difficult since a large number of patients and a long time frame are required. Also, since most of these products come under the umbrella of "cosmetics" rather than "medications," the companies that make them are not required or motivated to prove efficacy. They can say what they want, so they do.

The bottom line is this: buyer beware. There are only two appropriate criteria when deciding to use an alternative product: Is it safe? And does it really work beyond the 30 percent placebo effect? Too often, no one really knows. The only ones who consistently benefit from alternative products are the companies that sell them. Having said that, many women swear by these products, and if you want to try them, you can be comfortable knowing that at least they are not harmful.

> DOCTOR: How often do you try to have sex?
> PATIENT: We try to have sex three times a week. We tried on Monday, Wednesday, and Friday.

11

NOTHING'S HAPPENING

I'd like to buy a vowel—
the key to getting the big O back

Prior to the 1800s, it was believed that conception would not occur unless the female had an orgasm.

Then, during the Victorian era, most physicians began to assert that sexual pleasure did not exist for women in the marital bed. Intercourse was something to be "endured," female sexual excitement did not exist, and anorgasmia was declared the norm.

By the latter part of the nineteenth century, orgasms were finally medically recognized as a normal part of sexual response, but only if they occurred during coitus between a married couple. However, in the 1918 sexual guide *Married Love* by Marie Stopes, the wise doctor (and one of the rare women doctors!) described the importance of female orgasm, the problem of premature ejaculation, and its effect on achieving the goal of simultaneous orgasms:

> *Though in some instances the woman may have one or more crises*
> *before the man achieves his, it is perhaps hardly an exaggeration*
> *to say that 70 or 80 per cent of our married women (in the middle*
> *and intellectual classes) are deprived of the full orgasm through the*

excessive speed of the husband's reactions, i.e., through premature ejaculation. . . . So complex, so profound, are woman's sex-instincts that in rousing them the man is rousing her whole body and soul. And this takes time. More time indeed than the average husband dreams of spending upon it. Yet woman has at the surface a small vestigial organ called the clitoris, which corresponds morphologically to the man's penis, and which, like it, is extremely sensitive to touch-sensations. This little crest, which lies anteriorly between the inner lips round the vagina, erects itself when the woman is really tumescent, and by the stimulation of movement it is intensely roused and transmits this stimulus to every nerve in her body. But even after a woman's dormant sex-feeling is aroused and all the complex reactions of her being have been set in motion, it may take from ten to twenty minutes of actual physical union to consummate her feeling, while one, two or three minutes of actual union often satisfies a man who is ignorant of the art of controlling his reactions so that he may experience the added enjoyment of a mutual simultaneous orgasm.

Today we fully agree that arousal is critical if orgasm is to occur—and orgasm, even if not simultaneous, is the ultimate goal of any sexual experience. And why not? Orgasms make us feel good. Yet, with so much emphasis on the climax, *and getting to the top,* the trip up the mountain is perceived as unimportant if you don't make it to the peak.

It's time to acknowledge that while orgasms are wonderful, a woman can have satisfying and pleasurable sex without having an orgasm. In most cases, if you make the climb more enjoyable, the peak is not only more attainable but more gratifying as well. In fact, the practice of tantric sex places essentially no value on orgasm. The pleasure is in the pre–orgasmic state that leads to a richer, more intense experience. (More on tantric sex later!)

So while some women are able to consistently orgasm, and a lucky few enjoy multiple orgasms, others may experience no orgasm at all. All of these patterns are normal and may change from time to time. That is why it is important for women to keep in mind that by tapping into how they like to be stimulated, anyone can experience sexual pleasure.

Having said that, the rest of this chapter will explore how to make it happen—or make it better.

What's an Orgasm?

An orgasm is essentially the physical phenomenon that follows sexual arousal and stimulation. At the peak of sexual pleasure (the plateau phase) there is a muscle tension and congestion of tissues due to increased pelvic blood flow. The orgasm, which follows, consists of involuntary but coordinated rhythmic contractions of the pelvic muscles, uterus, vagina, and anus, lasting 15 to 20 seconds and resulting in an intense feeling of pleasure. Blood pressure increases, pulse quickens, and pupils dilate. Brain imaging shows that during an orgasm specific areas of the brain are activated. This intense reaction is followed by resolution, muscle relaxation, and contentment.

This describes an orgasm when everything is working correctly.

While some women experience fireworks during an orgasm, for others it's more of a flickering candle. Too many women are unable to achieve any kind of an orgasm. There was great hope that Viagra would totally solve the absent orgasm issue by increasing blood flow to the clitoris and thereby increasing sensitivity and pleasure. But it's not that simple. Yes, it's about blood flow, but it's also about neurology and hormones and neurotransmitters and anatomy and arousal and relationships and genetics and prior experiences and expectations.

> ### Dr. Streicher's SexAbility Survey
>
> When asked which movie title best describes their typical orgasm,
>
> 8.9 percent of women said *Much Ado About Nothing*
> 23.5 percent said *Mission Impossible*
> 35.7 percent said *Swept Away*
> 9.5 percent said *Toy Story*
> 22.3 percent said *Fast and Furious*

The Four Things That Need to Happen for Orgasm to Happen

Remember the fantasy scene that opened chapter 2, when Brad Pitt entered the room and it all started getting steamy? The sexual response cycle, if all is working well, can result in orgasm. Here's how.

1. Arousal

Arousal is triggered by both physical and emotional stimulation. While your body is better able to become aroused if both are present, it is totally possible to become aroused with just one. Just thinking about sex can sometimes cause the physical response of increased pelvic blood flow, vaginal lubrication, and hard nipples. Then again, our bodies can respond automatically in response to sexual touching. And though some women need an emotional connection for their bodies to follow suit, some women don't.

2. Stimulation

Regardless of which combination of factors works best for them, most women need some form of physiological stimulation to achieve pre-orgasm readiness. And some women do seem to have an easier time at this than others. Studies confirm that women who are easily aroused are less likely to have orgasmic disorders than women who are difficult to arouse. If someone is psychologically ready (perhaps because she's been reading an erotic book), she can easily become physically aroused. She will have hard nipples and wetness without any touching.

However, once a woman is aroused, there needs to be (except in rare situations) physical stimulation. Both the type of physical stimulation and the intensity of stimulation needed to induce orgasm can vary greatly throughout the life cycle. Physically touching the clitoris is usually required, but there is good evidence that orgasm can occur without clitoral provocation.

Is Clitoral Stimulation the Only Way?

Everyone agrees that clitoral stimulation in the form of pressure, massage, vibration, licking, or touching will generally trigger an orgasm. But is orgasm possible if there is *no clitoral stimulation?* Throughout history, there is good documentation that female orgasms can result from mental stimulation, anal stimulation, nipple/breast stimulation, cervical and vaginal stimulation . . . pretty much stimulation of any body part (including the brain!) The real proof is that women who have a spinal cord injury and cannot feel clitoral nerve touching can still achieve orgasm.

3. Intact Neurologic System

Clitoral stimulation results in over 8,000 nerve endings sending signals to the spinal cord and brain. This is the primary pathway by which women achieve orgasm. But there is a backup system. It appears that stimulation of some parts of the vagina and cervix can, in some women, stimulate the pelvic branch of the vagus nerve, which travels to the brain, but not via the spinal cord. The vagus nerve provides an alternate pathway and is the mechanism by which women with complete spinal cord injuries are able to climax from vaginal stimulation.

This backup system explains why women who experience both clitoral and nonclitoral orgasms report that these two kinds of orgasm are "different"—not more or less pleasurable, just different.

4. Adequate Blood Flow

In addition to being neurologically intact, a body cannot experience orgasm without adequate blood flow. An adequate blood supply is needed to lubricate vaginal walls and help in arousal, and it's also responsible for congestion of the muscles and clitoral tissues, which is necessary for the plateau phase just prior to orgasm. Those 8,000 clitoral nerves also require adequate blood to function properly.

The Great Debate: Clitoral Orgasms vs. Vaginal Orgasms

Clearly the vast majority of orgasms *not* associated with intercourse are from direct clitoral stimulation. The burning question is this: Is an orgasm *during* intercourse a result of vaginal stimulation? Or are "vaginal" orgasms not vaginal at all, but the result of clitoral stimulation during intercourse from pressure on the clitoris?

It was in 1905 that Sigmund Freud set the stage for the notion that not only should women expect to have vaginal orgasms, but that clitoral orgasms were "immature." This idea would cause generations of women to feel inadequate when they required clitoral stimulation to climax. This myth was propagated until the more realistic (and scientific) Kinsey team reported in 1953 that "sexual intercourse is an extremely inefficient way to stimulate the clitoris."

In the 1960s, William H. Masters and Virginia E. Johnson took things a step further and hypothesized, based on filming subjects having intercourse in their lab, that given the vagina's elasticity and poor innervation, orgasm could not be vaginal in origin. For that reason, they also said that penis size was irrelevant to triggering orgasm. In the often quoted *Hite Report on Female Sexuality,* published in 1976, Shere Hite revealed that only 30 percent of women climax during intercourse. More recent scientific studies show that 30 percent is probably a gross overestimation and that only about 5 to 10 percent of women are able to reach vaginal orgasm in the absence of clitoral stimulation.

Whether the number is 5 percent or 30 percent, plenty of scientific studies (and patients with spinal cord injuries) have shown that stimulation of many nonclitoral erogenous zones results in contraction of pelvic floor muscles, or orgasm. While the walls of the vagina have relatively few nerve endings, the roof of the vagina does have nerve endings, and either the G-spot, the internal root of the clitoris, periurethral nerves, or cervical nerves can be stimulated to result in an orgasm. There is no doubt that while clitoral stimulation is the most efficient and reliable way to orgasm, a non-clitoral-induced orgasm exists.

Orgasmic Disorders

An orgasmic disorder is defined as either persistent or recurrent absence, reduced intensity, or delay of orgasm *following a sexual excitement phase* that causes *distress or interpersonal difficulty.* And yes, some women have satisfying, positive sexual experiences and are okay not having an orgasm.

Notice that the definition says nothing about intercourse. Not having an orgasm during intercourse not only is common but is completely *normal.* The definition also includes adequate stimulation: if there is no sexual excitement, it is normal to not have an orgasm.

Someone who has never experienced an orgasm is described as having primary anorgasmia and is also referred to optimistically as "pre-orgasmic." Someone whose orgasms have disappeared has secondary anorgasmia, or acquired orgasmic disorder.

As you can imagine, it's hard to know precisely how many women suffer from orgasmic issues, but somewhere between 20 and 40 percent of women report problems with orgasm at some point in their life. After hypoactive sexual desire disorder, orgasm issues are the second most common sexual complaint. Many women who have difficulties reaching orgasm also have other sexual issues, such as decreased libido, diminished lubrication, and pain with sexual activity. With all that going on too, no wonder it is difficult to do research specifically on orgasms, making it a challenge to fix the problem.

What I can say with assurance is that lack of orgasm is a common problem and has the same prevalence in both lesbian and hetero-sexual populations. (I guess that means we have to stop blaming it on clueless guys who need a map to find the clitoris.)

Things That Get in the Way of the Big O
Lack of Arousal

If there is no arousal, there will be no orgasm, plain and simple. Psychological, social, and physical factors all have an impact on arousal. Essentially, everyone has "excitatory" processes and "inhibitory" processes that control sexual excitement and the ability to have an orgasm. Inhibitory things include difficulties with your partner, a high stress level, and guilt about feeling sexual. Medications or medical problems that inhibit blood flow, create pain, or compromise neurologic pathways are also inhibitors. Excitatory things include neurologic stimulation, positive emotional feelings, physical stimulation, and terrific blood flow. If each of these elements represented points, it would be easy to add them all together for a winning score . . . but it isn't so easy, right?

Limited Sexual Experience of Individual or Partner

Very often primary orgasmic disorders are a result of not knowing *how* to have an orgasm. Not every man and woman knows what to do. Some guys really have no idea what a clitoris is, where it is, and what they are supposed to do with it. Ditto some women. Sometimes the inability to have an orgasm has nothing to do with physiology and everything to do with education.

Anatomy—Hers and His

Intercourse is not a very efficient or effective way for most women to have an orgasm. The clitoris, while conveniently located for masturbation, is anatomically poorly positioned for stimulation during intercourse. When it comes to the guy's anatomy, contact between a man's pubic bone and the clitoris during intercourse seems to be a key factor. This is a consequence of his anatomy, your anatomy, and coital position.

While penis dimension has essentially no impact on clitoral orgasms, size does matter when it comes to the likelihood of a vaginal orgasm. Stimulation of the anterior vaginal wall (home of the internal part of the clitoral complex and G-spot) is dependent on the girth of the penis. Stimulation of the cervix, which fires the vagus nerve, is dependent on the length of the penis.

Psychological, Relationship, and Communication Factors (Inhibition, Cultural Factors)

Feeling guilty about sex owing to religious beliefs, a history of sexual abuse, or anything else can create a negative emotion about achieving orgasm that can and will impact your ability to do so. In fact, many studies correlate childhood sexual abuse or a violent rape with a very high incidence of inability to achieve orgasm in a loving relationship.

Women who cannot lose control, who are unable to "be in the moment," are often unable to focus on sensory stimuli enough to achieve orgasm. Not only do women have to feel safe and emotionally trusting, but they also cannot feel inhibited by how they may look or act during an orgasm. If a woman is worrying about her fat butt, or a funny vaginal smell, or the noise she might make when she climaxes, she is going to have a very hard time having an orgasm. And while we are talking about noises women make when they have sex, it's not always involuntary. A small 2011 study (that focused solely on heterosexual women) found that 66 percent moan during sex to speed up their partner's climax, while 87 percent did so to boost their partner's self-esteem.

Women who are able to achieve orgasm through self-stimulation but not with a partner may be harboring feelings of anger, dissatisfaction, and inability to communicate. And of course there is also the issue of the partner who doesn't know how to stimulate the clitoris effectively, and the woman who is not able to help him out because she is uncomfortable communicating this.

Medical Conditions

I hear it all the time. "I feel dead down there." "I have no sensation." "I can't even tell he's in me." There are many medical situations in which decreased genital blood flow or neurologic damage can decrease sensation in the pelvic area. Weak pelvic floor muscles are a huge, underappreciated issue. In one study, 60 percent of women with urinary incontinence due to a weak pelvic floor were anorgasmic.

Chronic medical conditions that affect blood flow or the neurologic system include heart disease, diabetes, multiple sclerosis, and spinal cord issues, and these all have an impact on the ability to have an orgasm. Hypothyroidism, which is present in 1 of 10 women over the age of 50, is also associated with decreased genital sensation. In addition, chronic illness, even if it has no direct impact on blood flow or nerves, is associated with orgasmic disorders. In many studies, about 53 percent of women with orgasmic issues also met the criteria for depression.

Menopause

Estrogen is actually not required to have an orgasm, and many women who have estrogen and progesterone levels of zero still climax regularly. Menopause does, however, affect the ability to become aroused. Low estrogen decreases blood flow to the vagina and leads to lack of lubrication. Dry, painful intercourse is not going to lead to pleasure of any kind.

In addition, studies show that estrogen is needed to have optimal clitoral blood flow. Testosterone has been found in some studies to be involved in arousal and the orgasm experience. So while estrogen and testosterone are not absolutely essential to achieve a satisfying orgasm, they certainly help, and low levels of these hormones explain why many postmenopausal women report having a more difficult time reaching orgasm and having orgasms of shorter duration and weaker intensity than before menopause set in.

Medications

It's often difficult to figure out if it is the medication that is causing the problem or the condition the medication is supposed to treat that is the problem. Having said that, there are some drugs that are specifically associated with orgasmic disorder. It has been well established that SSRIs not only have an impact on libido and can delay orgasm but also affect the ability to have an orgasm. (The details of the impact of SSRIs are covered in chapter 9.) The good news is that, in roughly 30 percent of cases, after taking the medication for a period of time (usually at around three months), your orgasms come back! It's worth sticking it out for a while before you talk to your doctor to see if there is an alternative option. This appears to be a dose-related phenomenon, so sometimes lowering the amount of the SSRI that you take will solve the problem.

Other medications that are known to squelch the ability to climax are antipsychotic drugs, cardiovascular medications, hypertension drugs, and chemotherapy.

Substance Use

Alcohol

As with libido, a little alcohol gets you in the mood, a lot gets in the way. And yes, intoxication does reduce the ability to achieve orgasm.

Tobacco

Since orgasms depend on an adequate blood supply and nicotine diminishes blood flow to the penis, guy smokers have a higher incidence of erectile dysfunction. This has not been well studied in women, but since the clitoris also depends on blood flow, it follows that orgasms in women who are heavy smokers may also be diminished.

Marijuana

I know you are out there . . . don't pretend you're not. And during the Summer of Love, marijuana was as much a part of "make love not war" as the pill. There are a number of anecdotal reports that marijuana enhances orgasm, but it's hard to say whether this is a direct effect of the drug or a result of women becoming more relaxed and able to let go. Large amounts of marijuana are known to decrease testosterone levels, which in turn may affect libido. There are actually no good studies looking at the effect of marijuana on female orgasm, which leaves the question wide open for some enterprising medical student.

Hysterectomy and Other Pelvic Surgeries: "It Just Isn't the Same"

Medical studies show that long-term orgasmic function is essentially unaffected by hysterectomy. However, many of my post-hysterectomy patients have reported that things seem different; their orgasms are less intense, and some women are unable to achieve orgasm. There are three possible reasons for these changes:

- While removal of the uterus does not change anything hormonally, some women enter menopause at the time of hysterectomy because they also have their ovaries removed. It is not the hysterectomy but menopause that creates the orgasm problem.
- Most women are only aware of pelvic floor contractions during orgasm, but some women are aware of uterine contractions when they climax. If the uterus is gone, that aspect of their orgasm will also disappear.
- Hysterectomy does not always include removal of the cervix. If it does, and if you are one of those women who have a vaginal orgasm from stimulation of cervical nerves, you will notice a difference. If you are going to have a hysterectomy,

you may want to consider preservation of your cervix if that is an option.

My 2012 SexAbility survey of over 2,000 women who had undergone hysterectomy reported that their orgasms after hysterectomy were:

No different than before surgery (56.4 percent)
More intense and more pleasurable (21.6 percent)
Less intense and less pleasurable (15.3 percent)
Still not happening (7.1 percent)

Women who have more extensive hysterectomies because of cancer are the most likely to have problems. Survivors of cervical and vaginal cancers appear to have orgasmic problems twice as often as women in the general population, probably because of pain or damage to pelvic nerves from the surgery. Hysterectomy is not the only pelvic surgery, of course, and any operation in the pelvis can disrupt the ability to have an orgasm. These issues are usually short-term and resolve in time as tissue heals and nerves regenerate.

And Then There's the Bicycle Problem...

Erectile dysfunction has long been linked to bike riding, but it wasn't until a 2013 study at Yale University that it was determined that this is not just a male issue. Whether it's frequent spin classes or 10-mile rides, prolonged clitoral pressure compresses nerve endings and blood vessels. Genital numbness, tingling, or soreness of any kind is an indication that an adjustment is in order. The position of the handlebars on your bike is far more important than the type of seat it has or the height of the seat. The lower the handlebars on your bike the more pressure on critical structures down there. Ideally, the handlebars should be as high as the seat to ensure minimal pressure.

Things That Help with the Big O
Don't Ignore the Relationship and Psychological Aspects of Orgasm

If you have identified relational or psychological issues that are impeding your ability to orgasm, they need to be addressed. Individual and/or couples therapy is critical, even while you are exploring other medical options. A therapist experienced in sexual issues is ideal, but any good therapist can address depression, anxiety, or other inhibiting factors that get in the way of sexual health.

In addition, the inability to have an orgasm in itself causes psychological anxiety, and that distress needs to be managed. Communication is key—you need to be able not only to discuss the relationship issues with a partner but to feel comfortable directing him or her to do the things that will give you a physical response. In addition to talk therapy and cognitive therapy, mindfulness meditation and yoga have been shown in some studies to facilitate the ability to "be in the moment."

Even if your relationship is terrific and you have no psychological issues, keep in mind that the brain is an amazing erogenous zone, not only with respect to libido but arousal as well. I rarely tell personal stories, but here goes. I love my husband. No, I adore my husband and find him to be an incredibly sexy, giving partner. But I don't always have sex with my husband. Sometimes I have sex with Mikhail Baryshnikov. I have actually never met Baryshnikov, but I have watched *The Turning Point* dozens of times and feel like I know him intimately. To clarify, I am not having sex with 65-year-old *Sex in the City* Misha. I am having sex with the 30-year-old incredibly hot guy I saw dancing in *Don Quixote* when I was in my twenties. And while I am having sex with him, I am also in my twenties. I have asked my husband countless times to put on a pair of tights, but he refuses. I do however yell "Bravo!" at the end, which he really likes. Just saying.

If fantasizing about a sexy dancer doesn't do it for you, find your own version of Misha. Erotic books, films, and fantasy go a long way toward helping with orgasm.

So let's assume that you do not have pain, you have no relationship or psychological issues, and you are physically able to have intercourse or self-stimulate, but you just simply cannot make "it" happen. Or when it does happen it takes so much work or is so unsatisfying that not only is it hardly worth the time and effort but it leaves you feeling frustrated or in an uncomfortable state of sexual tension.

What follows are specific strategies, products, medications, and devices to heighten arousal, increase genital stimulation, increase blood flow, stimulate the nervous system, and, ultimately, facilitate the ability to orgasm. And while I do believe that a vaginal orgasm is possible, go for the low-hanging fruit and focus on the clitoris— unless, of course, you are a woman who either has no clitoris, has suffered a spinal cord injury, or has scarring that makes the clitoris inaccessible.

Faking It: "I'll Have What She's Having"

While not every woman fakes orgasm, and most don't do it routinely, it's the rare woman who hasn't done it at least once. And if there were any doubt, the iconic scene in *When Harry Met Sally* is a testimony to just how convincing women can be. Why do women fake it?

- To make their partner happy
- To make him come faster
- Because orgasm is unlikely and she wants him to stop trying
- To get some sleep
- To not feel like a failure

A 2010 Indiana University study showed that while 85 percent of the men surveyed said that their latest sexual partner had an orgasm, only 64 percent of those women said that they climaxed the last time they had sex. So not only did 21 percent of these women fake it, but 100 percent of the time the guys believed it, proving that women are better actors than they think. In another 2010 study from the University of Kansas, 50 percent of women reported pretending orgasm, but women were not the only ones who faked it—25 percent of the guys reported pretending to come as well!

Instead of working on the Academy Award for Best Performance for Faking an Orgasm, it is probably a better idea to communicate to your partner that even if you don't have an orgasm, you are still having a really good time.

Masturbation U

While masturbation in women is still too often a taboo topic, we have come a long way from the early 1900s when doctors used to view masturbation as "self-abuse" that would "wreck" a woman's system. Facilitating self-stimulation is now considered to be part of normal sexual health. Yet for something so natural and healthy, doctors are unlikely to bring it up and mothers aren't exactly teaching their daughters this skill. We aren't yet that enlightened, and young women are left to figure it out on their own . . . or not. And unlike the penis, which stands up and announces itself to a young man, a clitoris, like most buried treasure, needs to be "discovered," so to speak.

So, if you have *never* had an orgasm, you are much better off eliminating the partner variable and figuring this one out on your own. Particularly in the case of primary orgasmic dysfunction (those who've never experienced orgasm), a technique known as "directed masturbation" solves the problem more often than not.

Directed masturbation refers to masturbation lessons, and yes, sex therapists facilitate this by telling you where to touch and how to touch. Not only does this eliminate all of the complicated dynamics that accompany a partnered sexual experience, but also it really does become "all about you." Literally. And who is going to be less judgmental about what it takes to get you off than you? Exactly.

In one study, anorgasmic women were assigned to a masturbation education group or a wait list. The women in the education group received explicit instructions, along with a vibrator. At the end of the study, 60 percent of the women in the masturbation education group were achieving orgasm as opposed to 0 percent in the wait-listed group. Another similarly designed study resulted in a 90 percent ability to have an orgasm with directed masturbation.

So if you have never self-stimulated, it's time to start. If you have, but have never used a vibrator, it's time to go shopping. (See chapter 20 for the full scoop on toys.) And if you are in the 99 percent of the population who don't have a personal sex therapist and you really aren't sure what to do with your new vibrator, pick up a copy of *Becoming Orgasmic* by Julia Heiman. Once you have figured it out for yourself, you can tutor your partner.

Another more couples-oriented educational tool commonly used by sex therapists is "sensate focus treatment." This is basically a series of biweekly home exercises to encourage intimacy, touch, and sensual pleasure. Intercourse is typically off the table during this treatment, and the emphasis is on touching other erogenous zones to give pleasure. While not as successful as directed masturbation, there is definitely an uptick in the number of women able to achieve orgasm with a partner after undergoing this treatment.

Anatomy Issues

If you are able to have an orgasm with self or digital stimulation but cannot during intercourse, *and* if having an orgasm during intercourse is something that is important to you, maximizing stimulation during intercourse by altering position may do the trick. People tend to fall into sexual patterns, and it rarely occurs to a couple that a change in position might be a game-changer.

Here are some ways to optimize clitoral stimulation during intercourse:

Option 1: *In the missionary position, the guy positions his pelvic bone right above the pubic bone of the woman. The woman wraps* *her legs around his legs. Thrusting should be downward rather than horizontal. Intercourse isn't as deep, but the glans of the clitoris will be stimulated more than if the guy is deep inside you. (This is known as the coital alignment technique.)*

Option 2: *There's a reason many women prefer the female superior position: it allows them to position themselves in such a way as to get maximum clitoral stimulation.*

Option 3: *"Spooning" allows intercourse (entry from behind), but also makes it easy for a woman to receive digital or vibrator clitoral stimulation from herself or her partner.*

Sometimes the clitoris is anatomically not accessible. This can occur if there is scar tissue that prevents the clitoral hood from retracting, or if the top of the labia has sealed together from atrophy or lichen sclerosus. Use a mirror and take a look down there. If you can't see your clitoris, there may be a medical problem that needs treatment.

Hormone Therapy

Obviously, appropriate hormone therapy is going to go a long way toward making intercourse more comfortable. (See chapters 12 and 13 for more on hormone therapy.) The question in regard to orgasm is whether the addition of hormone therapy is going to specifically enhance the ability to have an orgasm.

While not consistent, there are certainly some studies that have found that supplemental estrogen alone or with testosterone in a postmenopausal woman may facilitate orgasm by increasing blood flow and increasing sensitivity to the clitoris. Studies have consistently shown, however, that hormone therapy does not help premenopausal women.

Testosterone without estrogen is often recommended, but again, there is little science to back it up. Most studies on testosterone therapy do not specifically focus on orgasm but rather on libido or "satisfying sexual experiences."

What is known is that excess doses of testosterone result in enlargement of the clitoris, but a bigger clitoris doesn't necessarily mean a more responsive clitoris. It's also not clear what the best way is to deliver testosterone to enhance orgasm. Some women are advised to put testosterone cream directly on the clitoris, while others are prescribed systemic testosterone to apply to their thigh. To date, there is no data showing that one way is more effective than another.

My feeling is that while more studies are needed to determine if supplementation of estrogen and testosterone are efficacious, there is enough convincing data in postmenopausal women to give it a try.

Available by prescription from compounding pharmacies, vaginal DHEA, the precursor to estrogen and testosterone, increases vaginal lubrication. It may also help libido and orgasm, so this is also a reasonable approach.

Nonhormonal Prescription Pharmaceuticals

Going with the theory that the clitoris is just a little penis, many prescription drugs used to treat erectile dysfunction are now sometimes used for female orgasmic dysfunction. The problem is that a clitoris is not a penis, and erectile dysfunction is not the same as anorgasmia. Just because something works in guys doesn't mean it's going to work in women. Many of these drugs have not been adequately studied in women, and information is anecdotal, not scientific. Also, keep in mind that none of these prescription drugs are intended to be used for treatment of female orgasmic disorders, nor have they been approved by the FDA for such uses.

Phosphodiasterase (PDE5) Inhibitors (Viagra, Cialis)

It's so tempting. His little blue pills are sitting there and certainly seem to solve his problem. Why not take one and see what happens? It did wonders for Samantha on *Sex in the City,* who had earth-shattering orgasms after she took her guy's Viagra.

Not so fast.

It seems that taking a phosphodiasterase (PDE5) inhibitor would be a reasonable strategy, since these drugs are known to dilate blood vessels and increase genital blood flow. Sadly, multiple studies do not demonstrate a positive sexual effect in most women, despite increased blood flow.

There is one exception: some studies have demonstrated that women who are on antidepressants and women who have decreased blood flow because of diabetes, multiple sclerosis, or a spinal cord injury experience increased arousal and responsiveness.

A transdermal PDE5 inhibitor is in development. The behind-the-scenes word is that this gel works in women, has no side effects, and may even be available over the counter! Alas, it is at least three years away, but you heard it here first.

Yohimbe

Erex, Testomar, Yocon, Yohimar, and Yohimbe are all brand names for a mild monoamine oxidase inhibitor (MAOI) that was originally studied as a remedy for type 2 diabetes but was found to affect sexual stimulation and is now sometimes used to treat erectile dysfunction. Yohimbe, taken one to two hours before sexual activity to enhance female orgasm, has been shown to be effective in some studies.

Amantadine/Buspirone (Symmetrel)

This is an anti-Parkinson's and antiviral drug that increases dopamine levels. While sometimes recommended, it has not been found to be effective to treat anorgasmia in women.

Bupropion

Zyban, Wellbutrin, Budeprion, Prexaton, Elontril, and Aplenzin are all forms of bupropion, a well-known antidepressant that is also used for smoking cessation. Some studies show an increase in orgasmic responsiveness in women who use it. It is often prescribed with other antidepressants to counteract their sexual side effects.

Femprox

Femprox, a cream that is applied to the vulva and clitoris at the time of sexual activity, is another arousal-enhancing drug in development. In one very small study, it was shown to be beneficial in reaching orgasm. The active ingredient, aloprostadil (a prostaglandin), purportedly dilates clitoral blood vessels, increasing blood flow and arousal. Since it is already available for the treatment of erectile dysfunction, some women use it off-label.

Neutraceuticals

Women's magazines, health food stores, and, of course, the companies that sell them tout nutritional supplements and botanicals such as L-arginine, ginseng, and ginkgo biloba as products that enhance orgasm. None of these products require FDA approval to make their claims, and so, not surprisingly, none have been the subject of the kind of long-term, controlled study to prove efficacy that is required for prescription products.

It also should be noted that most of these products instruct the user to massage them onto the clitoris. Beyond the placebo effect, one has to assume that a nice long clitoral massage maybe—just maybe!—has a *little* something to do with "efficacy."

Zestra is a botanical massage oil made of biological ingredients such as borage seed oil, evening primrose oil, angelica extract, coleus extract, and vitamins C and E. According to the company that makes it, Zestra "naturally stimulates the body's own sensory nerve conduction, heightening sexual sensation and pleasure." It was first developed for patients with multiple sclerosis who, because of reduced sensation, were unable to have orgasms. While Zestra does increase blood flow, it primarily helps by sensitizing nerves to stimulation. Results are variable. In one study, there were statistically significant improvements in level of arousal, level of desire, satisfaction with arousal, genital sensation, and the ability to have orgasms. A temporary genital burning sensation (experienced by 15 percent of study participants) was the main side effect.

ArginMax is a dietary supplement capsule that contains ginseng, ginkgo, damiana, and L-arginine. In a small, randomized control study (of only 77 women), 73.5 percent of the ArginMax group reported improved satisfaction in overall sex life, compared with 37.2 percent of the placebo group. Improvement of clitoral sensation and orgasm was specifically noted.

Lubricants That Promise More Than Wetness

Vibrel, HerSolution, Sliquid Stimulating O Gel, KY Yours and Mine, KY Intense Arousal Gel, Intimate Organics Clitoral Stimulating Gel . . . a plethora of lubricants are available that promise to make things not only more slippery but also more orgasmic. None have been tested scientifically, but you wouldn't know that from the testimonials that populate the product websites. Most, at a minimum, cause the clitoris to "tingle" or cause a sensation of warmth or coolness, which evidently some women find stimulating.

Wet wOw is an example of a lube that promises lots of extra benefits. The active ingredient, methyl nicotinate (also used as a lip plumper, as in your face lips), creates a temporary inflammatory reaction that causes slight swelling and increased sensation. Vanillyl butyl ether has a warming effect. A dash of peppermint extract gives a cooling sensation. It sounds like there's a lot going on, and hopefully the poor little clit won't panic from feeling warm, cold, swollen, and excited all at the same time. On the other hand . . . that sounds a lot like love. In any case, the rave reviews the company touts are purely anecdotal at this point.

While additional studies are needed to determine the efficacy of herbal and other non-FDA-approved substances for treatment, neutraceuticals and lubes are low-risk options with potentially high return. If they work for you—lucky you! If they don't, you haven't lost much beyond the cost of the product. So, good luck!

Devices to Induce Orgasm

In Woody Allen's 1973 hit movie *Sleeper,* one simply has to enter the "Orgasmatron" to efficiently induce a mind-blowing orgasm. Alternatively, simply holding a cantaloupe-size orb can induce an orgasm in seconds without the bother of having to remove clothing or touch genitals.

The evil Dr. Durand in the 1964 film *Barbarella* invents the "Excessive Machine," which uses constant stimulation with a paddle device as a form of torture that induces death by orgasm. Barbarella survives with a smile.

Flesh Gordon, the 1974 parody of *Flash Gordon,* utilizes a "Sex Ray" to cause earthlings to become aroused. The Coneheads (remember them?) use "Sensor Rings" to give their partners pleasure.

Until someone invents an actual Orgasmatron, Excessive Machine, Sex Ray, or Sensor Rings, this is what is out there that you can try.

Pelvic Physical Therapy and Pelvic Floor Strengthening Devices

As you saw in chapter 6, pelvic floor strengthening and other techniques done with a pelvic physical therapist can do wonders for sexual response. Not only will these techniques help you have an orgasm, but they may also help make your orgasms stronger. This makes sense since a healthy orgasm requires a contraction and release of pelvic floor muscles. That is the premise behind many of the SexAbilitators discussed in chapter 6, including the Magic Banana and a variety of weighted balls, cones, and, yes, barbells. All of these products promise better orgasms when used regularly. No scientific studies have actually been conducted to prove this, and currently none are planned.

Intensity

Intensity is the newest and one of the more promising devices specifically designed to treat orgasmic dysfunction. At first glance, it looks like a giant rabbit-type vibrator, but unlike a vibrator, Intensity utilizes electrical muscle stimulation to strengthen pelvic floor muscles. The inflatable vaginal probe (designed to fit every vagina) ensures close contact with pelvic floor muscles.

And yes, there is also a clitoral stimulator with an ultra-intense vibration. Scientific studies on Intensity are in progress, and they are promising. Most of my patients, though, don't care about the studies. They just want to know where they can get it—right now this device is only available online (Pourmoi.com).

EROS

The EROS Clitoral Therapy Device was approved by the FDA in 2000 for the treatment of orgasmic disorders and female sexual dysfunction. This battery-powered device is applied to the clitoris and works by applying a gentle vacuum to increase blood flow and enhance engorgement. A number of well-designed studies on the EROS device have been published by sexual health experts, and they have demonstrated effectiveness, with up to 60 percent of women finding their ability to achieve orgasm enhanced. The device has also been studied and found to be effective in diabetics and in women who have had pelvic surgery or received radiation to the pelvis.

Slightest Touch Electro Sex

Best. Sex. Ever. That's what the company that makes Slightest Touch promises you, along with a "spectacular orgasm or your money back." Slightest Touch is a battery-operated device that stimulates nerve pathways to the genital area. Essentially a TENS (transcutaneous electrical nerve stimulation) unit, it requires that you apply electrode pads to the top of the foot, above the ankles, and on the buttocks. The premise is that stimulation of nerves in the back will trigger an orgasm. No studies have been published, but I did find a number of people on the Internet who were (unsuccessfully) trying to get their money back.

InterStim

This is a pelvic nerve stimulation system that must be surgically implanted. It is used to help treat urinary incontinence, but has also been found to increase women's orgasmic ability.

Vielle

This is a female massager. Designed for a single use, it is worn on a finger when providing digital stimulation. The company claims this will improve orgasm. Essentially, it adds little bumpy projections to the end of the stimulating finger. I'm skeptical, but it can't hurt to try.

Vibrators, aka "BOB" (Battery-Operated Boyfriend)

My advice is to start with what works for most women and is the most accessible. Even corner drugstores and airport gift shops (Come fly with me!) are selling vibrators these days. Over the years I have found that when the majority of my patients who have never had an orgasm try a vibrator, something wonderful happens. For many normal women, the intensity of a vibrator makes it the only way they are able to climax. A woman in her fifties who has lost the ability to have an orgasm may require a vibrator to get the same response that she easily achieved with digital stimulation in her thirties. And when I refer to a "vibrator," I'm not talking about that battery-operated long hard thing you got as a gag gift in 1982. Toss it and go shopping. But read chapter 20 first.

Surgery?

Every once in a while you will see a claim that a procedure such as G-spot augmentation with collagen injections, clitoral hood reduction, an injection, or a cosmetic procedure will facilitate orgasm. Don't do it.

Tantric Sex

Another approach is to forget the destination (orgasm) and focus on the journey (great sex). Tantric sex, which dates back 5,000 years, promises amazing climaxes that last longer than the average O. But that's actually not the point of the experience. While most only experience a transcendent state during an orgasm, people who engage in this ancient Eastern spiritual practice aim to extend arousal throughout the entire sexual experience. Much like yoga, the key to a tantric experience is in your breath.

If you hone in on your breathing, you can rid your mind of all things mundane and truly focus on how you're feeling. This can be applied to activities outside the bedroom as well. But during sex the participants add reverence to sex, taking time to appreciate each other's arousal. While you may have heard rumors about tantric sex lasting for hours and hours (I'm looking at you, Sting), that's not necessarily the goal. The objective should be to get yourself into the right frame of mind. How can you get there? For starters, spend time talking about having sex, enjoy just kissing, or give each other a sensual massage. If and when that orgasm happens, it will be worth the wait.

When Having the Orgasm Itself Is the Problem

While anorgasmia is the most common orgasmic disorder that plagues women, some have no problem climaxing but may experience orgasmic headache, pain with orgasms, incontinence, or a relatively rare but very distressing condition known as persistent genital arousal syndrome.

Not Tonight, Honey, I'm About to Get a Headache

The first time a patient came to me and told me that every time she had an orgasm she experienced a terrible headache, I advised her to see her internist, or maybe a neurologist. Quite frankly, I thought she suffered from migraines and the correlation with her orgasm was simply a coincidence.

Wrong! Now I know there is a specific phenomenon known as "orgasmic headache." Let me be clear, though: headache associated *with* sexual activity is not the same as headache *before* sexual activity, as in, "Not tonight, honey, I've got a headache."

This is an uncommon issue, affecting only about 1 percent of the population, but even if only one in 100 women experience a headache during sexual activity, that's significant. Fortunately, 75 percent of the time orgasmic headache is a onetime event.

I learned more about sexual headache when I heard a lecture by Dr. Robert Cowan, the director of the Headache Program at Stanford University. He emphasized that there are two very distinct categories of sexual headaches. Pre-orgasmic headaches occur during arousal and usually start as a mild dull ache in the head and neck. Many women describe a throbbing, pressure-like sensation in the head accompanied by a muscle contraction in the neck or jaw. Pre-orgasmic headaches get worse with increased sexual excitement and can last up to three hours. While a real romance killer, these sexual headaches are generally not an indication of anything serious. You can take a nonsteroidal anti-inflammatory drug (NSAID) like indomethacin 30 minutes prior to sexual activity (I know, it's not like you have a schedule for intercourse), and if that doesn't work, see your doctor for further evaluation and a prescription remedy.

A true orgasmic headache is a sudden explosive headache that is simultaneous with orgasm. It starts in one spot and quickly spreads. This is the important part. A true orgasmic headache has a very high correlation with a more serious problem, such as stroke or brain hemorrhage. In fact, 4 to 12 percent of patients with a subarachnoid brain hemorrhage report that their first indication that something was wrong was experiencing an excruciating headache during sex.

The bottom line is this: if you have a severe explosive headache simultaneous with orgasm, put on your clothes and get yourself to an emergency room immediately. A head CT scan or MRI will determine whether there is something serious going on. In many cases, it will turn out to be nothing serious. But if you have a ruptured aneurysm, your orgasm will have literally saved your life.

Incontinence

If you have no problem with your orgasms other than you wet the bed anytime you have one, you are not alone. Occasionally, it is not urine at all, but female ejaculation from a vestibular gland in the vagina. In most cases, however, an orgasmic pelvic floor contraction has combined with a penis pushing on the bladder to cause an involuntary loss of urine that is distressing to say the least. (Incontinence is covered in more detail in chapter 15.)

Painful Orgasms

It's bad enough to have pain in any circumstance, but to have pain when you are expecting pleasure is the equivalent of thinking you are about to get into a nice warm shower only to discover that there is no hot water.

Most women who have pain with orgasm are experiencing painful intercourse that continues or worsens if there is an orgasm. Since an orgasm is essentially a contraction and release of pelvic floor muscles, most pain with orgasm is a result of a hypertonic pelvic floor. Eliminating the source of the pain with pelvic floor physical therapy will alleviate this problem.

Pain-free pleasurable intercourse that culminates in a painful orgasm is a different matter.

The first step is to determine what hurts.

If the clitoris hurts, it may be that the nerves have continued to fire after orgasm. This is a likely scenario if the first orgasm is fine but during additional orgasms things get progressively more painful. You may need to just give it a rest!

Sometimes, if there is clitoral pain, there may be scarring from an old infection, or potentially a current infection. I once found that a patient who had excruciating orgasmic pain had an active herpes sore right on the tip of her clitoris. Sometimes the clitoral hood has adhesions from an old infection, or inflammation and engorgement of the clitoris causes the hood to "pull" on the clitoris, resulting in pain. Women from developing countries that still perform genital cutting also often have scarring that results in pain. In these cases, surgically removing the adhesions eliminates the pain.

If there is generalized pelvic pain and cramping in addition to the pain you experience during orgasm, it may indicate there is something amiss in your pelvis, such as endometriosis, an ovarian cyst, or other gynecologic problems. (See chapter 9 for more information on the possibilities.) In any case, an orgasm shouldn't be painful, and if the pain persists, a visit to your gynecologist is in order.

Persistent Genital Arousal Disorder: Too Much of a Good Thing?

What could be better! Constant orgasms! Constant pleasure! Your first thought might be, *Where can I get some of that?* Well, not so fast. For the women who have persistent genital arousal disorder (PGAD), there is nothing pleasurable about what they are experiencing.

I still remember my first exposure to persistent genital arousal syndrome. I had just completed the exam of a new patient. Everything was normal, but when I asked her if she had any issues she wanted to discuss, she began to weep. "I'm excited all the time, and I keep having . . . actually, orgasms. All day long. Constantly."

I must have looked puzzled, because she went on to say, "I mean, even when I am not sexually excited, like when my boss, who I can't stand, gives me extra work. It's constant, and I can't make it stop. Sitting on the bus, having my morning coffee. I don't know what to do." She wept harder.

I was at a loss. Didn't orgasms feel good? I saw patients all day who were desperate to have orgasms. Was she crazy? So I did what every doctor does when confronted with something they don't know. I told her to get dressed and I tried to look it up. The problem was that I didn't know how to look it up. The phrase "persistent genital arousal syndrome" didn't yet exist. I put "too many orgasms" in my computer's search engine. You can only imagine what came up. Constant orgasm? Even worse.

I gave up on the Internet and turned to my medical textbooks. My gynecologic textbook didn't even have "orgasm" in the index, much less "constant" or "too many." I was stuck.

So I did the other thing doctors do when they have no clue. I referred her to someone else, who probably didn't have a clue either. I don't even remember what specialty I picked. I think I probably considered that my patient might have been a little crazy, but she seemed so normal, so ordinary.

Fast-forward. Today I know a lot about this very real, very distressing syndrome.

PGAD has been around forever but was not described in the medical literature until 2001, as a condition in which there is constant genital arousal in the absence of sexual desire. The absence of desire is important and differentiates the person suffering from PGAD from someone who is hypersexual and feels desire all the time. It has been known to affect teens, young women, and postmenopausal women.

Pretty much anything that causes even slight clitoral pressure can trigger the symptoms. Sexual activities such as intercourse or masturbation can initiate an episode. Nonsexual situations such as bike riding, tight jeans, vibrations from a car, or even sitting can also set off feelings of arousal that last for hours, days, or weeks. Orgasms, when they do occur, do not always give relief; sometimes they can be painful.

Here are the specific criteria required to make the diagnosis:

1. Having feelings of sexual arousal (pre-orgasmic genital fullness and swelling) that last for a minimum of hours.

2. Having orgasms does not make the symptoms go away. In spite of constantly feeling like you are on the brink of an orgasm, there is no pleasure or relief when it happens.

3. Sexual arousal is unrelated to any subjective sense of sexual excitement or desire—for example, feeling pre-orgasmic while your smelly, overweight boss is yelling at you.

4. The symptoms are intrusive and unwanted. The moment when you are about to take an important test is not when you want to be thinking about your clitoris.

5. Having the symptoms causes distress. This seems a bit redundant, since anyone experiencing symptoms 1 to 4 is not going to be happy, but this criterion is meant to differentiate someone with this syndrome from a person who finds these symptoms pleasurable.

Even if they don't meet all these criteria, some women may still experience some of the symptoms, such as persistent vasocongestion, tingling, wetness, throbbing, and genital contractions.

Proposed Causes of PGAD

What causes PGAD is highly controversial, and in many cases it has multiple roots. While it is associated with a number of conditions such as depression, anxiety, sexual abuse, and panic attacks, "associated with" (and exacerbating the symptoms) is not the same as "causing." Many researchers believe that treating any underlying depression or anxiety is an appropriate first step. Other conditions linked to PGAD include cysts on the sacral bone that impinge on nerve endings, increased soy intake, and various medications. One theory is that PGAD is the female clitoral version of priapism, a condition in men who have a persistent erection caused by engorgement of blood vessels.

Neurologic problems such as epilepsy, overactive bladder, restless leg syndrome, brain arteriovenous fistulas, or stroke have also been described as potential causes of PGAD. Increased vascularity to the pelvis, as seen in pelvic varicose veins, is another possible link. Antidepressants such as SSRIs have been implicated in triggering PGAD, but obviously women who are starting SSRIs also have high levels of anxiety and depression.

Whatever the source of this condition—vascular, hormonal, physical—there is an inappropriate triggering and hypersensitivity of the nerve, or a branch of the nerve, that supplies the clitoris.

Therapy for PGAD

While having an orgasm will not eliminate the symptoms, sometimes *multiple* orgasms will relieve the discomfort. But women quickly discover that, in addition to providing only incomplete relief, going to the bathroom to masturbate multiple times before giving a presentation to one's colleagues is no way to live.

Most women go to several doctors before they find someone who can help. Sexual health programs that routinely treat PGAD are the best bet. These programs utilize a team approach that includes gynecologists, pelvic physical therapists, and psychologists.

The first step is to identify any potential causes that are reversible, such as a physical nerve entrapment, a sacral cyst, or a medication issue. Most pelvic examinations are normal, but they still should be done to determine if there is clitoral engorgement. A pelvic ultrasound will determine if there are any pelvic masses, and an MRI will show if there is a nerve entrapment, varicose veins, or a sacral cyst. Therapies to "quiet" the clitoral nerve include medications that alter neurotransmitters, nerve blocks, topical anesthetics, and ice. If pelvic varicosities are present, embolization can be considered.

Cognitive behavioral therapy has been a useful treatment, along with distraction techniques such as exercise.

Clearly, much research still needs to be done on this issue, but at least now the problem is recognized, it's been given a name, and therapies have become available that in fact often work.

And by the way, I would like to say to that first patient of mine, I'm so sorry I didn't help you. I am so sorry I didn't take your problem seriously enough to do additional research. I hope you found the help you needed.

part four

HORMONE HAVOC

12

PMS, pregnancy, postpartum, infertility, contraception—strap in, it's going to be a bumpy ride

Women stoically ride the hormonal roller coaster of life navigating the ups and downs of PMS, contraception, attempting conception, pregnancy, and postpartum. And even before perimenopause hits, it's pretty obvious that it too will be no day at the amusement park. Since the right balance of hormones is critical to maintaining a healthy sex life, anything that alters or has altered hormonal levels is going to have an impact or already has. So strap in . . . it's going to be a bumpy ride.

Premenstrual Syndrome

Prior to the 1970s, few people had heard of premenstrual syndrome (PMS). Today it's hard to browse through a greeting card section without being inundated with dozens of examples of PMS "humor." But for the 50 million women who suffer from monthly premenstrual mood swings, irritability, and weight gain, it's no joke. Premenstrual syndrome is different for everyone, but one thing is consistent . . . women who suffer from PMS experience at least one physical or emotional symptom that starts five days before menses and disappears within four days after a period starts. (If moodiness and bloating come and go throughout the month, PMS is not the problem.)

There are more than 150 premenstrual symptoms that a woman might experience during the premenstrual phase of her cycle. Seventy to 90 percent of reproductive-age women report at least one adverse symptom, and up to 40 percent feel that their symptoms are bothersome enough to qualify as PMS because they not only interfere with their ability to think clearly and feel good but affect their relationships with everyone around them. It goes without saying that most women are not feeling particularly sexual when PMS hits.

It takes only *one* of these premenstrual symptoms to have PMS:

Emotional symptoms
Irritability
Depression
Angry outbursts
Anxiety
Confusion
Social withdrawal
Physical symptoms
Breast tenderness
Abdominal bloating
Headache
Swelling in the extremities

Is PMS the Same as PMDD?

Premenstrual dysphoric syndrome (PMDD), by contrast, is a far more severe and debilitating version of PMS that affects 3 to 8 percent of reproductive-age women. While a diagnosis of premenstrual syndrome requires the presence of only one of the symptoms just listed that are associated with PMS, women who suffer from

PMDD have a minimum of five of those symptoms, and at least one of those five symptoms is depression, anxiety, or irritability severe enough to interfere with school, work, or relationships. Like PMS, PMDD symptoms are present five days before a period and are completely gone within four days of the onset of menses.

What Causes PMS?

The woman who lashes out at her family and friends the week before her period is not a wicked, nasty person—she is simply suffering from raging, out-of-control hormones. Women with PMS actually have normal estrogen and progesterone levels, but for reasons not really understood, they have an exaggerated response to normal cyclic changes. There does seem to be a genetic predisposition, but beyond that there is no way to predict who is going to have the most trouble.

Taming the Beast

Since PMS was identified as a specific phenomenon, many attempts have been made to control symptoms with progesterone, estrogen, vitamins, exercise, and dietary changes. Most women just live with the monthly misery, either because they think the symptoms are not severe enough to bother talking to a doctor or because they think nothing will help anyway. PMS is often accepted as another "natural" part of being a woman, like menstrual cramps and labor pain.

The data on diet changes and supplements is inconsistent, but some supplements, such as progesterone, evening primrose oil, and ginkgo biloba, have been definitively proven to be ineffective.

Some, but not all, studies show that vitamin B6 (100 milligrams a day), vitamin E (400 milligrams a day), calcium, and magnesium (200 to 300 milligrams a day) reduce PMS symptoms. And chocolate? Well, there is no question that women crave carbs during that time of month, so it's not unexpected that carbohydrate-rich food and beverages reduce symptoms by boosting serotonin production.

Proven Treatments

Only two treatments, one an antidepressant, the other a birth control pill, have been FDA-approved for the treatment of premenstrual symptoms. Three of the selective serotonin reuptake inhibitors—fluoxetine, sertraline, and paroxetine—have been proven to alleviate symptoms.

Since PMS is hormonally driven, it makes sense that suppressing the normal menstrual cycle by taking birth control pills would eliminate symptoms. Unfortunately, until recently, no traditional oral contraception has been shown to alter the incidence or severity of premenstrual symptoms. Yaz is the only non-antidepressant and the only oral contraceptive to be FDA-approved for the treatment of premenstrual symptoms. Unlike other pills, Yaz contains drospirenone, the only progesterone that acts as a diuretic, encouraging water elimination, which in turn reduces bloating and breast tenderness. Because Yaz is taken 24 days a month rather than the traditional 21, the effects are maintained during the four-day "off" interval. Studies show that Yaz reduces premenstrual symptoms in at least 50 percent of women . . . much better than in placebo groups or with other remedies.

The Contraception Conundrum: When Taking the Pill Takes Away Your Sex Life

For the sexually active woman who is done having kids, not interested in having kids, not ready to have kids, or in between kids, fear of pregnancy is a major libido killer. For the last 50 years, however, women have enjoyed the almost 100 percent certainty of preventing pregnancy with birth control pills. But in an incredibly unfair twist, for some women the very pill that allows such freedom can affect libido and vaginal lubrication and make them not even want to have sex.

Before I launch into the obstacles that the pill causes for some women, I do want to emphasize that for the majority of users the pill is a really good thing—not only for sexual health but for general health as well. The list of the pill's medical benefits for most women is a long one and includes:

Reduction in or elimination of heavy menstrual bleeding
Decrease in anemia
Reduction of pain during menses
Reduction of PMS symptoms
Reduction in perimenopausal hormonal swings
Prevention of menstrual migraine headaches
Reduction in the occurrence of acne
Decrease of facial and body hair
Control of bleeding from fibroid tumors
Decrease of pain in women with endometriosis
Decreased risk of uterine cancer
Decreased risk of ovarian cancer
Decreased risk of colon cancer

With a list like that, it's not surprising that 58 percent of women rely on hormonal contraception for purposes beyond the prevention of pregnancy. Actually, at least 14 percent of women taking hormonal contraception pills use them exclusively for noncontraceptive purposes.

Aside from the medical benefits that indirectly enhance sexual health, the pill also has specific sexual benefits. Separating procreative sexuality from recreational sexuality is a good thing. There is no doubt that removing cramps, PMS, heavy bleeding, and the fear of pregnancy from the equation goes a long way toward increasing the desire to have sex. Clear skin is also a proven esteem booster.

For the Lucky Majority, the Pill Actually Enhances Libido

Many large studies have shown that libido is enhanced in the majority of pill users: they have a higher frequency of sexual thoughts and fantasies, have better orgasms, and are more interested in having sex. Overall, women who use reliable birth control, including the pill, have increased sexual enjoyment.

The Pill's Negative Effects on Sexuality

It would be nice if this was the end of the pill story, but for a significant number of women, taking hormonal contraception has a negative impact on sexual health. It may seem odd that while estrogen increases sex drive, the pill, with relatively high levels of estrogen, can have the opposite effect. The explanation primarily lies in the other part of the hormone cocktail that's responsible for that lusty feeling—testosterone.

Birth control pills contain both estrogen and progestin. The progestin prevents pregnancy, while the estrogen stabilizes the uterine lining to prevent pesky breakthrough bleeding. All progestins have androgenic (testosterone-like) properties, but newer pills contain progestins that are less androgenic. That's a good thing if you are trying to reduce acne or excess hair growth (two of the negative side effects of androgenic progestins), but not such a good thing for your libido.

In addition, taking the pill inhibits your ovarian production of testosterone. The end result of the newer pills is that you are taking less androgen *and* making less on your own. Then comes the final blow. The estrogen in birth control pills increases the amount of sex-hormone binding globulin. As discussed in chapter 10, the more SHBG, the less active (unbound) testosterone is available to boost libido. So not only are your total testosterone levels lower, but what's there is in an inactive form.

Less Testosterone, Less Libido

A decreased libido is the most common and best known negative sexual side effect of hormonal contraception. While some research clearly shows that the pill has a positive effect on libido for some women, there is no question that for others it's a huge libido killer. If that wasn't bad enough, in addition to decreasing libido, low testosterone can lead to fatigue, lethargy, and moodiness—all symptoms that make you more likely to want to take a nap than to make love.

Recent large-scale studies have confirmed that some pill users have decreased desire, arousal, and sexual thoughts. One of the largest studies, published in 2010 in *the Journal of Sexual Medicine,* followed the sex lives of 1,000 German medical students, some pill users and some not. The pill users had significantly more libido and arousal issues.

Studies also confirm that women on hormonal contraception with decreased libido generally have lower free testosterone levels than women who do not take hormonal contraception. However, before you run off to get a testosterone blood test, be aware that taking a measurement is not helpful, since specific testosterone levels do not always correlate with sexual satisfaction. Many women with low numbers have a very robust libido.

Decreased Lubrication

While many women have heard about the libido issues associated with the pill, far fewer women are aware of the profound effect it can have on vaginal lubrication. Your gynecologist may not even be aware of this side effect. New studies show that a small but significant percentage of women on hormonal contraception have a reduction in vaginal lubrication due to both relatively low levels of estrogen and low testosterone. Women who take the pill stop making estrogen on their own since the pill takes over and suppresses natural estrogen production. Because the estrogen component of the pill is responsible for an increase in blood clots, most new pills have a very small amount of estrogen. Here's the problem. The estrogen in a very low-dose pill is high enough to suppress the ovaries (excellent for contraception!) but too low to provide lubrication for some women. Testosterone receptors in the vagina also contribute to lubrication, so the lack of androgenic activity can not only kill the libido but dry things up.

There also seems to be a genetic component to this response to the pill, which occurs in about 3 percent of the population. So, if you can't figure out why your vagina is like the Sahara Desert even though you are 30 years old, totally in lust with your partner, and feel great otherwise, you are not imagining it. It's real.

Vestibular Pain

Some pill users find that total lack of lubrication is the least of their problems. Seemingly out of nowhere, some women on the pill develop vestibular pain that precludes even getting to the gate. Acquired vestibulodynia caused by using oral hormonal contraception results in painful hypersensitivity when any area of the vestibule is touched. If you are frantically doing gymnastics with a mirror to see why you are suddenly having pain, you may see some obvious areas of redness, but in most cases everything looks completely normal (see chapter 8 on vestibulodynia). This appears to be more of an issue with newer pills that contain less estrogen, particularly in women who start the pill prior to age 19.

Anatomical Changes

And as if you needed any more convincing that the changes that occur on the pill are not just "in your head," a small study published in the *Journal of Sexual Medicine* in 2012 reported that measurements of the thickness of the labia minora and the vaginal tissue at the entry of the vagina showed that pill users had a significant decrease in thickness. In that study, the thin tissue was associated with an increased risk of pain during intercourse, decreased libido, decreased arousal, and a decrease in orgasms. Not really a surprise, is it?

And it's concerning that almost 70 percent of women ages 30 to 40 were the least aware of the negative effects of birth control on their sex lives.

The Fixes

So, if you are on the pill and find you would rather play Sudoku than play with your guy, what options do you have?

Yes, you can alleviate the dryness with lubes, moisturizers, and vaginal estrogens, as discussed in chapters 5 and 7, but since most women need contraception for an average of 25 years, you may want to consider a different option.

Try a Different Pill

Some pills may be better for you than others. One study showed that pills that contain newer progestins, such as drospirenone, desogestrol, and norgestimate, might have more impact on libido and vaginal dryness than other progestins.

Pills that contain a lower dose of estrogen seem to be more problematic, so consider switching to a 30-microgram pill, which is still low enough to minimize the risk of blood clots but may be high enough to eliminate sexual problems.

The Nuva ring and progestin-only contraception options, such as Depo-Provera or Nexplanon, appear to have fewer sexual side effects, but some studies show a negative impact with these methods as well.

> SHBG remains elevated until six months after you stop taking the pill, so don't expect instant improvement.

Switch to a Different Kind of Contraception

Birth control pills are not the only way to prevent pregnancy. Not every woman can use, or wants to use, hormonal contraception.

For them, an intrauterine device (IUD), with or without progestin, is a great solution.

The first IUD was reportedly a stone placed in a camel's uterus to prevent pregnancy during the long desert trek, when a camel pregnancy would have been catastrophic. (Evidently camels are pretty randy.) The modern IUD came along in the 1960s and hit its peak during the 1970s, when 10 percent of women used an IUD for contraception. The design of the original IUD, particularly the outmoded Dalkon Shield, increased the risk of pelvic infection, and many women who used IUDs in the 1970s had serious complications. Forty years later, mention IUD and words like "dangerous" and "infertility" still come to mind. It's no wonder that many women steer clear. Fortunately, the new IUDs are designed differently, do not have the same issues, and may in fact be one of the safest, most beneficial contraceptive options.

Currently there are three intrauterine options available. All can be placed in the uterine cavity during an office visit. All provide excellent contraception protection—about 99 percent.

The copper IUD, Paraguard, lasts for ten years and prevents pregnancy by preventing implantation of the fertilized egg in the wall of the uterus. The main downside to the copper IUD is that it may make your periods heavier than usual.

The other available IUDs, Mirena and Skyla, contain a small amount of progestin called levonorgestrol. While strictly speaking they are hormonal contraceptives, they are not in the same category as other hormonal options since the hormone is released in the uterus with minimal systemic effects. The primary way levonorgestrol IUDs prevent pregnancy is by making the mucous in the cervical opening so thick that even the most motivated sperm can't get through. If one hardy sperm does manage to get past the cervical barrier, implantation is unlikely since the progestin makes the uterine lining thin and inactive. Mirena offers many noncontraceptive benefits such as reducing menstrual bleeding by 95 percent, preventing uterine cancer, and treating endometriosis and other gynecologic conditions. Skyla, the newest IUD, is a lower-dose version of Mirena. It has an even smaller amount of progestin (causing fewer systemic effects) but provides contraception for only three years and may not have the same noncontraceptive benefits as Mirena.

All three IUDs give excellent contraception in addition to scoring A+ for convenience. This is not just my opinion. Women who use IUDs are usually the biggest fans, which is why there is an 86 percent continuation rate. Birth control pills have only a 55 percent continuation rate after 12 months of use.

The number-one group of women who choose IUD contraception for themselves? Female gynecologists. Need I say more?

Injectables and Implants

Injectable and implanted birth control is another option that many women choose over the pill. Nexplanon is a matchstick-size rod that is placed under the skin of the arm, where it slowly releases a progestin called etonorgestrol. It lasts for three years.

Depo-Provera is a progestin shot administered every three months. While some women love it, others find that it causes weight gain and irregular menses.

Barricading the Sperm Meets Egg Highway

If you have given your maternity clothes to Goodwill and used the crib for firewood, it may be time to consider permanent sterilization.

While "tubal ligation" and "getting your tubes tied" are the commonly used terms, the more appropriate term is "tubal interruption." That's because there is no actual "tying" involved in the techniques currently used to block the road between the ovary and the uterus.

The very first tubal interruptions were performed as major surgery requiring a large abdominal incision. By the 1970s, a woman requesting sterilization required only an outpatient laparoscopic procedure involving a small incision in the belly button and one or two other tiny incisions in the lower abdomen. The surgeon would then use clips, rings, or cautery to seal the fallopian tubes. No matter the method, the result was the same: an egg could no longer rendezvous with a sperm.

Today a new "no incision" sterilization can be performed in a doctor's office with local anesthesia and essentially no recovery time. "Essure" is a technique in which a slender scope is inserted through the cervix, enabling the gynecologist to place tiny coils inside the tubes as they enter the uterus. The coil doesn't block the sperm; instead, it stimulates scar tissue to grow around the coils, which eventually occludes the tube. An X-ray is performed a few months after the procedure to ensure that the tubes are completely closed.

The upside to sterilization? It is a onetime procedure with no hormonal changes and afterward there is no further need for contraception. Another bonus is that women who have undergone tubal sterilization have a decreased risk of developing ovarian cancer. Keep in mind that while these new methods of sterilization are *much* safer and easier than they used to be, small risks still remain.

The major downside to any permanent sterilization? It's *permanent*. That means you have to be completely, absolutely, totally, 100 percent sure that you don't want to become pregnant. That might sound obvious, but a lot of women who think they are sure change their minds. Studies have shown that 3 to 25 percent of women regret getting a tubal ligation. The most common reason is a change in marital status, particularly in young women. While post-sterilization pregnancy is possible utilizing in vitro fertilization (IVF) techniques, the expense is prohibitive and the procedure is not always successful.

Is It His Turn?

And then there's vasectomy. Before you skip over this section, think about this. Women willingly accept years of contraceptives, pregnancies, labors, deliveries, and postpartums. Yet, once the decision for permanent sterilization has been made, the men who have watched them experience all that often balk at the very notion of undergoing the comparatively minimal discomfort and inconvenience associated with having a vasectomy. That has always been the case, which is why it's the women who end up taking responsibility for permanent contraception 75 percent of the time. Every year 1.5 million tubal ligations are done in the United States, compared to only 500,000 vasectomies.

Since the women are the ones who endure the discomfort, risks, and inconvenience of years of contraception and/or pregnancies, it seems to me that by the time a couple is ready to call it quits, vasectomy is the perfect "thank you" gift. And if you are single and looking and not interested in having kids, you might want to think of adding "has vasectomy" to your perfect guy wish list along with "great sense of humor" and "likes pets."

I'm just waiting for Match.com to list "vasectomy" as a part of the profile. Talk about a popularity booster!

The Impact of Infertility on Sexual Health

After years of preventing pregnancy, it's a cruel turn of events when a woman finds that she can't get pregnant once she decides she is ready. Women who go through fertility treatments deal with not only astronomical expense but incredible stress, not to mention unpleasant physical changes as a result of being barraged with hormones. Did I mention the massive weight gain that many women experience as a result of fertility medications?

Nothing is more associated with having sex than actively trying to get pregnant, yet the difficulties that come with sex during fertility treatment are pretty much never discussed.

Sex on demand doesn't help make an already difficult situation any less so, and a woman can hardly expect to be aroused, moist, and "good to go" just because the ovulation predictor kit says it is the right time. There is an unspoken assumption that sexual pleasure is completely irrelevant for the infertile couple. This wouldn't be such a big deal if it lasted only a few months, but for many couples fertility treatment drags on for years, or over multiple pregnancy attempts. Recently, there has been some research about sexuality during fertility treatment. A 2012 study out of the Indiana University School of Public Health confirmed what most couples have already figured out—assisted reproductive techniques, especially IVF, cause problems with sexual desire, interest, and satisfaction. As expected, "mood-type symptoms" that could be attributed to the stress of going through fertility treatments, like sadness and anxiety, were huge, but the study also found that women had physical issues such as vaginal pain and dryness.

What Is the Solution for Couples Struggling with Infertility?

For couples who can't conceive, there aren't a whole lot of options when it comes to dealing with the sexual difficulties that sometimes accompany the process. (I know, since when did sex become a "process"?) A good lubricant can be helpful, but people trying to get pregnant often avoid using one, since lubricants can have a negative impact on sperm. The lube Pre-Seed, as I mentioned in chapter 5, does not have any impact on sperm count or motility. A long-acting vaginal moisturizer or local vaginal estrogen is also a solution to make all that sex on demand more comfortable.

Fortunately, for most couples treatment doesn't last long, and the sexual issues associated with infertility treatment will disappear right around the time the sexual issues associated with pregnancy start.

Pregnancy Pitfalls

Name a common medical condition, other than cancer, in which over the course of a year you go through major hormonal, cardiovascular, hematologic, metabolic, and pulmonary changes, not to mention a massive change in your body habitus. That "medical condition," of course, is not a disease, but the normal physiologic change most women go through at least twice in their life—pregnancy.

Yet in spite of the fact that women spend an average of two and a half years of their adult lives pregnant and others spend far longer (Mrs. Duggar!), little attention is paid to sex during pregnancy other than the advice to "follow the advice of your doctor." A 2012 study showed that only 17 percent of ob-gyn residents even asked their patients about sexual concerns during pregnancy, confirming that this is a conversation that most doctors don't initiate beyond, "It's safe," or "Please abstain."

I was once asked to go on *The Jenny Jones Show* (Remember that one? It was one of the first in the too-much-information-about-your-personal-life TV genre) to talk about sex during pregnancy. I declined (an excellent decision on my part), but one of my patients agreed to be a guest. Jenny asked her how her sex life was during her high-risk pregnancy. I had advised her to abstain from having intercourse because of preterm labor. She replied (on live national TV): "If I give one more blow job, my lips are going to fall off." As I said . . .

So here's the rundown: During the first trimester, most women have significant breast tenderness (as in they hurt so much you order your partner to not get anywhere near them), nausea, vomiting, extreme fatigue, and in some cases fear of miscarriage. Real aphrodisiacs, right?

The second trimester is when most women are told that intercourse is the most pleasurable and comfortable, and for many it is. It is also the time when it becomes physically obvious to your husband that you have an actual human being inside you. Now, some men are totally turned on by a pregnant belly and are not in the least bit freaked out by a little kick or reminder that there are now three people in the bed instead of two. Others worry that they are hurting the baby or feel like they are having sex with the children watching. This is particularly a problem as you get closer to delivery and a moving human being is obviously in your belly. Even if both of you remain interested, by the third trimester, in spite of creative arrangement of pillows and positions, intercourse is physically very uncomfortable for some women.

Comfort aside, there seem to be two groups of women . . . those who have an amazing libido and incredible orgasms during pregnancy (these are the women with really large families) and women who feel asexual and have zero interest (mostly parents of only children?!).

So, a few tips if you are currently pregnant or thinking about becoming pregnant:

Unless your doctor tells you otherwise, you can continue to do pretty much anything you would ordinarily do, as long as you want to. If it doesn't hurt, it's okay. If your doctor tells you to abstain, ask him or her to get specific. Should you abstain only from intercourse? Or should you abstain from any sexual activity that might result in an orgasm?

I still remember the woman who asked me, when I told her she should abstain from intercourse, if anal intercourse was acceptable. I was so taken aback by her question that I don't remember what I said. I think I mumbled something like, "I guess so." This was before I became an expert in medical sexuality! In retrospect, I should have told her no, since what I was trying to have her avoid were the uterine contractions that occur as a result of orgasm. I honestly don't think I was aware at the time that women can have orgasms from anal intercourse.

Most women are fine with giving up their sex lives for a few months for the sake of having a healthy baby, but be aware that if you are in that group experiencing no desire and no pleasure during pregnancy, you still have the postpartum to look forward to—and that's where the real trouble can start.

Postpartum: The Big Secret

Everyone assures you that you will be ecstatically happy once you are no longer pregnant and have a healthy baby. It's funny how everyone forgets to mention the part about peeing in your pants every time you laugh, cough, or sneeze after childbirth, the chronic exhaustion, and not being sure you even like, much less love, your baby. It doesn't help that your body no longer even remotely resembles your pre-pregnancy figure and shows no signs of returning to form anytime soon. Put that together with healing vaginal tears, a crying baby in the next room, and a useless husband *in* the room and many women wonder if they are destined to have only one child simply because they can't imagine ever having sex again. When you finally do try to revisit your sexual side, your vaginal walls are more often than not thin, dry, and nonresponsive.

What's going on down there, other than the obvious, is that nursing, postpartum women have low estrogen levels. The good news is that those low levels prevent ovulation and provide automatic contraception. The bad news is that it doesn't do you any good to have natural contraception if you can't have sex.

It's pretty clear that for at least the first three months postpartum the couple with a "normal" sex life is the exception, not the rule. By three months postpartum, 80 to 93 percent of women have resumed sexual intercourse, but in a study of over 400 first-time moms, 83 percent reported sexual problems at three months postpartum, and 64 percent reported that intercourse was still painful at six months postpartum owing to healing vaginal tears or decreased lubrication. Sexual problems were strongly correlated with poor body image, urinary incontinence, and painful intercourse for postpartum women.

The majority of studies that look at postpartum sexual issues look only at intercourse—who is having it, when penile-vaginal intercourse is resumed, and whether or not it hurts. But what about oral, digital, or self-stimulation? A 2012 study looked at postpartum sexuality in much broader terms, with really interesting results. An online questionnaire was sent to 300 women in a study out of the University of Michigan. These researchers found that the length of time it took before resumption of any kind of sexual activity after childbirth (not just intercourse) was variable and primarily driven by fatigue. Partner interest was the other driver behind earlier rather than later sexual activity. Men evidently have no postpartum sexual issues and expect that as soon as the doctor says a woman is "good to go," she *will* be "good to go." And most women comply. Variables that didn't seem to matter in terms of resumption of sexual activity were breast-feeding status, stress, and body image.

During the three-month postpartum period, 85 percent of the women surveyed had intercourse, 65 percent had oral sex, and 61 percent masturbated. The types of activities were initiated in the following order:

First: *Oral sex on partners (I feel sorry for the poor guy, he's been waiting forever)*
Second: *Self-stimulation/masturbation (I'm not ready for intercourse, but an orgasm might be nice)*
Third: *Intercourse, usually after six weeks, when most doctors give the green light*
Fourth: *Receiving oral sex (generally the last kind of sexual activity reinitiated)*

Engaging in sexual activity is not the same as enjoying it; the women surveyed in the University of Michigan study had the most pleasure from masturbation.

The Challenges of Postpartum Sexuality
Obviously, not every woman has difficulty with postpartum sexuality, and many are able to ignore a screaming a baby long enough

to engage in satisfying, pain-free sex. But for many women, primarily first-time moms, who are more likely to have vaginal tears (and less likely to be able to ignore a screaming baby), the following factors have the biggest impact on postpartum sexuality:

Fatigue

Multiple studies show an association between fatigue and libido in any circumstance. Postpartum is a time of extreme, chronic fatigue, since it's the rare baby that says, *No problem, tonight I'll sleep all night and give you a little break.*

This is where an otherwise overbearing mother-in-law comes in very handy. Enlist her to stay overnight, and splurge on a night in a local hotel. Get some sleep and maybe you will get some sex. Either way, you will be grateful for the sleep. Trust me.

Relationship Dissatisfaction

This kind of emotionally laden issue is often overlooked as a possible cause by women who don't want to have sex postpartum. It isn't hard to understand, however, that some women just aren't all that interested in having sex with the guy who was all over the idea of having a baby but has zero interest in changing poopy diapers, taking on the 2:00 AM feeding, or doing the mountains of laundry that are inexplicably generated by a tiny human with no job or social life.

Body Image

In most studies, women who perceive themselves to be attractive have more interest in sex. There's something about carrying around an extra 50 pounds, a belly that still looks like you are in your second trimester, and dark circles under your eyes that makes most women feel slightly less attractive than usual . . . you know?

Postpartum Depression

Postpartum is a difficult time, for so many reasons. With all the attention on labor and delivery (classes, books, birth plans), it has always been a mystery to me why virtually no attention is paid to the first couple of weeks postpartum, which is physically and emotionally a far more difficult time. (There is no equivalent of an epidural to numb you for the first two weeks after delivery!)

The typical new mom is sleep-deprived, has a painfully throbbing vagina and sore, leaky breasts, and may be secretly wondering why she was so anxious to have a baby in the first place. Not to mention it's a major miracle if at the end of the day she has had an opportunity to take an actual shower and brush her hair. And yet, the first two weeks after having a baby, you would think she's a movie star what with the constant taking of photos. Then there's the fact that she seldom gets out of her yoga pants. Oh, and on discovering that the scale is *not* broken and that, no, the weight doesn't all disappear after delivery, being less than ecstatically happy is not a surprising reaction.

Up to 80 percent of women develop mood changes shortly after giving birth. This temporary feeling of sadness, irritability, insomnia, and tearfulness, referred to as "postpartum blues," is almost always transient and does not require treatment. But that isn't true for everyone. Postpartum depression (PPD) affects up to one in ten women. The cause of postpartum depression is not entirely understood, but normal post-pregnancy hormonal fluctuations seem to affect certain women more than others. A family history of postpartum depression, a personal history of depression, and a difficult pregnancy are just a few of the underlying conditions that might cause a woman to develop PPD.

Women with postpartum depression suffer with all the symptoms of postpartum blues, but those feelings don't go away. Feelings of sadness not only persist beyond the two weeks after the baby is born but are accompanied by anxiety, panic attacks, intense anger, feelings of guilt, and a sense of being overwhelmed. Women with postpartum depression often do not feel as if they love their baby and even sometimes have thoughts of hurting their baby. This leads to *more* guilt and causes many women to avoid seeking the care they need. I can't emphasize how important it is to seek professional help, particularly if you are feeling hopeless, feel panicked, or have thoughts of hurting yourself or your baby. Start with your OB, who will refer you to a mental health professional, but if you are not immediately getting the help you need, it is totally appropriate to go to the emergency department of your hospital.

Breast-feeding

Yes, breast-feeding causes low estrogen and low testosterone, which in turn causes vaginal atrophy such that intercourse is as excruciating as it can be in a postmenopausal woman. But it doesn't end there. Women who breast-feed sometimes downplay their sexuality (breasts are for food, not stimulation) and take on the role of a feeder only, as opposed to a sexual partner.

Stress Incontinence

Many women panic when they discover that in addition to all the other new surprises that come with motherhood, they are also unable to make it to the bathroom in time, or cough, laugh, or sneeze without losing urine. Thirty to 50 percent of women experience incontinence at least once in their life, and for many it occurs during the first few months after delivery. Before running out and buying diapers in two sizes (newborn and adult), it's important to not overreact over this.

For most women this is only a temporary issue. Once your baby is weaned and your estrogen levels increase, your pelvic tissues will tone and you will once again only be buying one size of diapers. Kegel exercises or an Apex device are commonly recommended postpartum to help strengthen the pelvic floor. In the meantime, it's understandable that this involuntary loss of urine is a real libido killer (see chapter 10).

Your Vagina Has Gone to War!

Take a 22-hour labor, followed by three hours of pushing, resulting in a forceps delivery and an episiotomy, or vaginal tear, and throw in low estrogen from nursing . . . and the result is a vagina that's pretty much been through the war and is now in a refugee camp.

It goes without saying that women who have had difficult deliveries, vaginal tears, or episiotomies are going to need significant healing time before intercourse is even on the table.

Solutions

Fortunately, the physical and hormonal problems that present postpartum are generally temporary. Once your ovaries kick in and start producing estrogen again, you'll be fine. In the meantime, follow the advice for the postmenopausal women in regard to vaginal dryness (see chapter 13). And yes, you can use vaginal estrogen products while you are nursing, regardless of the gender of your baby. Your blood estrogen levels are far too low to show up in breast milk or affect your baby in any way.

Some women have vaginal scarring from a tear or episiotomy that remains painful despite time and a bucketful of lubricant. In most cases, pelvic physical therapy, along with vaginal dilators and local estrogen, will alleviate that problem. Some women will require a minor surgical procedure to remove scar tissue.

In the best of times, libido is complex and dependent on a lot of variables. Add in the extraordinary fatigue and stress associated with the arrival of an infant and sexual problems in the postpartum period can extend well beyond physical and hormonal changes. The fact that most women have more than one baby is the greatest reassurance that things will improve enough to have sex at least one more time. And yes, the second time will be easier.

13

How to turn back the clock on your vagina when your estrogen tank is on empty

Six years ago, I started dating a really nice man. I mentioned to him that I was scheduled to attend a three-day medical conference on menopause and vaginal dryness. Later I heard him on the phone talking to one of his friends. "Three days of lectures on vaginal dryness? I can't believe there is *that* much to talk about!"

I pointed out to him that if every man in America woke up on his 50th birthday to discover that his testicles had atrophied, his penis had shrunk to the size of a breakfast sausage, and ever having sex again was *completely* out of the question, there wouldn't be a mere three-day medical conference on the subject. A national emergency would be declared, and the surgeon general would be on network television to address the crisis. Men would be flocking to the pharmacy to stock up on testosterone. Internists would certainly not be suggesting to their male patients that they stop using their testosterone after a year to "see how it goes." Thankfully, he got it. I married him.

Menopause officially occurs when your ovaries permanently stop producing estrogen or are surgically removed. For many women, the onset of menopause represents freedom from monthly cramps, bleeding, and PMS. Sadly, for many it also represents the end of what was once a healthy, satisfying sex life. No matter what other issues you have that affect your sexual health, this is the one that is universal to every woman—if not now, then in the future. Hot flashes, vaginal dryness, insomnia, mood swings, brain fog. It's a very special time of life. But given increasing life expectancy, women today can expect to live almost 40 percent of their lives after the menopause transition. As far as I'm concerned, nothing less than symptom-free is acceptable.

> All female mammals, with the exception of humans and whales, die shortly after the onset of menopause.

In our culture, most women know that "the change of life" is associated with hot flashes, which while not exactly welcome are at least expected. And yet, a surprising number of otherwise savvy women are not aware of the association between lack of estrogen and the onset of symptoms such as painful intercourse and vaginal irritation. Surveys show that only about 50 percent of women are even aware that vaginal dryness is a direct result of menopause. They only know that, seemingly overnight, slippery sex has turned into sandpaper sex.

Flashes Are Fleeting, Dryness Is Forever

It's also surprising to me how many women assume that all symptoms of menopause are temporary and that once the hot flashes go away, menopause is officially over. A few years ago I was giving a lecture on postmenopause problems at a large women's convention. Before the talk, I was wandering around and heard many of the women say, "I'm done with menopause, so I don't need to hear that talk!"

Well, since postmenopause is defined as the time in a woman's life when she is no longer producing estrogen, no one is *ever* finished with menopause, until of course she is dead. She may not have hot flashes, insomnia, or brain fog anymore, but she will never produce estrogen again. In other words, while *some* symptoms of menopause are temporary, the inability to produce estrogen is permanent. The symptoms of menopause that will not go away without intervention are those associated with vaginal atrophy. In fact, vaginal atrophy only gets worse. Much worse.

In addition, while hot flashes occur early on in menopause, the symptoms of vaginal atrophy sometimes don't appear until years later.

When does the dryness hit?

For 4 percent of women, in perimenopause

For 21 percent of women, in the first year after menses stops

For 47 percent of women, within three years postmenopause

Many women don't even associate a new onset of painful intercourse with menopause, which explains why women were skipping my lecture on menopause. However, the ones who did attend the lecture were floored to learn that their vaginal dryness was a treatable, reversible problem shared by *many* other women.

What Happens to the Vagina When Estrogen Production Stops

Years before estrogen production completely shuts down, hormone levels start to fluctuate wildly during that special time of life known as perimenopause. While the average age to stop menstruating is 51, there are vaginal changes that begin long before you officially donate your tampons to your daughter.

Without estrogen to stimulate the estrogen receptors on the vulva, vestibule, and vagina, the lubrication normally provided by moisture from the cells that line the vaginal wall, the secretions of Bartholin's glands and of Skene's glands, and cervical mucus pretty much disappears. In addition to becoming dry, the collagen layer in the vagina diminishes, making the walls tissue-paper-thin. Changes also occur inside the individual cells. Vaginal cells produce glycogen, which is necessary for lactobacilli to survive. (Remember them, the good guys in your vaginal ecosystem?) The lactobacilli also convert glucose to lactic acid, which keeps the pH of the vagina at a healthy 3.5 to 4.5. It is only at this normal pH that there is protection from vaginal and urinary tract infections.

Diminished blood flow, especially if you smoke or have vascular problems, diabetes, or any of the other medical illnesses discussed in chapter 15, only make things worse.

In short, soon after you blow out the candles on your 50th birthday cake, your vaginal walls dry up and become thin and inelastic, the folds (rugae) in the walls disappear, and the vagina shortens and narrows. You become a frequent flyer at your gynecologist's office to figure out why you always seem to have a yeast infection, bacterial vaginosis, irritation, and odor. And this is all just about what is happening *inside* the vagina.

> If Mother Nature were really a woman, we would keep our vaginal wrinkles and lose our face wrinkles.

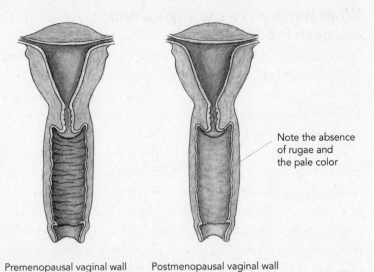

Note the absence of rugae and the pale color

Premenopausal vaginal wall   Postmenopausal vaginal wall

External Physical Changes

Sometimes the external physical consequences of low estrogen are subtle, but sometimes the changes are so striking that you can't help but wonder if you had a vulvar/vaginal transplant in the middle of the night. (Whose vagina is this and how did it get in my body?)

When estrogen levels decline, pubic hair is often diminished, but with the current hairstyle of minimal pubic hair, that's not something every woman notices or worries about. The vulvar skin often becomes pale, dry, and not as stretchy. Labia minora can become smaller (why oh why couldn't it be the hips!), and in severe atrophy actually start to fuse together. The labia majora often appear to be bigger, but in actuality that is an optical illusion. It's the labial fat that has diminished (why oh why couldn't it be the hips!), making the labia majora seem more pendulous, the labia minora less distinct, and sometimes the clitoris more prominent. The urethral opening also appears more prominent and sometimes looks red. The vaginal opening, yes, actually gets smaller. (Why oh why . . . oh forget it!)

The medical term for these physical changes is vulvovaginal atrophy, but I prefer the term genital dryness. (Remember chapter 1!) Symptoms of vulvovaginal atrophy, aka genital dryness, include:

Dryness
Burning
Painful intercourse
Vaginal discharge
Genital itching
Painful urination
Urinary urgency
Recurrent urinary tract infections
Bleeding after intercourse
Fissures after intercourse
Decreased lubrication

It's hardly shocking that for women with this condition inter-course can become excruciatingly painful, or simply impossible. Even a Pap test can cause bleeding and inflammation.

> Before Botox, one look at a woman's face told her age. Now you have to rely on the appearance of the inside of her vagina to know if she is in the over-50 club. The vagina doesn't lie.

Other Consequences of Atrophy (It's Not Just About Sex)

Atrophy from lack of estrogen is not just about sex: it's about having a healthy vagina. No one wants her vagina to emit an odor or con-stantly be irritated and uncomfortable, but that's what can happen as a consequence of the higher pH and an altered ecosystem.

Estrogen is also intimately tied to bladder health. That's right—since there are estrogen receptors in the bladder and urethra, a lack of estrogen is also responsible for an overactive bladder, urethral discomfort, urinary frequency, and recurrent urinary tract infec-tions.

> Sylvie came to see me because she kept getting yeast infections. She mentioned that she needed to take a lot of antibiotics be-cause of frequent bladder infections. Her frustration was obvi-ous, and she mentioned that she had an appointment with a third urologist to figure out what was going on. She had already had a cystoscopy, a CT scan, and too many cultures to count, but so far no answers as to why she kept getting bladder infections. She was shocked when I told her all she needed was a local vaginal estrogen to eliminate the UTIs. Sure enough, when I saw her six months later she reported that she'd had no further problems.

The Scope of the Problem

The current life expectancy for women in the United States is 81. The average age of menopause is 51. Right now in the United States, more than 50 million women are no longer producing estrogen.

Not every woman has vaginal atrophy as a result of menopause, but over 50 percent report that they have symptoms of atrophy such as painful intercourse and "vaginal discomfort." The number of women who have issues is doubtless higher, since the number of women who discuss those symptoms with their doctors and seek care is astonishingly low—at best, around 20 to 30 percent.

> By 2030, 1.2 *billion* women will be postmenopausal.

Making the Diagnosis

It's not rocket science to figure out what's going on when a 52-year-old patient tells me that six months after her period disappeared her vagina became like the Sahara Desert and sex was suddenly a nightmare. I'm pretty sure what the problem is about 90 percent of the time after just talking to my patient. I still need to do an exam to confirm the diagnosis, since other things could be causing similar symptoms, but vaginal atrophy is generally the culprit. More important, I need to determine the degree of the problem to know what the solution will be.

During the exam, I pay specific attention to the external tissues of the vagina, noting whether they are thin and dry. Sometimes I see splits in the skin. The speculum exam clinches it when I see vaginal walls that are pale with no rugae, no lubrication, and sometimes even bleeding just from inserting the speculum. I also routinely measure vaginal pH, so that I have an objective indicator of the degree of the atrophy and can monitor improvement over time.

With rare exception, I don't need to measure blood estrogen levels to diagnose a lack of estrogen. A nonexistent estrogen level in a 53-year-old woman who has not had a period in two years and has a vagina that looks like the surface of the moon is expected, just like getting a sky-high pregnancy test in someone who is nine months pregnant. It doesn't tell you anything you don't already know.

The Fix

It makes me totally crazy when I read magazine articles that tell women who have stopped having sex after menopause that all they need to do to solve the problem is to "plan a special date night," "try sex in the kitchen," or even worse, "watch a sexy movie together" to rekindle the magic and perk things up. These articles are generally written by someone in her twenties who has absolutely no idea what is actually going on in a 50-year-old vagina. I know because I am frequently interviewed for these articles.

Some women, especially if their atrophy is mild, only need to use a good vaginal lubricant to get back in the saddle. Having read chapter 5, you are now an expert on the different types of lubes. But choosing the right lubricant is only the first step. You need to know how to use it correctly. (Please refer back to chapter 5 for that lesson!)

Estrogen

It would be nice if lubricants always solved the problem, but sometimes the ravages of menopause make the vaginal walls so thin and dry that the only way to reverse the vaginal clock and make intercourse comfortable is to use estrogen. I know . . . *estrogen*. Everyone thinks breast cancer, blood clots, bad stuff. And if you weren't thinking that, you will when you read the FDA-required package insert that comes with the prescription.

There are two general categories of estrogen therapy:

Systemic estrogens are intended to work throughout the body to alleviate symptoms such as hot flashes. The blood level you achieve with estrogen therapy is not intended to be as high as when you were 20 (which is why it is called estrogen therapy as opposed to estrogen replacement), but high enough to alleviate symptoms. Sometimes systemic estrogen relieves vaginal dryness, but not always. A systemic estrogen may be oral (a pill), or it may be transdermal in the form of a spray, patch, gel, or cream. One vaginal product, Femring, delivers systemic-level doses in the same range as transdermal and oral products. (For the details about systemic estrogen therapy, see chapter 14.)

Local vaginal estrogens are products that are placed in the vagina to specifically alleviate the symptoms of vaginal atrophy. While some vaginal estrogen is absorbed into the bloodstream, the amount is minimal and its effects are local rather than systemic. For that reason, vaginal estrogen has no impact on your hot flashes, bones, or brain.

Vaginal Estrogen—Creams, Rings, and Other Things

There are three types of local vaginal estrogen products to treat postmenopause vulvovaginal atrophy, all of which meet the following strict criteria imposed by the FDA.

For starters, women enrolled in any studies must actually have documented vaginal atrophy, as demonstrated by three medical criteria:

1. *A vaginal pH greater than 5*
2. *A thin vaginal wall*
3. *Bothersome symptoms, such as painful intercourse*

For a product to prove efficacy, three changes must be met after 12 weeks of treatment:

1. *Vaginal pH must decrease to less than 5*
2. *The vaginal wall must become thicker*
3. *The initial bothersome symptom (such as painful sex) must be reduced*

In addition, the products must also prove to be safe. Often the FDA requires far longer than 12 weeks of use to ensure safety, since treatment of vulvovaginal atrophy generally takes place not over weeks or months but over years. While we are on the topic of safety, let's talk about that product insert that essentially makes you feel like it would be prudent to update your will before you start to treat your vaginal dryness.

FDA class labeling requires all products with the same ingredient to have the same warning, even if it has never been demonstrated in that product. For example, in some circumstances, taking systemic estrogens can increase the risk of developing a blood clot. That risk has *never* been demonstrated in the use of a local vaginal estrogen product; nevertheless, the FDA requires that warning to be on every product that contains estrogen. In fact, every single one of the warnings on local vaginal estrogen labels is based on the risks associated with systemic *oral* estrogen. Not one single complication listed on the package insert has *ever* been shown to result from using vaginal estrogen. Currently there is a movement among scientists to get these dire warnings off the label since there is no evidence of truth to them and many women who would benefit from using vaginal estrogen are too frightened to do so.

All of the following FDA-approved local vaginal estrogen products have met the same safety and efficacy criteria. While there are differences among them, usually the decision as to which product to use comes down to personal preference or, sometimes, finances.

Vaginal Estrogen Creams

There are currently two FDA-approved vaginal estrogen creams. Estrace contains a plant-derived 17-beta estradiol. Premarin contains conjugated estrogens derived from horse urine.

Research has shown that, with *systemic* hormone therapy estrogens, there seems to be an advantage to a plant-derived estradiol product over conjugated estrogens. As far as *vaginal* estrogen creams are concerned, however, there doesn't seem to be any significant difference in efficacy or safety between the two. Many women object to the treatment of the horses that are used to manufacture Premarin and for that reason prefer the plant-derived therapy.

How to Use Vaginal Creams

Creams come in a toothpastelike tube. You squeeze the cream into a reusable applicator, insert the applicator into the vagina, and use a plunger to release the cream. The typical recommended dosage is one-half to one full applicator. Women who prefer not to use the applicator can put a strip of cream on their finger and insert their finger in their vagina. This way is environmentally friendly, and there's no applicator to wash and reuse!

Advantages of Creams over Other Vaginal Estrogen Products

Creams are generally the least expensive form of vaginal estrogen, since they have been around for a long time.

Another advantage is being able to control the amount you use. You can taper the amount of cream you insert to determine the lowest amount you need to get results. This is important, since the recommended amount of estrogen cream results in blood levels that are slightly higher than those with other vaginal estrogen products. Many of my patients require only a tiny amount of vaginal estrogen to keep things lubricated and elastic. It doesn't take much.

While cream is intended to be used inside the vagina, a major advantage to the cream is that it can also be applied directly to the opening or outside of the vagina to help reverse thinness and dryness of *external* tissues such as the vulva, vestibule, and clitoris.

Disadvantages of Creams over Other Estrogen Products

Creams tend to be messy. They tend to "drip" out of the vagina. The reusable applicator, while environmentally friendly, has to be washed after every use. You also need to measure the cream as you load the applicator. Most women find estrogen cream to be a lot less convenient than other products, even though they pack a slightly stronger estrogen punch.

The Vaginal Estrogen Ring: What Is It?

Currently there is only one *low-dose* vaginal ring, Estring, a soft, flexible, nonlatex ring that contains 7.5 micrograms of a plant-derived beta estradiol.

How to Use It

Estring sits in the vagina and must be replaced every three months. Kind of like the filter in your Brita. One size fits all, and unlike a diaphragm, this ring does not need to fit a certain way. You simply fold the flexible two-inch ring and give it a little push so that it slips into the back of the vagina. Once it is in, you will not feel it or be aware of it in any way. It does not need to be removed during intercourse (although you can if you want to), and it is the rare guy who can feel it.

Advantages of the Ring over Other Vaginal Estrogen Products

Convenience, convenience, convenience. There is no dripping cream, and no applicator to wash. You only need to think about this product four times a year.

Disadvantages of the Ring over Other Estrogen Products

An internal ring offers some of the external benefit of estrogen creams, but not as much. Also, you cannot control the amount of estrogen being delivered the way you can with estrogen creams. The ring is expensive, and not every insurance plan will cover it. Some women just don't like having something inside their vagina all the time, and some have difficulty putting it in place, then taking it out. I do have a handful of patients who come in and have me do it for them, but only rarely. Most patients who try the ring like it and continue to happily use it.

Vaginal Estrogen Tablets

Vagifem is a vaginal tablet that contains 10 micrograms of plant-derived beta estradiol. This tiny tablet (about the size of a baby aspirin) comes preloaded on a slender disposable applicator. You insert it a few inches into the vagina, push the plunger, and throw away the applicator. The tablet magically sticks to the wall of the vagina and slowly dissolves. It sticks so well that you can insert it anytime.

Even if you go for a brisk walk just after inserting it, you will not find your vaginal tablet sticking to the toe of your shoe!

Advantages of Tablets over Other Vaginal Estrogen Products

Like the ring, vaginal tablets offer a consistent dose of estrogen. There is no mess with tablets and no applicator to wash—in fact, most women find tablets to be the easiest product to use. You can also taper the dose by using it less often. Vagifem delivers the lowest dose of all the vaginal estrogens. That doesn't make it any safer (they are all equally safe), but for women who desire the lowest dose of estrogen, this is the one.

Disadvantages of Tablets over Other Estrogen Products

Like the ring, vaginal tablets primarily deliver internal benefits. There is some external benefit, but some women find that they still need external help. Environmentally conscious women don't like that the applicator is disposable. Also, with tablets you have to remember to insert one every few days. Unlike the ring, you can't "set it and forget it."

Which Vaginal Estrogen Product Works Best?

Again, studies show that every single estrogen product on the market works equally well. All are safe. All normalize vaginal pH. All restore the vaginal walls to premenopause status so that intercourse is comfortable. All help with bladder symptoms and eliminate irritation and odor. Your decision as to which product you choose is completely based on personal preference, convenience, ease of use, and, in many cases, what your insurance will cover. It's not unusual for someone to start with one product and find that she prefers another.

The Best of Both Worlds

I find that many of my patients need a combination approach when it comes to vaginal estrogen. I advise them to use the ring or the tablet to get rid of the internal sandpaper feeling and apply estrogen cream on the outside once or twice a week to increase the elasticity of the external tissues.

When treating external tissues, you should apply a dab of estrogen cream using your fingers once a day, focusing on the opening of the vagina and the vestibule. Once normal elasticity is restored (usually after about two weeks), once or twice a week is generally adequate for maintenance.

Here are some more questions you may have:

How Often Do I Need to Use a Vaginal Estrogen?

If you are using a cream or tablet, you need to use it every night for 14 days (the "repair" part of the treatment). Twice weekly is recommended for maintenance if you use the cream or tablet, but I find that many of my patients do just fine if they use it only once a week. Some need to use it twice a week, and I have the occasional patient who is dry unless she uses it three times a week. The key is consistency! If you stop your estrogen treatment, it doesn't take long for atrophy to set in again. In other words, skipping your estrogen for months and then deciding to use it the night before you leave on a cruise is not a good plan. Vaginal estrogen products are not lubricants—they restore lubrication.

How Quickly Will I See Results?

Within two to four weeks of initiating estrogen therapy, most women are able to have comfortable intercourse. In fact, a look at vaginal tissue under a microscope shows that normal thickness is often restored to the vaginal walls in that amount of time and the tissue is indistinguishable from premenopausal vaginal tissue. Some women need a longer "repair" time, and the effects are cumulative.

Many women are reluctant to try a local vaginal estrogen. But once they do, they rarely stop.

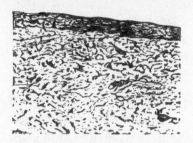

Vaginal biopsy showing
atrophic changes

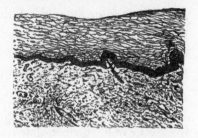

Vaginal biopsy from the same patient
after local estrogen therapy

How Much Estrogen Is Absorbed into My Body?

When you use vaginal estrogen, the amount of hormone that is absorbed into your bloodstream is minuscule, and even though it sounds counterintuitive, the longer you use it, the less estrogen gets absorbed.

You read that right. Dry, thin vaginal walls are like tissue paper, so when estrogen is first applied, it doesn't stay in the vagina but seeps right through and gets absorbed into the bloodstream. Within a short time of starting therapy, the thin vaginal tissue thickens enough that the estrogen stays in the vagina instead of getting absorbed into the bloodstream. If you measure blood estrogen levels in a woman who routinely uses small amounts of vaginal estrogen, her levels would be *no higher* than the normal postmenopausal range. That's great news for the woman who is concerned about any risks that might be associated with using estrogen.

> The amount of systemic absorption of estrogen in a year of using the vaginal tablet Vagifem is the same as if you took two oral estrogen tablets a year.

In the case of the ring and vaginal tablets, levels are essentially in the same range that you would find in menopausal women who do not use vaginal estrogen. The cream does have a slightly greater absorption rate than the ring or tablets. Since women use highly variable amounts, serum levels are variable as well.

Are There Ever Systemic Side Effects?

It is possible in the first couple of weeks, when absorption of vaginal estrogen is slightly higher, to have some systemic side effects. In the first two weeks, remember, you are using Vagifem tablets every night, the Estring releases a little more estrogen when it is first placed, and vaginal creams are more absorbed at the start of use. Some of my patients note a little breast tenderness or some alleviation of hot flashes at the onset of using these medications. Stick with it and the breast tenderness will go away. Don't get too excited if your hot flashes are diminished, because that will probably not last either.

What Changes Can I Expect?

Local vaginal estrogens reverse essentially every one of the genital changes that occur when estrogen levels go down. The increased blood flow will cause the vaginal tissues to thicken and have a pinker appearance, and it will also improve the ability of those tissues to heal if there is a scratch or tear. Lubrication will increase. Elasticity and rugae will return, and the vagina will be able to expand and accommodate even a jumbo penis. (You should be so lucky!) The increase in collagen fibers will make external vulvar skin thicker. In short, your vagina and vulva will be as they were prior to menopause. Well, not exactly. Your pubic hair will still be sparse and gray.

> Most women think that if they are not having intercourse, there is no reason to use vaginal estrogen. Think again! Fewer bladder infections, less urinary urgency, less odor, less irritation, and fewer vaginal infections are all really good things.

Local Estrogen: True or False?

You name it, I've heard it. So, for the record: If you use vaginal estrogen, your husband will not grow breasts, you do not need to abstain from intercourse for 24 hours, and no, the cream should not be used at the time of intercourse. The biggest myth is that you cannot use a local vaginal estrogen product if you have breast cancer or are at risk for breast cancer (see chapter 16). Then there's the question about using a little on your face to eliminate the wrinkles where you don't want them. I'm not allowed to answer that one. (Smile.)

How Long Can I (or Should I) Continue to Use Vaginal Estrogen?

Estrogen does not accumulate over time. The blood level of estrogen in a woman who has been using local estrogen for two years is the same as it is in the woman who has been using it for ten years. So that recommendation that you might have heard about using estrogen at the lowest amount for the shortest period of time? That doesn't apply to vaginal estrogen. In fact, the North American Menopause Society (NAMS) recently proclaimed that "Vaginal Estrogen Therapy should be continued as long as distressful symptoms remain." Not only is there no time limit, but you need to remember to consistently use it since, if you stop, it's pretty much a guarantee that the dryness will return.

So, you can use vaginal estrogen as long as you're interested in having intercourse and maintaining vaginal health—in other words, until death. Women in their eighties can still enjoy intercourse. The real challenge is finding a partner who is still "good to go."

Do You Know?

Forty-two percent of women are not aware that local estrogen prescriptions are available, and only 7 percent of women seeking treatment for sexual problems are offered a prescription to relieve any of their symptoms. Most never fill it.

Local Estrogen Alternatives

Some women have been told not to use a local vaginal estrogen for various medical reasons, or they simply prefer not to. Many of those women will see similar results from using a long-acting vaginal moisturizer. (Refer back to chapter 5 for information on buying the right product!) Another strategy is to initially use a local estrogen to treat atrophy, and then continue with a long-acting moisturizer for maintenance.

Ospemifene

Ospemifene (Osphena) is a daily pill to be taken by mouth. (Now that you know some pills are taken by vagina, I need to be specific!) This pill is not estrogen but is classified as a SERM, or selective estrogen receptor modulator. SERMs are drugs that either block estrogen pathways or activate estrogen pathways in specific tissues. SERMs used to be called "anti-estrogens," but since they can have either estrogen-like or anti-estrogen-like activity, that term is no longer used. Tamoxifen is a SERM that blocks estrogen pathways in the breast, which is why it is useful in the prevention of breast cancer. Raloxifene is another well-known SERM that activates estrogen pathways in bone (to treat osteoporosis) but blocks estrogen pathways in the breast (to prevent breast cancer).

Ospemifene activates estrogen pathways in vaginal tissue to lower pH, thicken vaginal tissue, and alleviate painful intercourse from vaginal atrophy. It essentially has the same effect as local vaginal estrogen. Further good news—ospemifene activates estrogen receptors in bone and blocks estrogen receptors in breast tissue!

Ospemifene does weakly stimulate the tissue that lines the uterus, but there is no evidence that this will increase the risk of uterine cancer. Of course, any woman, whether she takes ospemifene or not, should evaluate any postmenopausal spotting or bleeding. About 7 percent of women have a few more hot flashes when using this product. Women with breast cancer are advised not to use this drug, not because there may be problems with it for them, but because it hasn't yet been tested in women with breast cancer. In fact, since ospemifene blocks estrogen receptors in breast tissue, most experts feel that it is the perfect option for the woman with breast cancer. It has even been shown to shrink breast tumors in rats! It is also ideal for the 50 percent of women who, according to the 2013 *Revive* survey, prefer to swallow a pill than to put something in their vagina.

Like local estrogen, ospemifene is not a cure-all, and many women will still need to use a lubricant or a long-acting vaginal moisturizer with this medication. But since only 7 percent of the 32 million women who need help with painful intercourse are getting it, another option is always a welcome addition.

Vaginal DHEA

Vaginal DHEA (didehydroepiandrosterone) is one of the most promising products soon to arrive (hopefully!) in your neighborhood pharmacy. DHEA is the precursor hormone to estrogen and testosterone that is naturally secreted by the adrenal glands in low amounts. DHEA decreases by roughly 60 percent at menopause and continues to decline over time. DHEA is often recommended to enhance libido, but what many women don't appreciate is that multiple well-designed scientific studies have proven that vaginal DHEA can reverse vaginal dryness in menopausal women as well as vaginal estrogen does. Daily intravaginal DHEA improves pH, thickens vaginal walls, and decreases pain during intercourse. DHEA supplementation appears to be safe and does not stimulate breast or uterine tissue.

Currently, vaginal DHEA ovules can be obtained only by prescription in a compounding pharmacy. Dosages vary but are generally in the neighborhood of 0.25 milligram a day twice a week.

What About Vaginal Testosterone?

You know by now that the standard hormonal treatment for vaginal dryness is local estrogen. This makes sense since we know that vaginal tissues are loaded with estrogen receptors in desperate need of fuel to function and that local vaginal estrogen, for most women, alleviates this problem.

While testosterone has long been recognized as an essential requirement for an intact libido, we now also understand that vaginal and vulvar tissues are rich in testosterone receptors that play a role in normal lubrication. Some sexual health experts are now treating vulvar and vaginal atrophy with a combination of estrogen and testosterone, and preliminary studies indicate that the combo works much better than either hormone alone. If you are still dry despite local estrogen therapy, you may want to consider the addition of a compounded testosterone to get things slippery.

Your Cheat Sheet for a More Slippery Sex Life After Menopause

I've given you a lot of information, and I know it's confusing. Clearly, there are a lot of tools out there to alleviate vaginal dryness and pain—lubes, moisturizers, local estrogens, DHEA, ospemifene, systemic estrogens, pelvic physical therapy, dilators. Where to begin?

It really depends on the severity of your issues. There is a huge difference between the woman who says, "Gee, it doesn't feel as wet as it used to," and the woman who hasn't had anything even approach her vagina for 20 years because it was so excruciatingly painful the last time she tried. What follows are some general guidelines—and the heart and soul of the book.

Group 1: Mild Dryness

I can have intercourse, and sometimes it's okay, but more often than not it feels a little dry and scratchy. Sometimes it really hurts.

Apply a generous amount of lubricant to the outside of your vagina and all over his penis. If intercourse is pain-free and pleasurable, there is no need to do anything else other than having frequent intercourse. And have plenty of lube on hand.

Some women find that even if a lubricant works, they don't want to use one just at the time of intercourse and would rather do something that will keep things wet and ready to go anytime. If that's your preference, try a long-acting vaginal moisturizer, a local vaginal estrogen product, ospemifene, or vaginal DHEA. You are not required to have severe atrophy to be prescribed one of these solutions.

Group 2: Lube Isn't Doing the Job

The lube helps a little, but only a little. I'd rather just skip sex instead.

In spite of making things slippery, lube is not enough if your vaginal tissue is thin and has lost its elasticity. You need to start with either a long-acting moisturizer or a medication to get the tissues in shape. If you want to try a local estrogen product, DHEA, or ospemifene, you will need to see your doctor to get a prescription. No matter which product you choose, use it for at least 14 days before you attempt intercourse again.

Use a lubricant even if you are using a long-acting moisturizer or prescription product. In one study, 40 percent of women discontinued using their local estrogen product because "there wasn't enough relief." Just because you are using estrogen doesn't mean you don't also need a lube.

If things are fine once he is inside but the entry still feels tight and dry (and if the lubricant doesn't help), use a vaginal estrogen cream on the outside daily for two weeks, and then taper to one to two times per week.

If intercourse is pain-free and pleasurable, great. Do not stop using the moisturizer or prescription product! I guarantee you that things will get dry again if you do. You are not suddenly going to start making estrogen.

After a few months, it is fine to increase the time between doses. If your atrophy is not severe, and most important, if you are having intercourse on a regular basis, some women are able to use the local vaginal estrogen only once a week or the long-acting moisturizer only once a week. That is great—not because it is safer, but because it is cheaper and more convenient. But if you taper down to once a week and things start to get dry, obviously you need the estrogen and/or moisturizer twice a week and there is no getting around it.

Group 3: Things Are Bad . . . Really Bad

He can't even get it in there. Cleaning toilets sounds infinitely more appealing than attempting intercourse.

There is no getting around it: you are going to need to get a prescription for a local vaginal estrogen product, DHEA, or ospemifene. Your vagina is broken and needs to be repaired. Don't panic. Just get a prescription.

Before you try intercourse with an actual penis, start with dilators (remember chapter 6?). Once you are successful with dilators, continue to work with them until you are able to get a dilator in that is slightly larger than the penis in your life. When you first attempt to have intercourse, use a generous amount of lubricant and be in a position that puts you in control if things are not going well. A warm bath beforehand will help relax you and your vagina.

If things are going well, keep using whichever product is keeping your tissues healthy. Twice weekly is recommended for maintenance if you use the cream or tablet, but I have the occasional patient who is dry unless she uses it three times a week. The key is consistency! It doesn't work if you stop using your estrogen for months and then decide to use it on date night.

If you are not making progress with the dilators, if you are unable even to get a small dilator in, or if you are still having pain, you need to be evaluated by a gynecologist who can determine if the tissues are healthy, or if there is another issue going on. If everything checks out, you probably have pelvic floor pain and dysfunction from muscle memory and will need pelvic floor physical therapy.

I know you are frustrated, but this is fixable! It is just no longer a do-it-yourself project.

Use It or Lose It

Don't underestimate the importance of having intercourse on a regular basis once vaginal elasticity is restored. "Use it or lose it" is one of those phrases that actually has some truth to it. If no ready or able partner is available, a toy is a good substitute, both for your own pleasure and to keep things alive until a priapic prince comes along!

14

THE COLD TRUTH ABOUT HOT FLASHES

*Vaginal dryness is not the only issue
that sabotages your SexAbility*

For hundreds of years, women have struggled to find solutions for menopause symptoms such as hot flashes and sleep disturbances that affect not only their SexAbility but also their overall quality of life. In the 1870s, Lydia Pinkham's Vegetable Compound was a popular remedy for virtually every gynecologic ailment, including menopause-related problems. Roving salesmen (the 1870 equivalent of the health food store clerk) would go house to house selling the stuff. The ads claimed the compound was a "positive cure for all those painful complaints and weaknesses so common to our best female population and is particularly adapted to the change of life."

No doubt, its 18 percent alcohol content had something to do with its efficacy—even proper ladies could remain happily inebriated while dealing with difficult menopausal hot flashes and sleeplessness. Another key ingredient in Pinkham's remedy was none other than black cohosh, an extract of dried underground roots derived from a plant used by Native Americans. Today black cohosh remains one of the most widely used alternative therapies for treatment of hot flashes despite research questioning its effectiveness.

Estrogen therapy entered the scene in 1941 when Premarin came on the market. A 1948 *Reader's Digest* article proclaimed, "The melancholy sickness that blights the happiness of some women at their change of life [can be] controlled by female hormones; yet most women have gone on suffering. . . . But now at last they are ready to transfigure the stormy afternoon of life . . . into a time of serenity and vigor." By the 1960s, the estrogen boom was in full swing, in large part thanks to *Feminine Forever,* a book written by Dr. Robert Wilson (and funded by the company that sold estrogen!). Proclaiming that menopause was a disease that required estrogen as treatment, this best-seller stated on its cover that "every women, regardless of age, can safely live a full sex life, for her entire life." Sales soared.

A slight bump in the estrogen road appeared in the 1970s when it was discovered that women who took estrogen were at increased risk for developing uterine cancer. The addition of a progesterone pill, to protect the lining of the uterus from a buildup of abnormal tissue, solved that problem, which is why a progestin (a form of progesterone) is now routinely prescribed along with estrogen for anyone who has not had a hysterectomy.

Despite the claims of *Feminine Forever,* estrogen was originally intended for—and in fact was only FDA-approved for—the treatment of hot flashes and vaginal dryness. But in the 1980s some studies suggested that in addition to helping with bothersome symptoms, postmenopause hormone therapy was also beneficial to prevent heart problems, osteoporosis, and Alzheimer's disease. As a result, women were advised to routinely take estrogen after menopause, even if they were asymptomatic.

The Women's Health Initiative: The Flush Heard Round the World

The Women's Health Initiative (WHI) was a large study initiated in 1997 with the purpose of definitively determining whether long-term hormone therapy could prevent heart disease and prolong life in addition to controlling postmenopausal symptoms. The 27,000 women between the ages of 50 and 79 who enrolled were divided into three groups. One group took estrogen and progesterone, the second group took only estrogen (these were women who did not need a progesterone to protect the lining of the uterus because they'd had a hysterectomy), and the third group was given a placebo pill. The women were not told what they were taking, and they were all monitored for side effects and potential benefits. The study was intended to run for eight years but was abruptly ended prematurely at five years when it appeared that the group taking estrogen and progesterone had a higher incidence of breast cancer, blood clots, and stroke. When the results of the study were released to the media, the news immediately went viral.

On July 22, 2002, women all over the United States woke up to the news that the hormone therapy their doctors had recommended was in fact dangerous, increased the risk of breast cancer, increased the risk of blood clots, increased the risk of stroke, and should be discontinued *immediately*. Millions of hormone pills were flushed down the toilet in anger and fear. Sales dropped by 70 percent. Most media outlets forgot to emphasize that 97.5 percent of women taking hormone therapy had no problems and that the number of women who had problems was actually quite small.

Breaking news in 2002:

"Red Flag on Hormone Replacement"
—CBS News

"Hormone Replacement Is Riskier than Advertised. What's a Woman to Do?"
—*Time*

"New Study Raises Fears About the Risks for Millions of Women"
—*Newsweek*

Putting the WHI in Perspective

The WHI showed that for every 10,000 women per year who used estrogen and progesterone (compared to the women who were not taking any hormones or were taking estrogen alone), there were:

Seven additional myocardial infarctions
Eight additional strokes
Eight additional breast cancers
Eighteen additional blood clots
Six fewer colorectal cancers
Five fewer hip fractures

There were no additional deaths.

Despite the fact that the absolute number of women who had problems from hormone therapy was quite small, results from the WHI study have continued to contribute to a great deal of concern and confusion regarding the safety of hormone therapy.

> Over 80 percent of women who have breast cancer have never taken hormone replacement of any kind. In addition, the risk of developing breast cancer from hormone therapy is lower than the risk associated with daily alcohol use or obesity.

Why WHI Shouldn't Be a Source of Panic for Women Who Take Estrogen

Since the initial release of the WHI findings in 2002, the data has been revisited, and it is now clear that both the design of the study and the initial interpretation of the data were problematic. There were three striking issues.

Issue 1: Age Matters

The average age of women in the study was 63, and over 70 percent of the women enrolled were over the age of 60. Since most women go through menopause between the ages of 50 and 55 (representing only 10 percent of the study population), the overall results were not reflective of most women who take hormone therapy. A reevaluation of the study looking only at women in the 50–60-year-old range showed completely different and very reassuring results. There was a *decrease* in coronary heart disease, fractures, and overall mortality. There was no increase in breast cancer, and in fact there was a slight decrease.

Issue 2: Taking Estrogen Alone Is Not the Same as Taking Estrogen and Progesterone Together

Many women were also unaware that the results released in 2002 applied only to women taking estrogen and progesterone. The study group that included women who took estrogen alone was not discontinued until March 2004 and had strikingly different results. Women in the 50–60-year-old WHI group who took estrogen alone had a 37 percent decrease in heart disease, an 11 percent decrease in stroke, a 12 percent decrease in new-onset diabetes, and a 30 percent decrease in fractures.

There appears to be a "critical window" to start hormone therapy in order to avoid other health problems.

And then there is the breast cancer issue. The news flash that didn't make it to the media was that in the estrogen-only group there was an 18 percent *decrease* in breast cancer. *There were six fewer cases of breast cancer per 10,000 women per year of estrogen use.* It is now clear that the modest increase that is sometimes seen in breast cancer in women who take hormone therapy is due to the *progestin, not the estrogen.*

In fact, total mortality in the 50–59-year-old age group was a whopping 30 percent lower than in women who did not take hormone therapy. Blood clots were the only remaining concern. Blood clots that form in the veins of the legs can travel through the body and block blood vessels that supply the heart, lungs, or brain. The 50–60-year-old group in WHI did have a 37 percent increase in venous blood clots, which sounds alarming. Keep in mind, though, that since the number of blood clots occurring in that age group is very small, even a small increase translates into a huge percentage increase. In absolute numbers, there were four additional blood clots per 10,000 women per year of estrogen therapy.

In spite of the fact that results for the estrogen-only group were very reassuring, they received essentially no media attention. (And I'd even waxed my eyebrows in preparation for explaining the good news on TV.)

Issue 3: Transdermal vs. Oral Estrogen: There Is a Difference
The third issue with the WHI was that it studied only one kind of hormone therapy, Premarin (conjugated equine estrogen) and Provera (medroxyprogesterone acetate). Many newer types of hormone therapy are metabolized by the body differently and are therefore significantly safer. Specifically, transdermal estrogens do not appear to have the adverse consequences of the oral estrogens.

In the 1980s, transdermal estrogen patches were developed as an alternative means of delivering estrogen. The primary advantage to the patch was that, since the skin absorbed the estrogen, it went directly into the bloodstream and didn't have to pass through the gastrointestinal system, as oral estrogen does. This was intended to benefit women who had liver or gallbladder disease that was known to be aggravated by oral estrogen. It soon became clear that the benefits of avoiding the trip through the liver were not limited to women with liver or gallbladder problems, but were available to all women. The main benefit was the elimination or lowering of the increased risk of blood clots and stroke. Here's why.

Blood clots are more likely to occur in the deep veins of the legs of women who have high cholesterol and triglycerides. All estrogens decrease cholesterol, but oral estrogens increase triglycerides, while transdermal estrogens decrease triglycerides.

Also increasing the chance that blood will form into dangerous clots is the presence of high levels of clotting factors such as fibrinogen and factor 7. Transdermal estrogens decrease fibrinogen and factor 7. In addition, a protein produced in the liver called C reactive protein causes blood clots to grow larger and more prone to breaking away and traveling to distant blood vessels. Oral estrogens increase C reactive protein. Transdermal estrogens do not.

At this point, hormone therapy is not recommended to treat or prevent cardiovascular disease. But since a transdermal product decreases the likelihood of developing a clot, transdermal estrogen therapy is unlikely to increase and may actually decrease a woman's risk for heart disease, stroke, or heart attack.

It's also important to keep in mind that anyone can get a blood clot or develop heart disease even if they are not using hormone therapy. Every postmenopausal woman should minimize her risk by maintaining a healthy body weight and sticking to a heart-healthy diet.

Transdermal estrogen is now available in a variety of forms other than patches, including spray, lotions, and gels. The active ingredient, a plant-based beta estradiol, is found in all transdermal products.

Unlike pills, which must be taken daily, patches offer the advantage of only needing to be used once or twice a week. The disadvantage is that many women don't like to wear a patch; it can irritate sensitive skin, and while it generally does not come off in the shower or the pool, sometimes it does. You also can't alter the dose on your own since it is not recommended to cut the patch. Sometimes the patch leaves behind a sticky residue and faint marks on your skin.

Estrogen sprays, gels, and lotions are applied to the arm or thigh on a daily basis. The major disadvantage to these products, compared to orally taken pills, is that they tend to be more expensive. They are also alcohol-based, and there is a chance that you will burst into flame if you light a cigarette—yet another reason to quit smoking.

Despite the Media Hysteria, Estrogen Is Not Poison

While subsequent reinterpretation of the WHI results has been very reassuring, most women (and sadly many doctors) are not aware that low-dose postmenopause estrogen therapy is appropriate and safe for most, if not all, women. The FDA label still inexplicably reflects the original concerns. Which is why, 12 years later, most menopausal women are suffering from hot flashes, insomnia, and sexual problems under the misconception that taking estrogen will cause breast cancer, strokes, heart disease, and ultimately death. A Yale study published in July 2013 suggested that continued sensationalism in the media about the WHI study and concerns about estrogen have caused thousands of needless deaths. The authors estimated that up to 48,835 fewer women would have died between 2002 and 2012 if they had not avoided estrogen. Fortunately, the estrogen pendulum is swinging again, and many women can feel a lot more comfortable about taking systemic estrogen to not only relieve symptoms but maybe even to prolong life.

It's always interesting to me when I have a patient who is sailing through perimenopause on her birth control pill but will balk when I tell her it is time to stop the pill and start hormone therapy. When I point out that the pill she has been happily taking for the last 20 years has a far higher level of estrogen than standard postmenopausal hormone therapy, she is usually shocked. She is also shocked when I discuss the results of the Women's Health Initiative study in detail and is relieved to hear that taking hormone therapy for relief of menopause symptoms is a safe, viable option.

It's also important to note that the WHI studied only hormone extension, that is, giving hormones to women who were in the typical postmenopausal age range. Hormone replacement in young women who have gone through a premature menopause is an entirely different matter. Unfortunately, the two are usually lumped together. As a result, the 36-year-old who takes estrogen feels she is putting herself at the same risk, and has the same issues, as the

52-year-old who takes estrogen supplements. No one worries about a 36-year-old woman taking birth control pills, but if the same woman goes through menopause, many erroneously believe that taking estrogen therapy (which provides dramatically less hormone than in a typical pill) is dangerous.

The Progestin Problem

If a woman is using *systemic* estrogen and has a uterus, it has been well established that a progestin is needed too, since there is an increased risk of uterine cancer if estrogen is taken alone. If the uterus has been removed, there is no reason to take a progestin. But now that it appears that there is no increase in breast cancer in women who take estrogen unless there is a progestin in the picture, this presents a real dilemma for many women.

In addition, some women don't tolerate taking a progestin and experience bloating, depression, and bleeding no matter what kind of progestin they use. It's really tempting to skip taking a progestin altogether, but it's not a good idea. Uterine cancer is the most common gynecologic cancer in this country and is significantly increased in women who take estrogen without a progestin.

Progestin Alternatives

Some gynecologists place a progestin IUD in the uterus instead of prescribing an oral progestin. While standard in Europe, this is not yet FDA-approved in the States and is therefore an off-label practice.

The vaginal progestins used in the fertility world to stabilize the uterine lining in early pregnancy have not been tested in postmenopausal women, and it is unknown whether they provide adequate uterine protection.

Progestins are generally given in pill form, since the molecule is too large to be absorbed through the skin. Although a couple of FDA-approved patches that have both estrogen and progestin are available, many women don't like those products because the patch is on the large side and comes with a higher rate of breakthrough bleeding.

While compounding pharmacies offer transdermal progestin creams, to date no scientific studies have demonstrated that they protect the uterine lining. In fact, there is data to support just the opposite. Using a compounded progestin cream is essentially the equivalent of using nothing. The same goes for over-the-counter products synthesized from yams that claim to offer protection.

While it sounds drastic, some of my patients have opted to have their uterus removed and take estrogen alone rather than deal with the risks and side effects of progestin.

Some women skip the progestin and monitor the uterine lining to make sure there is no abnormal buildup. While this approach is not currently recommended, in the future it may be a reasonable alternative for women at low risk of uterine cancer who are taking very small doses of systemic estrogen.

A new product, Duavee, may be the best bet for the woman with a uterus. Duavee is an oral estrogen pill that is combined with a unique SERM, bazedoxefene, which blocks estrogen pathways in the uterine lining. As a bonus, it also builds bone! Women who choose Duavee get the benefit of estrogen without the risk of taking a progestin.

Is a Progestin Needed with Local Vaginal Estrogens?
Since only systemic estrogens increase the risk of uterine cancer, there is no need to take a progestin if the only estrogen you are using is a vaginal product. Not one study shows the same risk with a local estrogen, which is why the North American Menopause Society made the position statement in 2007 that a progestogen is not necessary, in spite of the FDA warning label that says otherwise.

Why Take Estrogen?
To Put Out the Fire

The number-one reason most women start systemic estrogen is to treat hot flashes once they realize that taking yoga, carrying a portable fan, and dressing in layers are not real solutions. Toughing it out works for some women (like the ones who live in Alaska), but others who have severe hot flashes throughout the day and night are totally blindsided by just how debilitating hot flashes can be. While hot flashes last for two to four years in most women, some will experience them for up to 10 years. In ten percent of women they *never* go away.

Every once in a while, someone will say, "My grandmother didn't take anything for hot flashes, why should I?" Well, Grandma was more likely to be home baking cookies than doing a job that required a good night's sleep and the ability to think clearly. Grandma may have been having occasional sex with Grandpa (there's a visual I didn't need to give you!) but was unlikely to be starting a second marriage or a new relationship in her fifties. And Grandma probably did not live nearly as long as you will.

Hot flashes occur in 75 percent of menopausal women and typically begin as a sudden sensation of heat on the face and upper chest that becomes generalized. A severe flash can be pretty intense (I call it "the furnace inside you"), lasting between two and four minutes with profuse sweating, followed by chills and shivering.

Physiologically, a hot flash happens for the same reason you sweat in a sauna: the body is trying to cool down. The difference is that you don't really need to cool down, but your menopausal brain thinks you do. Let me explain.

The human body is meant to be roughly 98.6 degrees. If you go outside in the winter without your coat, you're going to shiver to generate heat. You sweat when you exercise to cool the body down. The part of the brain that keeps your body at the right temperature is known as the thermoregulatory zone. During menopause the thermoregulatory zone gets too sensitive, resulting in a hot flash even when the body doesn't really need to cool down.

For some women, hot flashes are extremely debilitating. For others, less so. Women who get warm a few times a day don't understand why some women need help to get through menopause. The woman who flashes twenty to thirty times a day can't sleep, can't get through a business meeting fully clothed, and probably coined the bumper-sticker-worthy phrase, "I'm out of estrogen and I've got a gun." Estrogen, even in very small doses, is the most effective treatment of hot flashes and sweats. Period. Estrogen not only works for hot flashes, it works fast. Women who start oral or transdermal systemic estrogen replacement generally experience relief within the first few weeks of treatment.

I am well aware that in spite of the reassurances of menopause experts like me, many women choose not to take estrogen or have been advised by their doctors to steer clear. In fact, *only 7 percent of women with hot flashes ultimately accept a prescription for estrogen*. For women who prefer not to take estrogen or have been told they should not, there is an FDA-approved alternative.

Brisdelle, the first and only FDA-approved *nonhormonal* option for hot flash relief, is a low dose (7.5 milligrams) of paroxetine, one of the SSRI antidepressants that years ago was serendipitously found to significantly reduce hot flashes in menopausal women. In the past, like many physicians, I prescribed paroxetine off-label. There are two reasons why I am glad I can now prescribe a low-dose, FDA-approved version as opposed to generic paroxetine.

Paroxetine at higher doses is intended for, studied for, and FDA-approved *only* for the treatment of depression, not hot flashes. Many of my patients have received a prescription and then also had the experience of their insurance company giving them a diagnosis of depression even though they are not depressed. Just hot. One patient for whom I prescribed Paxil for hot flash relief (as clearly documented on her electronic medical record) was contacted by her insurance company to see if her "depression" was improving and to offer psychotherapy!

Brisdelle is FDA-approved *only* for the treatment of moderate to severe hot flashes as a result of menopause. It cannot, and should not, be prescribed for the treatment of depression and therefore is not interpreted as a treatment for depression on your medical record.

The doses of generic paroxetine available for the treatment of depression are higher than needed to relieve hot flashes. With higher dosage comes a greater risk of side effects. For example, Paxil and other SSRIs are associated with an increase in sexual problems and an increase in pounds. The last thing a menopausal woman needs is a drug that might sabotage her diet or an already waning sex drive. In clinical trials, Brisdelle, with only 7.5 milligrams of paroxetine, did not demonstrate a decrease in libido or an increase in weight.

If nothing else is working to eliminate your flashes, you may want to check out a new procedure that appears to reduce hot flashes by at least 50 percent called the stellate ganglian block. The stellate ganglion is a bundle of nerves in the cervical spinal column. It appears that if a long-acting local anesthetic is injected into this ganglion, hot flashes are reduced for months. Something about getting a shot in the neck, however, makes all but the truly desperate a little leery.

To Alleviate Vaginal Dryness

Yes, local vaginal estrogens treat vaginal atrophy, but systemic estrogens can often alleviate vaginal dryness too. However, up to 25 percent of women taking systemic hormone therapy still have atrophy and still have problems with dryness and painful intercourse. The reason is simple. Estrogen therapy is not intended to give you the same kinds of estrogen levels you had when you were 20; it is only intended to alleviate symptoms such as hot flashes, and the amount of estrogen that alleviates hot flashes is sometimes not enough to alleviate vaginal atrophy. That's why it is called estrogen *therapy* instead of estrogen replacement.

The truth is that many women who use either systemic or local vaginal estrogen assume that they will no longer need a lubricant. That is not the case. Systemic and local estrogens are now so low-dose that their use is not always going to resolve significant vaginal atrophy. And let's face it—sometimes sex is more exciting or more stimulating than at other times, and you may need a little help to get things going. So, even if you are taking a systemic estrogen or using a local vaginal estrogen product, don't toss your bottle of lube.

To Get Some Sleep

Menopausal women generally have very little trouble falling asleep. It's the staying asleep that's the problem, which is why, when you send an email to 15 menopausal friends at 3:00 AM, you immediately get at least 12 replies. Nighttime awakening happens not only because of hot flashes. Even in the absence of hot flashes, menopausal women are plagued by insomnia because estrogen and progesterone influence multiple factors that control sleep. Hormone therapy is known to improve rapid-eye movement (REM) sleep and sleep quality, even in women who have no problem with flashes. As discussed in chapter 10, a decent night's sleep is essential not only to avoid getting fired from your job but also to have a decent libido.

To Protect the Heart?

Heart disease is the number-one killer of women. While most women perceive breast cancer as their greatest health threat, an American woman is ten times more likely to die from heart disease than from breast cancer. In addition, women who are overweight, smoke, and don't exercise or eat right are increasing their risk of heart disease far more than they would by taking estrogen. The WHI was quite clear that women between ages 50 and 60 who take estrogen do not increase their risk of cardiovascular disease and that, in the case of transdermal estrogen, may in fact decrease it.

To Reduce Brain Fog

This is another area that is still controversial. Many studies show an improvement in memory and cognitive function in women who start estrogen during that 5–10-year critical window at the onset of menopause. Estrogen receptors involved in cognition have been identified in many areas of the brain, and increased blood flow to the brain is known to occur in women on estrogen. In addition, sleep disturbances caused by lack of estrogen significantly contribute to an inability to think clearly. What is clear is that if estrogen is going to help cognitive function or decrease the risk of Alzheimer's, it needs to be started early. Studies consistently show that estrogen initiated more than 10 years after menopause not only doesn't help but also may actually make cognitive function worse.

To Protect the Bones

Every year 1.3 million women suffer from fractures as a result of osteoporosis, the bone loss that is usually a "silent" disease. There are no symptoms unless you break a bone, which is why bone density screening (a specialized X-ray) is recommended to find out if you are at risk. Any women can have bone loss leading to osteoporosis, but women at particular risk are women who are thin, smoke, take steroids, or have a genetic predisposition. By age 80, 50 percent of women have osteoporosis and are at significant risk of fracture if they fall. Thirty percent of women hospitalized for treatment of a hip fracture die. Osteoporosis is a life-threatening disease with consequences well beyond losing height or suffering the inconvenience of a fracture.

Low-dose systemic estrogen therapy reduces the risk of postmenopausal fractures, including hip, spine, and all nonspine fractures, *even in women without osteoporosis!* This protection only lasts while you are taking estrogen. Within a few years of discontinuation, the risk of hip fracture is the same as it would be if you had not taken estrogen.

To Decrease Wrinkles?

Women on estrogen have better skin. It's not your imagination that women on estrogen have fewer, shallower wrinkles. Just as estrogen increases collagen in your vulva, it also increases collagen in your face. Certainly other factors contribute to the skin changes associated with aging, such as sun, smoking, and genetics, but estrogen plays a part as well. This is not to suggest that vanity is a valid reason to take estrogen—it's just a fact! And one that explains why many women in the 1950s used estrogen-based face cream.

To Alleviate Nasty Mood Swings

Depression is one of the more complicated symptoms of menopause. Are you depressed because low estrogen has changed your chemical balance in such a way that you experience a chemical depression? Or are you depressed when you go through menopause because of sleep deprivation and the sudden lack of libido that has destroyed a formerly terrific sex life? There is also the issue of the extra pounds that have magically appeared on your belly and thighs, despite the fact that your eating and exercise routine is exactly the same as it was ten years ago. Remember too that your last child is probably about to leave for college, you may have been passed over for the promotion, and your husband is going through his own midlife crisis. Good times, right? No wonder you're depressed.

It's really not fair that a major hormonal plunge occurs at the same time as a lot of less-than-pleasant life changes. It's hard to know how much depression is a direct result of estrogen deprivation as opposed to external factors. The change in hormones is certainly a contributing factor, and many women find that estrogen replacement helps. Evidence is mixed about the effect of estrogen on mood. Getting rid of hot flashes and getting a full night's sleep are definitely going to cheer you up. The question is, if your only symptom is moodiness, will estrogen help? Probably not. It has also not been shown to be useful for the treatment of depression. Go see a therapist or your primary care physician in addition to your gynecologist if depression creeps in with menopause.

To Improve Your SexAbility!

Although many patients tell me otherwise, estrogen therapy has not been proven in scientific studies to improve libido or orgasms. However, for women who have vaginal dryness and painful sex and are exhausted from sleep disturbance and hot flashes, relief of those symptoms has been proven to improve desire, arousal, and orgasms.

part five

YOU'RE SPECIAL

MEDICAL CONDITIONS

Add low SexAbility to your list of symptoms

Up until now you may have been thinking, yes, these solutions may be the answer for other women, but I have a different problem. Perhaps you have problems from surgery . . . or heart disease . . . or diabetes . . . or multiple sclerosis . . . or any one of a number of medical conditions that might be affecting your sexual health and sexual experience. Virtually every acute or chronic disease can be accompanied by fatigue, anxiety, pain, or insomnia—all of which are culprits that can easily destroy a healthy sex life.

Anything that alters hormones, such as hypothyroidism, adrenal dysfunction, diabetes, and of course menopause, can be problematic. Hormones and neurotransmitters need to get to the right place, which is why any medical problem that compromises blood flow can have an impact on vaginal health, arousal, and orgasm. In addition, your nerves need to fire and your muscles need to contract (and relax!), which is why neurologic problems such as spinal cord injury, herniated discs, and multiple sclerosis have an impact.

To make matters even more complicated, many women have not one but two or more medical problems at the same time. Many women with heart disease also have diabetes or hypertension and are smokers. In addition, since most of these conditions are more common as women age, the majority of women are also dealing with postmenopausal hormonal changes. The drugs used to treat many disorders often create bigger problems than the illness itself.

There are over 50 medical conditions and classifications of medications that have been identified as having an impact specifically on the ability to have a normal sexual response and/or the ability to have intercourse. And over 50 percent of midlife women are coping with at least one of those issues.

Conditions and Medications That Have an Impact on Sexual Health

Medical Conditions

Hypothyroidism
Graves' disease
Adrenal dysfunction
Diabetes
Menopause
Spinal cord injury
Neuropathy
Herniated discs
Multiple sclerosis
Cardiovascular disease
Incontinence
Epilepsy
Hypertension
Atherosclerosis
Sickle cell disorder
Cancer
Pulmonary disease
Depression
Anxiety

Post-traumatic stress disorder
 (PSTD)
Eating disorders
Parkinson's disease
Stroke
Chronic pain
Kidney failure/dialysis
Psoriasis
Arthritis
Vascular disease
Heart failure
Pituitary tumors
Ulcerative colitis
Crohn's disease
Anemia
Endometriosis
Adenomyosis
Pelvic organ prolapse
Interstitial cystitis

Fibroids

Metabolic syndrome

Insomnia

Movement disorders

Sleep apnea

Hearing impairment

Physical disability

Surgery

Medications

Antidepressants

Anti-anxiety drugs

Antihypertensives

Antipsychotics

Hormonal contraception

Beta blockers

Lipid-lowering drugs

Histamine blockers

Narcotics

Anti-epileptic drugs

Anticholinergics

Antihistamines

Barbiturates

Comprehensive information on the impact on sexuality of each of the illnesses listed here would take up not a chapter but an encyclopedia. I discuss some of these conditions, such as endometriosis, in other chapters. I focus on the medical issues discussed in this chapter not because they are the most important, but because they are the most *common* conditions that have an impact on sexual health. (Cancer has its own set of issues and is covered in the next chapter.) Don't worry if your medical issue is something other than what is discussed here—the concerns are often the same.

While every medical situation is unique, the one consistent feature is that no matter which condition you have, chances are that your doctor has not adequately addressed, or even mentioned, its impact on your sex life. For example, according to a 2013 University of Chicago study, only 35 percent of women who had a myocardial infarction (commonly called a heart attack) received information about resuming sexual activity after treatment—and then only if the patient initiated the discussion.

Heart Disease

Heart disease is the number-one killer of women in this country. It is also one of the top killers of sexual health. There are really three basic questions for women with heart disease when it comes to sex:

> **Issue 1:** Do you have the physical strength and respiratory capacity to engage in a sexual workout?
>
> **Issue 2:** Will your body have a normal sexual response such that you are able to become aroused and have a pleasurable sexual experience?
>
> **Issue 3:** If you have fabulous sex and an explosive orgasm, is your heart going to be able to take it? What is the risk that if you "come," you might "go"?

Issue 1: Do You Have the Physical Strength and Respiratory Capacity to Engage in a Sexual Workout?

Women who have a damaged or compromised heart often experience fatigue, weakness, or shortness of breath at the slightest physical activity. They may indeed have reduced capacity for some sexual activities, which is why every woman who has a condition such as congenital heart problems, severe coronary artery disease, unstable angina, vascular disease, arrhythmia, or pericarditis, or who has had heart surgery or a myocardial infarction, must be evaluated and advised individually. Keep in mind that there is a difference between what is *safe* to do and what you are *able* to do. The safety of having sex depends on the specifics of your cardiac capabilities, and while the guidelines given here are useful, you still need to check with your cardiologist. Don't be afraid to be specific.

If your cardiologist has given you the green light but you simply feel like you don't have the physical strength to engage in sexual activity, you may need to adjust your expectations given the reality of your limitations. You can have sex more comfortably, for instance, by using pillows and props (as addressed in chapter 6). In other words, if you don't have the strength to prop yourself up and give oral sex for ten minutes, adapt your surroundings so that you can try, or enjoy other avenues for mutual pleasure.

Issue 2: Is Your Body Able to Have a Normal Sexual Response? Can You Become Aroused and Have a Pleasurable Sexual Experience?

Whether or not your body is capable of normal sexual response, to me, is the crux of this issue. With heart disease, it all comes down to blood flow—or more accurately, lack of blood flow. Women with coronary artery disease have plaque that builds up in blood vessels, reducing the amount of blood that is delivered to the heart. This condition is known as atherosclerosis. If there are changes in the blood vessels that supply the heart, there are also likely to be changes in the blood vessels that supply the genitals.

Reduced blood flow to the genitals may compromise genital engorgement. It's not just about the clitoris and labia—the blood supply to the vaginal walls must also be intact if lubrication and smooth muscle relaxation are to occur. If the muscles don't relax properly, the vagina's ability to lengthen and dilate will be impaired.

And then there is the orgasm issue. While it's fairly well known that men with cardiac disease often have erectile dysfunction, it's less well appreciated that up to 50 percent of women with significant coronary artery disease have a reduced ability to reach orgasm. Of course, it makes sense that if there is limited blood flow to the clitoris, not much is going to happen. This reduction in blood flow will not only impair engorgement and keep erectile tissue from responding but also inhibit the proper flow of blood needed to ensure that nerve endings are healthy and responsive. Indeed, the impairment of clitoral blood flow in women with vascular disease has been demonstrated not only by blood flow studies but also by microscopically looking at the clitoris at the time of autopsy in women who die from heart disease. Not surprisingly, by far the worst impairment in clitoral blood flow is in women with heart disease who are also heavy smokers.

Issue 3: Is Your Heart Going to Be Able to Take Fabulous Sex and Explosive Orgasms?

Nelson Rockefeller died while having sex with his mistress. Even the mighty Attila the Hun fell victim to a heart attack that caused his early demise—on his wedding night no less. And while people might kid about a heart attack during sex being a great way to go, fear of this happening significantly reduces the amount of sexual activity of patients with known heart problems. In one study, 71 percent of women avoided sexual activity after a heart attack specifically because of their own fear or the fear of their spouse. Fear is not exactly an aphrodisiac, and it's hard to relax or lubricate during sex if you don't know if you are going to come . . . or go.

Other than making your heart go "pitter-patter," what are the cardiac effects of sexual activity? Volunteers having sex in a laboratory setting (that must have been interesting!) have a significant increase in pulse, blood pressure, and respiratory rates. In other words, the heart works harder during sex, pretty much at the same level as a moderate workout.

What's really interesting is when similar studies are conducted among married couples in their own bedrooms—heart rates *don't* increase during sex! In fact, on average, married couples have heart rates that are *lower* during sex than the rates recorded during their normal daily activities. It's actually somewhat depressing (and re-assuring at the same time) that having sex with your spouse in your own bedroom requires only the same amount of exertion as a two- to four-mile-per-hour stroll on a level surface for a few minutes. This is probably why studies show that sexual activity is rarely responsible for a myocardial infarction. Risks are even smaller in men and women who are routinely sexually active and have regularly participated in a post-heart-attack exercise program.

An article published in the *Journal of the American Medical Association* in 2011 confirmed this. Researchers looked at 14 studies regarding risk of cardiac death during sex. They found that death was 2.7 times more likely to occur, but *only* for someone who rarely had intercourse or exercised. In fact, engaging in some form of exercise once a week decreased the risk of cardiac death during sex by 45 percent. The authors concluded that the risk of death during sex with your spouse is small, especially if you exercise and/or have sex regularly.

If you continue to avoid intimacy from a fear of dying or having another heart attack, it may help to have an exercise stress test to assure you that your heart can take it. In general, most cardiologists say that you are safe to have sex with your regular partner if you can climb up two flights of stairs without having chest pain or becoming out of breath. Obviously, it's important to check with your own doctor before initiating exercise or sex after a heart attack, but in general, patients who have no symptoms, have mild, stable angina, have controlled hypertension, and do not have exercise-induced reduced blood flow or chest pain should feel free to have sex with a partner six to eight weeks after a heart attack.

Do, however, keep this caution in mind: immediately after a heart attack is not the time to have an affair or join the mile-high club unless you are willing to suffer the fate of Nelson Rockefeller.

The Fixes
Once you are good to go and convinced that you are not going to die in the sack, it's really disheartening if you find that things are dry and nonresponsive. Here's what will help:

Enhance Vaginal Wall Lubrication
If your vagina isn't responding, remember, it's not that you are not emotionally aroused or feeling in the moment. No matter how turned on you may be, your genital blood supply may be inadequate to produce moisture right now. You need not only a good lubricant but a local vaginal estrogen as well, especially if you are peri- or postmenopausal. All of the options offered in chapter 13 are safe and appropriate if you have heart disease.

Try an Orgasm Booster

If there is nerve damage, it may take more clitoral stimulation than required in the past to achieve an orgasm. This is the time to revisit chapter 10. The fixes offered there also apply in this case. That being said, PDE5 inhibitors have been only minimally studied in women with heart disease, with mixed results, so until there is more information, it's best to steer clear.

If you have a pacemaker, there is no reason to believe that using a vibrator will cause it to malfunction. It's probably best, however, not to put your vibrator directly on your pacemaker.

Evaluate Your Medications

Medicines commonly prescribed to treat cardiovascular problems, such as thiazide diuretics, beta blockers, and lipid-lowering drugs (not to mention antidepressants), have generally been associated with sexual problems. However, according to a study published in the *Journal of Hypertension* in 2013, there are no significant associations between most antihypertensive medications and sexual dysfunction. If the sexual issues appeared at the same time you started taking a new drug, the drug might be the problem. Let your doctor know what's happening, so you can see if there is an alternative medication.

Face the Fear Factor

Make an appointment to talk specifically to your doctor about the appropriate level of sexual activity for you. Often women will ask these questions as the doctor is headed out the door and get only a cursory answer. By letting your doctor know that this is an important issue, not just something you're throwing out there at the end of your post-heart-attack checkup, you will get more information. Exercise regularly, take off any excess weight, stop smoking if you do, and do everything else your doctor has been encouraging you to do, since not only will it save your life, it will save your sex life.

If your doctor doesn't suggest a stress test, you might request one in order to prove to yourself that you are not going to die during sex. Bring your spouse or partner along to your appointment so that he can be reassured that you are not going to drop dead if you have a decent orgasm. Many cardiac rehab programs also have psychologists specifically trained to help you address anxiety about resuming your sex life.

Diabetes

Every diabetic woman is at risk for damage to her circulatory and nervous systems, which in turn makes every diabetic woman at risk for low libido, diminished arousal, sexual pain, and the inability to have an orgasm. While it is recognized that any woman with diabetes is likely to have some sexual issues, it's hard to group all women with diabetes under the same umbrella. There is an enormous difference between the overweight woman who was diagnosed with type 2 diabetes at age 60 and manages her condition with oral medication and diet, on the one hand, and a type 1 diabetic who has taken insulin her entire life, on the other.

While up to 75 percent of women with type 1 diabetes report at least one sexual problem, by far the most common issue they cite is decreased vaginal lubrication. Diabetics, even if they don't have atherosclerosis (and they often do), frequently have capillary damage. Capillaries, the smallest blood vessels, are the blood source in the vaginal wall and are therefore required to produce lubrication. This is not an estrogen issue, so even a young diabetic woman with more than adequate estrogen levels can have severe vaginal dryness. Dyspareunia becomes the norm, and decreased libido follows.

In the case of type 2 diabetes, all of these conditions apply, and more often than not other medical issues present that can affect sexuality, such as obesity and heart disease.

Vaginal Health Is a Challenge

Diabetics often have painful sex because of increased rates of vulvo-vaginal infection and inflammation. *Candida albicans* (yeast) colonize the vaginal walls of diabetics and multiply like crazy if they are surrounded by sugar, so even glucose levels that are only slightly out of balance can lead to chronic vaginal yeast infections for diabetics. In addition, decreased blood supply in the vaginal walls compromises the ability to fight off infection. And we're not even talking about what happens once menopause hits.

Neuropathy Doesn't Just Affect Feet

Both type 1 and type 2 diabetics, and even prediabetics, can suffer from neuropathy—nerve damage that causes pain, burning, numbness, and tingling, particularly in the feet and calves. But it's not just the nerves in the lower extremities that are damaged; the genital nerves may be vulnerable as well.

Many diabetics have decreased genital and clitoral sensation and in some cases an inability to have an orgasm. Clitoral biopsies from diabetic women (yes, done under anesthesia) have shown abnormalities of smooth muscle cells, increased glycogen deposits, and vascular abnormalities. In other words, there is damage to not only the nerves but the blood vessels and tissue.

The Fixes

Not surprisingly, the rates of low desire in the diabetic population are sky-high. A high proportion of women with diabetes simply give up. But keep reading! If you're diabetic, there *are* things you can do to keep your sexual health intact.

Control Your Blood Sugar

Add vaginal health to your already long list of reasons why tight control of glucose is critical—not only because elevated blood sugar levels increase the risk of vaginal infection, but also because out-of-control glucose increases the likelihood of damage to genital blood vessels and nerves.

Balance Your pH

An over-the-counter *vaginal* (not gastrointestinal) probiotic such as Pro B helps populate the vagina with healthy lactobacilli and keep things in balance. Just to be clear, a vaginal probiotic goes in your mouth, not in your vagina.

While diabetics are at increased risk for yeast infections, do not assume that every discharge is yeast. If there is a persistent odor or discharge despite treatment with an over-the-counter antifungal, see your doctor.

Use a Lubricant

Any lubricant used during intercourse, whether silicone- or water-based, should be glucose/glycogen-free. (See chapter 5 to refresh your memory.) In addition to using a lubricant to reduce friction, restoring vaginal moisture with either a long-acting moisturizer or a local vaginal estrogen is essential to reduce infection for diabetic women.

Try Vaginal Estrogen

Many diabetics are told that they can't use estrogen because it will make their diabetes worse. It is true that oral systemic estrogens increase insulin resistance. Transdermal systemic estrogens, however, do not increase insulin resistance, nor do vaginal estrogens affect blood glucose levels. Even diabetic women who are not postmenopausal may benefit from using a local vaginal estrogen or any of the other products discussed in chapter 13.

Investigate a Device

The EROS Clitoral Therapy Device, discussed in chapter 11, has specifically been tested in diabetics, and though some data suggests that it helps increase the possibility of having orgasms, the numbers were too small to make a definitive conclusion. In any case, no negative issues have been noted. So why not give it a try?

Essentially all of the solutions discussed in chapters 5, 9, 10, and 11 are not only appropriate for diabetics but pretty much mandatory.

Metabolic Syndrome

Metabolic syndrome refers to a constellation of symptoms that indicate a predisposition for heart disease and diabetes. To be identified as having metabolic syndrome, you must have central (abdominal) obesity and at least two of the following: hypertension, elevated fasting blood sugar (but not diabetes, also known as glucose intolerance), high triglycerides, and low HDL cholesterol (the good cholesterol). While women with metabolic syndrome may not have actual heart disease, diabetes, or coronary artery disease, they are predisposed to develop those conditions. And yes, since high blood pressure, a bad lipid profile, and glucose intolerance can all damage blood vessels and impair blood flow, the impact on sexual function can be the same as in women with fully diagnosed coronary artery disease or diabetes. Many women with metabolic syndrome are also menopausal, but studies indicate that metabolic syndrome is an independent risk factor for sexual dysfunction, independent of estrogen levels.

Obese but Otherwise Healthy

Obesity is generally associated with sexual problems because it is common for obese women to have at least one medical condition that has a negative impact on their sexual health. But not every woman with a BMI over 30 (the marker for the obese range) has medical issues. It is entirely possible to be significantly overweight and have normal cardiac function, normal cholesterol, and no diabetes. In the absence of medical problems, studies are inconclusive as to the impact of obesity alone on sexuality. What is probable, however, is that obesity in some women has a direct impact on poor body image and depression, which lead in turn to impaired libido and arousal.

Incontinence

The 30 percent of adult women who suffer from some sort of incontinence, or involuntary loss of urine, are not just afraid to laugh, sneeze, cough, or run without wearing a diaper or a pad—they are also afraid to have sex. Sexual dysfunction is reported by 26 to 47 percent of women with urinary incontinence. It's the combination of an awareness of constant odor and the fear of losing urine during intercourse that makes most women with incontinence go into avoidance mode. Eleven to 45 percent of women with incontinence lose urine during sexual intercourse, typically during penetration or orgasm—a disincentive and libido killer if there ever was one.

Stress incontinence is the loss of urine with coughing, sneezing, laughing, or anything that increases abdominal pressure. This is the incontinence that makes you grab your crotch when you cough. This is the incontinence that prevents you from playing tennis without at least considering wearing Depends. The problem with stress incontinence is that the bladder sphincter doesn't stay closed enough to prevent urine from exiting the bladder. This is caused by weakness of the pelvic floor tissue that supports the lowest portion of the bladder where it connects to the urethra and is often brought on (though not always) by childbirth. Any increase in abdominal pressure causes the bladder neck to funnel, the urethra to droop down, and urine to escape. Pressure against the bladder and bladder neck during intercourse can also trigger urine loss.

Urge incontinence, or overactive bladder, is a sudden, irresistible urge to pee. In urge incontinence, the bladder muscles contract when they should not. The woman with urge incontinence is fine until she puts her key in the door. If she is lucky, the door will open, she won't drop her packages, and she will make it to the toilet and get her pants down within the next four seconds. The cause of urge incontinence is not usually known, but it's attributed most commonly to age-related changes in the urinary tract. It is also caused by bladder irritation from infection, cancer, or inflammation. Urge incontinence can also be caused by neurologic problems, such as stroke or multiple sclerosis.

It is not unusual to have elements of both stress incontinence and urge incontinence, otherwise known as mixed incontinence. (Sounds fun, right? Not!) Successful treatment of mixed incontinence depends on treating the major issue and, in some cases, both components.

Keep in mind that the same pelvic floor weakness that is responsible for urine loss may also be responsible for many of the pelvic pain syndromes discussed in chapters 8 and 9. There is a very high association between urinary issues and deep dyspareunia. So, incontinent women avoid sex not only because they might pee on their partner, but also because it hurts.

The Fixes for Stress Incontinence

Approximately 80 percent of the estimated 15 million women who suffer from stress incontinence do nothing about it because they assume that it is a normal part of aging. They often also assume that their only option is to have a surgical procedure, which inherently involves potential complications and recovery time. But common is not the same as normal, and just because something is common does not mean you have to live with it.

Once your type of incontinence has been established, treatment options can be explored. A number of nonsurgical options are available to treat women who don't want surgery but would like to eliminate diapers, pads, and thick dark clothes as key wardrobe accessories.

Strengthen Those Muscles

The first step in the treatment of stress incontinence is to train the muscles that support the urethra and bladder. Kegel exercises have traditionally been recommended to strengthen muscles and improve the ability to hold urine. They rarely work in the woman with severe incontinence, but there can be some improvement in highly motivated women who do the exercises properly and consistently. (See chapter 6 for more information.)

Pelvic Floor Training

Total Control Programs are actually body fitness and lifestyle classes designed to strengthen the pelvic floor and abdominal wall muscles that are necessary for bladder control. Behavior modification is a key component of this comprehensive program that goes way beyond Kegels. Up to 20 percent of women who participate report that their stress incontinence symptoms are eliminated at the end of the seven-week program. For more information, go to www.totalcontrolprogram.com.

Pelvic floor muscle training with an experienced pelvic physical therapist can be highly effective. Some physical therapists also utilize electrical stimulation, with cure rates of 70 percent or more. (Go back to chapter 6 for more information on this.) Most women, however, do not have access to a pelvic physical therapist, which is why a new home device, InTone, is a welcome option. InTone is a silicone vaginal device that you get from your doctor and use at home to strengthen your pelvic floor and eliminate or greatly reduce incontinence. Once placed in the vagina, InTone is inflated to ensure comfortable but close contact with the vaginal walls. Two electrode contacts are designed to rest against pelvic muscles.

During 12-minute daily therapy sessions, a gentle electrical stimulation (the appropriate level is determined in the doctor's office) enables you to learn to contract and relax your pelvic floor muscles. A hand-held control unit provides voice coaching and visual biofeedback. Over two to four months, as the pelvic floor muscles gain strength, the electrical stimulation is gradually increased. The electrical stimulation also trains the muscles in the wall of the bladder (known as the detrusor muscles) to relax in order to alleviate urge incontinence. Once the incontinence is eliminated, a maintenance program of one session a week keeps the muscles toned. The bonus to eliminating incontinence, of course, is possibly alleviating dyspareunia as well.

If you fail to respond to pelvic floor strengthening techniques or would simply prefer a "quick fix," surgery will almost always correct stress incontinence. While there are many procedures, all incontinence surgeries have the common goal of correcting inadequate urethral support and restoring the urethra to its proper position. One of the most commonly done procedures is known as a TVT (tension-free vaginal tape), a urethral sling procedure that is performed on an outpatient basis. Essentially, a small piece of mesh tape that will sit underneath the urethra is inserted through a tiny vaginal incision. Over time, scar tissue forms around the tape, which "firms up" the tissue that supports the urethra. The cure rate is over 90 percent, complications such as bleeding or infection are rare, and the recovery is short. Women who have this procedure are thrilled that they no longer need to laugh with their legs crossed or worry about peeing on their partner.

The Fixes for Urge Incontinence

In contrast, the treatment of urge incontinence is never surgical, unless there is also a component of stress incontinence. While a wide range of commonly prescribed drugs are beneficial, most women are reluctant to take a medication that has side effects and is intended to be for lifelong use. Biofeedback, pelvic physical therapy, and InTone have been used very successfully for the treatment of urge incontinence and as far as I'm concerned should be the first line of treatment. Behavior modification, such as avoiding bladder irritants and urinating frequently, are commonly suggested. There are even apps for your phone that will identify not only the closest public bathroom but the cleanest!

In the meantime, empty your bladder prior to sex and, to be on the safe side, throw down a waterproof throw blanket to protect against accidents. Trust me, he won't mind.

Fecal Incontinence

Urine is not the only thing that can leak without warning. Nothing puts a black cloud over romance like underwear with poop on it or feces on the bed. Most women have at least heard of urinary incontinence, but fecal incontinence, a reality for at least 18 million Americans, is not exactly a topic that comes up at cocktail parties. People who suffer from fecal incontinence not only don't discuss it with family or friends but don't even bring it up to their doctors. With no apology to the $500 million a year adult diaper industry, I happen to believe that unless there is no other solution, the only diapers adults should be buying are those for their children or grandchildren.

Fecal incontinence pretty much heads the list of taboo topics, but until we get the conversation going, women who are secretly washing their soiled underwear have no way of knowing that there are a number of solutions beyond stocking up on diapers. Colon-rectal surgeons treat fecal incontinence, but surgery is not always needed or even the best option. Pelvic floor physical therapy and biofeedback are often successful. A cutting-edge treatment now available involves the surgical placement of a pacemaker-like device that decreases or eliminates the problem. Many women who use InTone to treat urinary incontinence find that it decreases fecal incontinence as well. While this is promising, clinical trials are pending.

Crohn's Disease and Ulcerative Colitis

Any type of inflammatory bowel disease can present challenges beyond the pain and fatigue that accompany every chronic medical problem. At the top of the list is deep pelvic pain from the same pelvic floor issues that accompany gynecologic conditions such as endometriosis. Everything in chapter 9 pertains to the woman with inflammatory bowel disease. In addition, women who have had extensive pelvic bowel surgeries can form adhesions or suffer with nerve damage, which has an impact on genital blood flow and sensation.

Sexuality and Stomas

Crohn's disease, ulcerative colitis, and gastrointestinal cancers are but a few of the reasons why some women end up with a temporary or permanent ileostomy or colostomy. A stoma is an artificial opening on the surface of the body for the purpose of eliminating waste when the normal route is no longer viable. A plastic pouch on the abdomen holds stool (and sometimes urine) and must be emptied throughout the day.

Every woman has concerns about looking attractive to her partner. Women with a stoma are especially apprehensive, particularly with a new partner, about revealing a bag with stool hanging off their body. Add to that the fear of odor or leakage or the pouch coming off during sex.

The Fixes

Most partners don't notice an ostomy bag any more than they notice other parts of your body. The typical sexual partner is far more interested in *you* than in a pouch that happens to be there. But if your bag is not an accessory you want to show off, hide it. Leave on a beautiful, long, sexy camisole or a short nightie after you slip your panties off. A tube top not only hides the pouch but also holds it in place. When you pull the tube top down just below your breasts, trust me, he won't be looking at your pouch. Use an opaque pouch or add a cover. You can also choose positions that are not directly face to face, such as spooning or rear entry. Turn down the lights and use plenty of candles.

The pouch is odor-proof, but if you are worried, there are pouch deodorizers. Devrom is an oral tablet that removes odor from stool. (This works for anyone who worries about odor from flatulence, not just women who have ostomies.) Of course, to minimize odor or leakage concerns, empty your pouch just prior to getting things going.

Stomas can make unexpected noise, but guess what? So can a functional anus. Farting happens during lovemaking for everyone. Everyone. If your stoma has a tendency to announce itself, avoid carbonated beverages, try a little Beano to decrease gas, and turn up the music.

Surgery

Any surgical procedure can cause fatigue and pain, which in most cases are temporary. Hysterectomy is the most common major surgical procedure that women undergo and is covered in chapter 9. Issues related to menopause as a consequence of ovary removal or changes in orgasms are discussed in chapters 11, 13, and 14.

It's not unusual for a physician to caution a patient about having sex after surgery for a particular period of time. The length of that period of time is not always based on anything scientific, nor is it always written in stone, so if you are feeling well and are interested in resuming your sex life before you have been given the official go-ahead, don't hesitate to ask. It is also important to be specific about what you can and can't do. Just because you are told you can't have intercourse doesn't mean you can't self-stimulate or receive oral sex. If in doubt, ask your doctor. In the case of abdominal surgery, a pillow clamped on the belly is a great way to protect an incision that's still sore.

Sometimes, particularly after orthopedic surgery, the primary issue is finding a comfortable position and protecting your new knee, hip, or shoulder. Talk about an opportunity to try new positions! If you are generally on top, trade places. Cushion your knee/hip/shoulder with a few strategically placed pillows and go for it.

You may find that even after your joint or broken bone heals, the new perspective is the preferred perspective!

Sexual Dysfunction and Psychiatric Disease

Throughout this book, I have discussed the impact of depression and antidepressants on libido and arousal. It's also important to note that a loss of libido can be the first sign of depression.

Depression is not the only psychiatric illness; women with bipolar disorders, schizophrenia or psychosis often have issues, usually directly related to medication. Many drugs that are used for treatment increase prolactin levels, a known libido-squelching hormone. Interestingly, prolactin levels do not necessarily correlate with the level of sexual dysfunction. Substitution of drugs or a PDE inhibitor may be an option, but you need to talk to your doctor on this one.

Multiple Sclerosis and Other Neuromuscular Conditions

Multiple sclerosis (MS) is a chronic disease that strikes young adults, with a predilection for women over men. This inflammatory process damages the protective coating (myelin) around nerves, causing impairment to nerve cells in the brain and spinal cord. A variety of symptoms, depending on the severity and progression of the illness, range from tremors, visual problems, fatigue, cognitive difficulties, numbness, tingling, and muscle spasticity to an inability to walk. Urinary incontinence and chronic constipation are common. So is depression.

Fortunately, most cases of MS progress very slowly, and there has been a great deal of progress in treatment, including medications to prevent attacks.

The sexual effects of MS and other neuromuscular conditions can be profound. Sensory and arousal issues are the result of neurologic damage, and there may be side effects from the medications.

In addition, many women with MS are also dealing with urinary incontinence.

As a result, among women with MS:

62 percent report loss of genital sensation
33 percent report loss of orgasm
36 percent report loss of vaginal lubrication
27 percent report loss of libido

Fifty percent of adults with MS are sexually inactive.

The Fixes

The savvy woman with MS learns to *plan* for intimacy. Timing is everything. For many women, morning is better than evening, not only because of general fatigue issues but also because spasticity intensifies as the day goes on.

Strategies like taking a warm bath to relax muscles to reduce spasticity, taking bladder control medications, and peeing just prior to sex will reduce the chance of incontinence. In addition to the incontinence solutions discussed earlier, a beautiful waterproof throw blanket will protect both the sheets and your pride.

Make sure the room temperature is not only comfortable but conducive to nakedness! Sensitivity and muscle spasms may be alleviated by cold packs applied to the genitals. A large bag of frozen peas is not only inexpensive (and available) but molds to a crotch perfectly. EROS or the other products discussed in chapter 10 should be explored to enhance clitoral sensitivity. As with diabetes, PDE5 inhibitors seem to be helpful in women with MS.

Hormones, including estrogen, progesterone, and testosterone, seem to be protective of nerves and promote myelin formation, which is one of the reasons why some researchers think that women with MS do better than men. In fact, pregnancy, with its sky-high estrogen levels, has a positive effect on women with MS.

Clinical trials are ongoing to see if estrogen, testosterone, or selective estrogen receptor modifiers are valid treatment options for MS. It stands to reason, however, that systemic hormone therapy in postmenopausal women might be beneficial. A transdermal preparation is preferable over an oral medication, not only because of its positive effects on libido but also because it reduces the blood clot risk (see chapter 14).

With or without systemic estrogen therapy, vaginal dryness caused by MS can be treated using a local vaginal estrogen or any of the other products discussed in the vaginal dryness section in chapter 13.

Arthritis

While many may not think of arthritis as an issue when it comes to sexuality, consider how difficult it is for someone with severe joint pain and limited mobility to accomplish simple day-to-day tasks such as opening jars, climbing stairs, or getting dressed. Then consider how difficult it would be for that person to get into and hold common sexual positions. Even separating their legs wide enough to have intercourse is an impossible feat for some women. Like many other medical conditions, however, arthritis is all about being creative, altering positions, and using pillows and other SexAbilitators to minimize pain or work around any mobility or strength impairments. And treat yourself to what I consider a brilliant invention: a neoprene glove that is specially designed to hold a vibrator. The glove allows a woman who cannot grasp anything to comfortably and easily self-stimulate. Genius!

Other Physical Disabilities

While true for any relationship, it is particularly important for the woman with disabilities to embrace the idea that sex is less about mechanics and more about psychological and emotional connections. Having said that, the mechanics of sexuality are a challenge for the 10 percent of the adult population with some sort of physical incapacity, whether it is severe arthritis, a spinal cord injury, missing limbs, blindness, deafness, or any other physical challenge. Sometimes, as in other gynecologic conditions, traditional intercourse is difficult or impossible and physical sexuality must be redefined in ways that are equally pleasurable. Mutual masturbation, creative masturbation, oral sex, and nongenital touching are only a few of the ways to have sexual pleasure.

In addition, planning for intimacy, as discussed before, is critical. Specific physical challenges call for disability-friendly accessories to facilitate the action. Sex doesn't always involve a bed. If you are more comfortable in a chair, have sex in a chair. Prefer the shower? That's what the hand-held nozzle is for. And if you want to splurge, forget the pillows and other supports and consider the Love Swing, which attaches to the ceiling and elevates you above the bed or ground. You don't have to do a thing. Let your partner do all the work while you are gloriously suspended!

The Fixes
Review the SexAbilitators section in chapter 6 and refer to the resources section for strategies and devices to facilitate sexuality no matter what your specific physical challenge is. Sometimes all it takes is the right pillow, the right device, and a little creativity to eliminate frustration.

Hire a Helping Hand
If you have a caretaker who helps you bathe, dress, or prepare meals, add "sexual health facilitator" to that person's job description. Expressing your need for sexual stimulation to your caregiver is not the same as expressing sexual desire *for* a caregiver. Be clear so your caretaker won't be uncomfortable.

The assistant need not stay in the room, but she can certainly attach the toy to your glove or arrange pillows. And whatever you do, don't forget to make sure the toy is charged or has fresh batteries before you send your assistant away! And, to make things even easier, invest in a vibrator with a remote control so your assistant need not even be in the same room to turn it off and on.

There is no way I can do justice to this topic in such minimal space, but fortunately a number of excellent resources are available with detailed information about enhancing sexuality in the face of physical challenges. At the top of the list is *The Ultimate Guide to Sex and Disability* by Miriam Kaufman, Corey Silverberg, and Fran Odette. This is a complete sex guide for people who live with disabilities, pain, illness, or chronic conditions. Whether it is chronic fatigue, back pain, spinal cord injury, hearing or visual impairment, multiple sclerosis, or pretty much any other physical issue, there is no end of websites with information and resources to help. Check out the resources section at the end of the book for a list of the many sites with inspiring ideas!

16

I'M GLAD TO BE ALIVE BUT . . .

The impact of cancer on SexAbility

For the woman who is newly contending with a diagnosis of cancer and facing the overwhelming stress of surgery, chemotherapy, and radiation, sex is usually the last thing on her mind. The emphasis is, and should be, on treating the cancer. But even after the cancer is gone, the physical scars have healed, and the hair has grown back, the consequences for a woman's sexuality are often minimized.

It's striking that every guy who gets diagnosed with prostate cancer is given detailed information about the potential post-treatment impact on sexual function. It is the rare oncologist who initiates a complete discussion about the possible sexual conse-quences of a woman's cancer treatment. From the time of diagnosis to the survivor stage, issues of sexuality and intimacy are rarely addressed, or at best they are underdiagnosed and undertreated. Up to 90 percent of cancer patients will experience sexual side effects, such as decreased libido, affected arousal, limited orgasmic abil-ity, and dyspareunia. Sadly, many cancer survivors feel reluctant to complain about something as "trivial" as the loss of their sex life. The woman who is brave enough to bring it up to her doctor typi-cally receives little advice beyond "buy a lubricant." With more and more women surviving cancer, this is a critical discussion to have. To be alive is great. To enjoy a good quality of life is even better.

There are currently approximately 13.7 million cancer survivors living in the United States. That number is likely to increase to 18 million by 2022.

Poor body image, fatigue, depression, and loss of independence are only some of the consequences of cancer treatment that can have an impact on sexuality. While many issues are directly related to the treatment, the psychological impact of a cancer diagnosis is also a huge factor. Many women benefit from antidepressants during this trying time, but as discussed, these drugs come with their own set of issues that can affect sexual health. One thing is consistent: good general health and an optimistic attitude translate into better sexual function after illness, regardless of the type of cancer and the type of therapy a patient receives. And if intercourse is off the table, never underestimate the power of genital touching, massage, kissing, and self-stimulation.

Treatment is dictated by the type of cancer and the stage and aggressiveness of the cancer. For example, some women with breast cancer require only a surgical removal of the cancerous tissue, others need a mastectomy, and still others undergo radiation and/or chemotherapy. Everyone's treatment, and response to treatment, is different. Breast and pelvic cancers present unique challenges and will be addressed later in this chapter. What follows are the general issues associated with chemotherapy, radiation, stem cell transplants, and cancer surgeries that all cancer patients must contend with, regardless of the type of cancer they have.

Chemotherapy

Losing her hair and her energy, not to mention the fear of losing her life, goes a long way toward pushing sex and intimacy to the bottom of a woman's list of priorities during chemotherapy. Add in nausea, diarrhea, weight fluctuations, and other side effects from chemo and it is hardly a surprise that it is the rare woman who has an interest in sex or feels like being sexually intimate. Having said that, if a cancer patient is feeling up to it, there is no reason to abstain from intercourse. Many women find that pleasurable physical sensations, intimacy, and the continuation of routine activities, including sex, "normalize" a very abnormal time. Those who do attempt intercourse, however, often are unaware that one of the possible side effects of chemotherapy is dyspareunia.

Here's why. The purpose of chemotherapy is to kill rapidly dividing cancer cells, but other cells in the body that rapidly divide can get caught in the cross fire. That's why the skin, hair, and nails often change during chemotherapy. The tissue that lines the mouth and gastrointestinal tract is also vulnerable. Sores in the mouth, pain, and inability to eat or drink, known as chemotherapy-induced oral mucositis, are really nasty side effects but usually not a total surprise, since most doctors mention them as a possibility. Those same doctors often forget to alert their patients, however, that similar changes can occur in the genital tract. It's a less than welcome surprise when sores, inflammation, dryness, and a really unpleasant burning sensation develop in the vagina. These changes are not limited to the vaginal walls but can occur on the vestibule and vulva as well. The medical term for this condition is vaginal mucosal erythrodysesthesia.

Chemotherapy can also reduce not only sensations in the hands and feet but pleasurable sensations in the genital and clitoral area as well. As if your vagina didn't have enough to worry about, a weakened immune system, which is unavoidable during chemo, increases the tendency to vaginal yeast infections and bacterial vaginosis and makes it more likely that dormant herpes or genital warts will become active.

But for many women, and particularly younger women, the big impact of chemotherapy comes not during treatment but after it's finished. Many chemotherapy protocols, particularly the ones used to treat Hodgkin's lymphoma and breast cancer, harm ovarian tissue and induce menopause.

The likelihood of permanent menopause depends not only on the type of chemotherapy but on the dose and age at time of treatment. Often, particularly in young women, the ovaries make a comeback and the plunge in estrogen is temporary. But ovarian function can be expected to return in only 10 percent of women over the age of 40 who become menopausal as a result of chemotherapy.

The Fix

Keep in mind that most of these effects are temporary and will resolve after chemo ends. If you have chemotherapy-induced vulvar erythrodysesthesia, you may benefit from compounded gabapentin cream (a prescription drug to desensitize nerves), lidocaine gel (to numb the burning sensation), and Neogyn vulvar soothing cream (see chapter 8). Keep your vaginal pH balanced with a probiotic and see your doctor if you have an abnormal discharge. Women with a history of genital herpes benefit from a daily dose of an antiviral drug, such as valcyclovir, to reduce the chance of an uncomfortable outbreak.

Dry vaginal tissues should be managed according to the recommendations in chapter 13, but it's particularly important that you choose your lubricant carefully. Silicone lubes are by far the most slippery. Pre-Seed (the lube recommended for couples trying to conceive) is not quite as slick but is the least irritating and often the best tolerated by cancer patients with inflamed tissue.

The suggestions in chapter 11 concerning orgasm are all relevant if decreased sensation is an issue.

Pelvic Radiation

Women with uterine, cervical, vulvar, rectal, or anal cancer often require radiation therapy to shrink the tumor before surgery or just after surgery to ensure that microscopic cancer cells are eliminated.

Pelvic radiation therapy does a wonderful job of eliminating cancer cells (a good thing), but unfortunately, it also sometimes destroys healthy cells in the neighborhood (a bad thing). As a result, a shrunken tumor is sometimes accompanied by a shrunken vagina. That's right—tissue damage from radiation can make the vagina shorter and smaller, decrease its sensation, diminish its elasticity, and render it unable to lubricate. In addition, some women have diminished estrogen levels as a result of the radiation treatment zapping their estrogen-producing ovarian tissue.

The combination of tissue changes from radiation and dryness from inadequate estrogen can make intercourse out of the question without some repair work.

Radiation can also result in skin changes and decreased sensation. But no, despite your partner's concerns, you are *not* radioactive.

The Fix

A program involving estrogen cream, lubricants, pelvic physical therapy, and vaginal dilators can treat the effects of radiation and make your vagina "good to go" again, but since the reversal of radiation changes can take months, patience is essential. Neogyn is particularly helpful for vulvar radiation effects. Some researchers have suggested that Viagra could be beneficial for cancer patients—not to increase blood flow but to facilitate response in the genital area post-radiation. However, no legitimate study has yet been conducted to examine this possibility.

Stem Cell Transplants

Fortunately, stem cell transplants have increased the survival rates for patients with leukemia, lymphomas, and other tumors, but sexual problems are common as a result of this lifesaving treatment. Fatigue, body changes (mainly from the use of steroids in treatment), and emotional issues can affect libido. Women who undergo a stem cell transplant are also at risk for chronic "graft-versus-host" disease, which can affect the vagina. In simple terms, in graft-versus-host disease the donor immune cells identify the cells of the body as foreign and attack them. The tissues involved might be the skin, liver, eyes, mouth sinus, intestines . . . and the vaginal mucosa. Symptoms such as pain, bleeding, irritation, and dryness are typical with this disease and can develop long after issues resolve in other organs.

The Fix
Local estrogen therapy and dilator therapy are appropriate and helpful for treating the effects of graft-versus-host disease, along with vulvar soothing cream. Cyclosporin is used to decrease the immune response to minimize the reaction.

Cancer Surgery
In general, no matter what body part is involved, cancer surgery in the best of circumstances has a profound impact on sexuality for all the obvious reasons: post-op pain, fatigue, and anemia from blood loss. Even after a full recovery from surgery, there can sometimes be long-term consequences from chronic pain or debilitation.

However, pelvic surgery for cancer has its own set of challenges. For one, removal of the uterus for treatment of some gynecologic cancers, unlike hysterectomy for noncancer problems, sometimes also requires removal of the upper portion of the vagina. This can result in a noticeable shortening of the vagina. Fortunately, vaginal tissues are amazingly elastic, and in the motivated woman these changes are almost always reversible. Once your surgeon gives you the go-ahead, ask your doctor if he or she thinks you will need dilators (chapter 6) prior to trying the real thing. If so, you will probably need to focus as much on length as on diameter. It's important to not force things but to use gentle pressure, especially at first. Over time the vagina will expand in order to allow comfortable placement.

> Modification of sexual positioning is important for patients who have a shortened vagina from radiation or surgery, since deep penetration may be particularly uncomfortable. Be creative! Positions such as spooning or female superior are generally more comfortable because depth of penetration can be controlled. A Comeclose collision ring (see chapter 9) is really helpful.

The Specific Problems of Specific Cancers
Breast Cancer

The 2.5 million women who are breast cancer survivors comprise the largest number of cancer survivors in the United States—not just because breast cancer is common, but also because treatment of breast cancer is increasingly successful.

It's not unusual, however, for a breast cancer survivor to attempt intercourse, only to find that what was once satisfying and enjoyable is now intolerable and upsetting.

In addition to the issues associated with recovery from cancer surgery, chemotherapy, and radiation, 26 percent of breast cancer survivors go through menopause as a result of treatment. Other women who are already menopausal at the time of their diagnosis discontinue their estrogen therapy, adding hot flashes, vaginal dryness, and insomnia to their list of challenges.

Following initial treatment, many women are advised to take a long-term oral medication to reduce the likelihood of recurrence of cancer. Women who have not yet gone through menopause and are still making some estrogen are generally prescribed tamoxifen, a selective estrogen receptor modulator (SERM) that specifically blocks estrogen receptors in the breast. Vaginal estrogen receptors are not blocked, but since overall estrogen levels are lower, it is not unusual for some women to experience vaginal dryness and painful intercourse while taking tamoxifen.

Women who are postmenopause are often prescribed an aroma-tase inhibitor such as Arimidex or Femara to completely block the formation of estrogen throughout the body. Zero estrogen in the body means zero estrogen in the vagina. Severe vaginal atrophy, with irritation, itching, frequent urinary tract infections, and sometimes even bleeding, while not universally experienced, is common.

Breast Cancer and Vaginal Atrophy

As a result of all this, up to 90 percent of breast cancer survivors develop sexual problems, the most common of which is vaginal atrophy. In a 2011 study out of the University of Chicago, more than 40 percent of breast cancer survivors expressed interest in receiving medical help for sexual issues, but only 7 percent had ever sought such care.

So, if you are post-breast-cancer and ready for sex, start with a silicone lubricant.

If sex is still dry and painful, don't give up. Most women assume that vaginal estrogen, the most successful way to reverse vaginal dryness, is just not an option if they have had breast cancer. Even if an enlightened doctor does give you the go-ahead to use a local vaginal estrogen product, many women take one look at the package insert that comes with this medication and decide it just isn't worth the risk.

As discussed in chapter 13, the "black box warning" that lists the dangers of using estrogen is not based on data that has anything to do with vaginal estrogen, much less women who have had breast cancer. Given that the minuscule amount of absorption from vaginal use doesn't even increase blood estrogen levels above the normal menopausal range, there is no reason to think that use of the product will lead to enough circulating estrogen to have any impact on breast cancer recurrence.

A paper published in *Breast Journal* calculated the total amount of estrogen delivered in one year of using a local vaginal estrogen product. Vagifem delivered 1.14 milligrams, with an average blood level of 4.6 picograms per milliliter. Estring delivered 2.74 milligrams, with an average blood level of 8.0 picograms per milliliter, and Estrace cream had a maximum yearly average of 7.1 milligrams, with a variable average blood level (since doses vary). As a point of reference, the average serum estrogen level in a post-menopausal woman who takes no estrogen is 10.0 picograms per milliliter or less. Women who take systemic estrogen therapy take 1 milligram each day. Women who use a vaginal estrogen take 1 to 7 milligrams per year.

Many women require even less than the recommended dose to reverse atrophy. I have many patients who use only tiny amounts of vaginal estrogen once or twice a week for maintenance and find that it does the job just fine. Others need to use vaginal estrogen to initiate post-treatment intercourse, but if they are regularly sexually active, they need not continue it over the long term.

Knowing that women who use vaginal estrogen have just as low a blood level of estrogen as women who don't use vaginal estrogen is very reassuring to women with breast cancer who want to use vaginal estrogen. There is essentially no actual evidence that using estrogen can increase the risk of cancer recurrence if placed directly on vaginal tissues. One study followed 1,472 breast cancer patients who routinely used vaginal estrogen. These patients were found to have a lower recurrence rate than women who did not use vaginal estrogen. This is why most breast surgeons and oncologists are comfortable allowing women with breast cancer to use vaginal estrogen.

In 2013 the North American Menopause Society issued a position statement that, for "a woman who is a survivor of breast or endometrial cancer, the choice of treatment depends on her preferences, needs, understanding of potential risks, and consultation with her oncologist." Essentially, the subtle message was that, in spite of FDA warnings, there is no reason not to prescribe vaginal estrogen for women with breast or uterine cancer.

In 2011, I conducted a poll of board-certified female gynecologists about decisions they make regarding their own health care. One of the questions I asked was, "If you had breast cancer and had problems with vaginal atrophy, would you personally use vaginal estrogen?"

Ninety-three percent of female gynecologists said yes: they would use a vaginal estrogen product even if they had breast cancer.

Ultimately, you need to do what you are comfortable with, but if you do decide to use vaginal estrogen, it should ease your anxiety a lot knowing that your gynecologist would more likely than not make the same decision for herself.

Non-Estrogen Options for Breast Cancer Survivors
Ospemifene

In spite of reassuring data, many women with breast cancer prefer to avoid estrogen. The only FDA–approved non–estrogen treatment for postmenopause vaginal atrophy is ospemifene, the SERM described in chapter 13.

The FDA warning on the package insert for ospemifene clearly states that this drug is not to be used in women with breast cancer. That is puzzling, because ospemifene blocks estrogen pathways in breast tissue just like the breast cancer drug tamoxifen. Reassuringly, in preclinical studies, ospemifene was shown to shrink breast tumors in rats. Why does the FDA make this warning? Because there were no women with breast cancer in the clinical trials! There were also no women with colon cancer, or any other kind of cancer for that matter, in the clinical trials, and yet the FDA has inexplicably insisted on this warning language. While I would not go so far as to say that ospemifene prevents or treats breast cancer, I am very comfortable saying that there is no reason to believe it would accelerate or cause breast cancer, and it will help women with breast cancer or breast cancer survivors to have better sex.

One downside is that ospemifene increases hot flashes in 7.5 percent of women, making it a nonstarter for many women who already feel like their internal furnace is going full blast. Also, keep in mind that ospemifene, like local vaginal estrogens, is not a magic bullet; many women will still need to use a lubricant or a long-acting vaginal moisturizer with this medication.

DHEA

Another non-estrogen option is compounded vaginal DHEA, which is discussed at great length in chapter 13. Didehydroepian-drosterone (say that five times fast!) is a precursor to estrogen and testosterone that has been shown to have all the effects of a local vaginal estrogen, including improved pH, lubrication, and elastic-ity. Some studies even show that women who use vaginal DHEA have an increase in libido and orgasm beyond what is expected from eliminating painful intercourse.

Breast Cancer and Hot Flashes

Vaginal atrophy is not, of course, the only consequence of lack of estrogen.

Some women find that their hot flashes after breast cancer are so severe that they are unable to function. While a case can be made that many women can safely take systemic estrogen even if they have breast cancer, in the absence of studies, most doctors advise women with breast cancer to not take systemic estrogen.

Alternatives to estrogen to relieve hot flashes are discussed in chapter 14. Be aware that paroxitene (Brisdelle) should not be used if a woman is taking tamoxifen since metabolism of the Brisdelle may speed up the metabolism of tamoxifen and potentially make it less effective. Venlafaxine is an SNRI (serotonin and norepi-nephrine reuptake inhibitor), as opposed to an SSRI, and has also been shown to decrease hot flashes and can be given together with tamoxifen.

Don't underestimate the value of exercise. Multiple studies demonstrate that women who work out regularly have fewer hot flashes owing to exercise-induced endorphin production. Losing that extra weight and eliminating cigarettes also make a huge difference. Dry Babe cooling pajamas also help, but the better solution is sleeping without pajamas . . . helps with hot flashes and encourages cuddling.

Breast Cancer and Altered Body Image

For some women, the adjustment to life after breast cancer goes beyond the physical changes and menopausal symptoms. Breast cancer survivors have to face a huge range of surgery and treatment options. From simple lumpectomy to double mastectomy, radiation, and chemotherapy, the effect on a woman's body from breast cancer is vast.

Many women who lose their breasts, particularly if they decline reconstruction, struggle with the feeling that they are no longer "feminine" or a true woman. The impact of an altered body image and the perception that they are less sexually attractive tends to be higher in younger women, but most women with breast cancer experience this to some degree. A post-mastectomy woman who counted on breast and nipple stimulation to get things going in the bedroom may need to discover new erogenous zones. Women without nipples can attach one, if that makes them feel more attractive. It goes without saying that purchasing beautiful lingerie is a required prescription.

Gynecologic Cancers

The most common gynecologic cancers are uterine (53 percent), ovarian (25 percent), and cervical (14 percent). All generally require hysterectomy.

In a 2004 study conducted at the University of Chicago, only 38 percent of women diagnosed with cervical or uterine cancer said their physician warned them that they might have sexual side effects.

Uterine Cancer

Uterine cancer, also known as endometrial cancer, is the most common gynecological cancer and the fourth most common cancer to occur in women. Most invasive uterine cancer is diagnosed in its early stages, when a woman first experiences abnormal bleeding. Since uterine cancer is usually diagnosed early, relatively few women die from it. The five-year survival rate for women diagnosed when their cancer is stage 1 is 96 percent. While most cases of uterine cancer occur after menopause (the average age is 61), 25 percent of cases are diagnosed in women who are premenopausal. Interestingly, the use of birth control pills or a progestin IUD for at least 12 months decreases the risk of uterine cancer by a whopping 50 to 80 percent. This protection lasts for 15 years after pill use is discontinued.

Treatment for uterine cancer is generally a robotic-assisted laparoscopic or abdominal hysterectomy with removal of tubes and ovaries and pelvic lymph node sampling. Women with early cancers usually require no further treatment beyond surgery, and intercourse can generally be resumed six to eight weeks after surgery. In more advanced cancers, or some less common cancers, postoperative radiation and/or chemotherapy is recommended, and side effects from these treatments, as discussed earlier, may be an issue. Women are often given conflicting advice as to the safety of estrogen therapy after treatment of uterine cancer, but most experts feel it is safe and will not influence recurrence of uterine cancer.

Ovarian and Fallopian Tube Cancer

One in 70 women will develop ovarian cancer during her lifetime. Contrary to what most people think, only 10 to 15 percent of ovarian cancer is hereditary. This is a cancer that is difficult to detect at an early stage, which is why most ovarian cancers are diagnosed and treated when they have already advanced. Treatment of ovarian cancer is almost always total abdominal hysterectomy, with removal of both fallopian tubes and ovaries and a lymph node sampling, followed by chemotherapy.

Fallopian tube cancer is extremely rare, representing only 0.2 percent of gynecologic cancers. Like ovarian cancer in many ways, it also is not symptomatic until it is at a late stage. Many experts now feel that most ovarian cancer actually starts as fallopian tube cancer, which would be why tubal ligation and tubal removal dramatically decrease the risk of developing ovarian cancer. The treatment is the same as for ovarian cancer.

Up to 57 percent of survivors report sexual issues after treatment for ovarian and fallopian tube cancer. The most common problem is dyspareunia from menopausal changes, as opposed to anatomical problems from surgery. Low libido is also prevalent and is no doubt a result of hormonal changes, concern about recurrence, and painful intercourse. Estrogen therapy is not contraindicated for women with ovarian or fallopian tube cancers.

What About Ovarian Cancer Screening?

Anyone who spends any time on the Internet, particularly if they get a lot of email from "helpful" people, has received the message touting the benefits of a blood test to see if they have elevated levels of CA125 and suggesting that every woman should demand this test from her doctor.

CA125 is a substance that ovarian cancer cells shed. But normal cells that become inflamed also make CA125. The majority of women with a slightly elevated CA125 do not have ovarian cancer but have a noncancerous condition, such as endometriosis or fibroids. In addition, CA125 levels don't increase until the disease is well established. Fifty percent of women with stage 1 ovarian cancer have normal CA125 levels! If the results of annual screening in symptom-free, low-risk women decreased the death rate for ovarian cancer, every gynecologist would recommend it, but no such benefit has been proven.

Cervical Cancer

The plummet in invasive cervical cancer rates is one of the cancer success stories of the 20th century. With the detection of treatable precancerous lesions on Pap tests, the rate of cervical cancer has dropped by 75 percent, so that cervical cancer currently accounts for only 1.7 percent of cancer deaths in women. Cervical cancer can occur in any sexually active age group but is most common in women 45 to 49 years of age, with a rate of 16.5 per 100,000 women per year. Forty percent of invasive cervical cancer is diagnosed in women under the age of 45. Early cervical cancer generally doesn't have any symptoms, which is why regular Pap tests are recommended.

Women with invasive cervical cancer often require a radical hysterectomy, a more extensive surgery than simply removing the uterus. The upper part of the vagina and pelvic lymph nodes are usually removed, along with the uterus, cervix, tubes, and ovaries to ensure that any cancer cells in adjacent tissue is removed. Removal of the ovaries is not always mandatory in young women. However, even when the ovaries are not removed, premature menopause is common due to the surgical impairment of ovarian blood flow, radiation, or chemotherapy. Many women require radiation and/or chemotherapy postsurgery.

After radical hysterectomy, the vagina may be shortened, making intercourse particularly challenging. If this is the case, pelvic physical therapy and dilators are an essential part of sexual rehab. In many cases, disruption of the blood and nerve supply in the genital area can affect sensation, lubrication, arousal, and the ability to have an orgasm. Many women who are initially unable to have an orgasm will regain the ability to do so six to twelve months after treatment. Lubrication will also improve with time. Nerve-sparing radical hysterectomy, a technique that limits damage to pelvic nerves, seems to have less impact and is an option to discuss with your surgeon.

There is no evidence or reason to believe that estrogen therapy, either vaginal or systemic, will increase the risk of cancer recurrence and is an option both to relieve symptoms and to improve vaginal dryness and elasticity.

Other Gynecologic Cancers
Vulvar Cancer

Vulvar cancer is the fourth most common gynecologic cancer, comprising about 5 percent. The mean age of the woman with vulvar cancer is 65; however, over the last 20 years the incidence of pre-vulvar cancer has tripled for women under the age of 50 as a result of HPV infection. (See chapter 18 for more information.) Vulvar cancer accounts for 800 deaths per year. Most vulvar cancer manifests itself as a vulvar lesion that doesn't go away. Frequently the skin involved is very itchy, which is why any suspicious sore or patch of skin should be biopsied.

Vulvar cancer treatments range from excision of a small area of the vulva to a radical vulvectomy. Radical vulvectomy includes removal of the entire vulva, pelvic lymph nodes, and in some cases the clitoris or part of the urethra. In other cases, a less radical procedure known as a skinning vulvectomy is performed. A skinning vulvectomy removes only the top layer of vulvar skin in order to preserve function and appearance. Sometimes radiation therapy is also required.

There are very few studies that look at sexuality after vulvar cancer, but it is clear that sexual problems after vulvar cancer treatment can be significant and appear to be related to a woman's age, general health at the time of diagnosis, and the extent of surgery.

Removal of the clitoris obviously will decrease, but not eliminate, the ability to have an orgasm. It is also common to have significant post-op numbness and narrowing of the vaginal opening. A topical estrogen is safe and appropriate for those who have completed vulvar cancer treatment, along with vaginal dilators and pelvic floor physical therapy.

Vaginal Cancer

Vaginal cancer comprises 3 percent of gynecologic cancer cases and occurs in 1 in 100,000 women per year, with the mean age of those women affected being 60. However, young women can also get vaginal cancer. Most women experience vaginal bleeding or an abnormal discharge as a symptom of vaginal cancer. Vaginal cancer is diagnosed when an abnormality is seen by the gynecologist or detected on a Pap test. Vaginal cancer is one of the reasons why you should continue annual visits with your gynecologist even if you have had a hysterectomy.

The location in the vagina, the extent of the cancer, and the age and general health of the patient determine the right treatment, which could include radiation, excision of part of the vagina, radical hysterectomy, lymph node dissection, and removal of at least the upper part of the vagina. Complete removal of the vagina is necessary in rare situations. Removal of the ovaries is not necessarily required if vaginal cancer occurs in a young woman, but radiation-induced menopause is common.

The ability to have vaginal intercourse after this cancer is dependent on the extent of the surgery. Generally, women who have faced this diagnosis require local estrogen therapy and vaginal dilators. If removal of the vagina is necessary, alternatives to vaginal intercourse are obviously required. So keep in mind that the clitoris is intact and functional!

Prophylactic Surgery for Women at Genetic Risk of Gynecologic Cancer

Many women don't have cancer, but because of a genetic predisposition to develop ovarian cancer because of a BRCA mutation, they may be advised to undergo lifesaving treatments that could have an impact on their sexual health.

In the early 1990s, BRCA1, or breast cancer gene 1, and BRCA2, breast cancer gene 2, were identified as gene mutations responsible for the majority of hereditary breast and ovarian cancer. (Remember that joke that circulated during seventh grade? If a kid has long hair, how do you know if it's a boy or a girl? You pull down the genes!) Genes, of course, are the parts of each cell that contain the hereditary information that determines whether you are destined to inherit your mom's curly hair and your dad's high cholesterol. Every gene has a job. The job of a normal BRCA gene is to stop cancer. A mutation is a misspelling of the gene that changes or impairs its function. If a BRCA mutation occurs, certain cancers are more likely to grow. Like any other gene, BRCA mutations can be passed on to subsequent generations.

Hereditary breast and ovarian cancer syndrome (HBOC) refers to men and women who have inherited a BRCA genetic mutation that increases their susceptibility to developing not only early-onset breast and ovarian cancer but also fallopian tube, prostate, and pancreatic cancer.

Anyone can have a gene mutation, but certain ethnic groups are at increased risk. Ashkenazi Jews who come from eastern European countries are one group that has been identified as particularly high-risk, with 2.5 percent of the population carrying BRCA mutations. But I want to emphasize that this mutation is not limited to Ashkenazi Jews. One in 200 people in the general population have this gene mutation. Since the majority of the population is not Jewish, neither are the majority of people who carry the BRCA gene.

Who Should Be Screened for BRCA Mutations?

The presence of a BRCA mutation can be detected in a blood sample. Not everyone needs to be tested for the presence of this mutation, but there are certain risk factors that should prompt a discussion. Family history is the primary tool in determining the likelihood for hereditary cancer. Both your mother's and father's histories are equally relevant. Sometimes this is hard information to get, especially if you come from a family that, unlike my family, doesn't regularly broadcast their gynecologic problems at the dinner table. Sometimes all you have to go on is, "Aunt Tilly died from *(whisper)* female trouble," or, "Grandma Rose had problems down there," or the very specific "Cancer . . . all over!"

Older generations may not be as forthcoming with their medical issues, and you may hear conflicting stories depending on who you ask. Be that as it may, your first step is to get as much information as possible about your not-too-distant relatives. If your first-degree (mother, sisters, daughters) or second-degree (grandmothers, aunts) relatives did not have ovarian or breast cancer, you don't need to know if your relatives who came over on the *Mayflower* did.

> A few years ago, I flew to New York to give a talk on menopause. Given the way we are smashed in like sardines, it's not unusual for whoever is sitting next to me to get an eyeful of whatever I'm working on. So on the flight over I was working on my presentation . . . lots of pictures about vaginal dryness, lubricants . . . you get the idea. The guy next to me was fascinated. At one point I thought he was going to take notes.
>
> On the way home I was working on a presentation about BRCA. I have a fear of flying, and it was pretty turbulent. Miraculously, we landed, and as I emerged from crash position I heard a voice say, "I'm at risk." I turned to the woman next to me. "Excuse me for reading over your shoulder, but I'm at risk. " I said, "Oh, so you're familiar with BRCA?" She said, "No, I never even heard of BRCA before. But now I know I am at risk, and I am going to talk to my doctor about being tested."

Do You Really Want to Know?

Each year 200,000 women are diagnosed with breast cancer, and roughly 22,000 are diagnosed with ovarian cancer. Of those, 5 to 10 percent are carriers of a BRCA mutation, which is responsible for their cancer. Half a million women in the United States have this gene mutation, but only 4 percent are aware of it. In other words, 96 percent of woman who are at very high risk for developing breast or ovarian cancer don't even know it.

Throughout my gynecologic career, I have told women many times that they have ovarian cancer. It's not easy. I also routinely tell women they are BRCA positive. Trust me, it is much less difficult to talk about strategies to decrease or eliminate the risk of cancer than to tell someone they already have it.

Women with a BRCA mutation have up to an 87 percent risk of developing breast cancer. These breast cancers occur at a much younger age, often before women are advised to get their first mammogram. The only way to completely eliminate your risk is to prophylactically remove the breasts, and many BRCA carriers choose mastectomy and reconstruction. Women who choose to have prophylactic mastectomies to reduce risk can opt for a nipple-sparing mastectomy with reconstruction. Since there is no radiation, aesthetic results for this kind of surgery are generally fabulous. In fact, the result is essentially the same as a woman gets when she chooses breast implants for cosmetic reasons.

If you have a BRCA mutation and do not opt for surgery, or you're not ready for surgery, a first mammogram should be done 10 years before the age at which your youngest relative was diagnosed or by age 25. Breast MRI and ultrasound are often recommended in addition to mammography.

Women with a BRCA mutation also have a 44 percent risk of developing ovarian cancer as opposed to the 1.4 percent risk found in the general population. The best way to significantly decrease your chances of developing cancer is to surgically remove your ovaries before cancer cells start to grow. For the many women who choose not to do that or who want to wait until they have completed their families, there are a number of risk-reducing strategies.

Women who are BRCA positive should have a CA125 test every six to 12 months, beginning at age 25, along with a transvaginal ultrasound. Taking birth control pills for five years or longer reduces the risk of developing ovarian cancer by as much as 60 percent. It's a mystery to me why pharmaceutical companies, which have made millions by advertising that birth control pills reduce acne, don't advertise that fact!

It appears that because the fallopian tubes are often the source for ovarian cancer cells, tubal ligation, or removal of the tubes, reduces rates of ovarian cancer as much as 40 percent.

So yes, a strong family history of cancer creates a lot of stress and anxiety. Contrary to what you might think, knowing your carrier status reduces stress. You can slay the monster you see coming, but not the monster that is invisible.

The Effect of a BRCA Mutation on Sexuality

Even in the absence of prophylactic mastectomy, sexuality can be impacted when there is a known BRCA mutation. According to Lindsay Avner, the founder of Bright Pink (www.bebrightpink .com), a national support group for young women at risk for genetic cancers, women with a known BRCA mutation sometimes experience discomfort with their healthy breasts and express that they don't enjoy having them touched in a sexual way. It's almost as if they have already become subconsciously reconciled to losing them, or perhaps they think of their breasts, not as a source of pleasure, but as a potentially life-threatening part of their body.

After mastectomy and reconstruction, even though breasts look perfect, the loss of nipple sensation can be distressing. Again, this calls for attention to other erogenous zones!

Menopause at 35?

You may be thinking that it would be better to face the risk of ovarian cancer than go through a surgical menopause. However, when ovaries are removed at a young age, taking hormone replacement is not a problem, since it's not the hormones that created the risk for cancer but the ovarian tissue. Just as it is fine for young women with a BRCA mutation to take birth control pills if they still have their ovaries, it is fine to take hormone therapy to alleviate menopause symptoms once the ovaries are removed. There is no data to suggest that young women who take estrogen and progestin are at higher risk for developing breast cancer. Keep in mind that many women who undergo prophylactic removal of their tubes and ovaries also have a prophylactic mastectomy, essentially eliminating the risk of breast cancer too.

One approach for the young woman who requires ovary removal is to start birth control pills during the years before surgery (to decrease the risk of ovarian cancer) and then to keep the pills going after the ovaries are removed. That way, she goes through no hormonal change as a result of surgery and can decrease her birth control dosage gradually until she is at a comfortable replacement dose. In her fifties, she can then decide if she wants to continue hormone therapy. Keep in mind that a woman who has surgical removal of her ovaries as opposed to a natural menopause may also need testosterone therapy. (For more information about the place of testosterone in a woman's hormone balance, see chapter 13.)

Lynch Syndrome

Just as some women have a familial predisposition to breast and ovarian cancer, some families have a genetic mutation that increases the risk for uterine cancer.

Lynch syndrome, also known as hereditary nonpolyposis colorectal cancer (HNPCC), is a genetic disorder associated with familial colon cancer. Up to 60 percent of women with Lynch syndrome also develop endometrial (uterine) cancer. Prophylactic hysterectomy should therefore be considered in patients who test positive for Lynch syndrome. Fortunately, the consequences of hysterectomy for women who have the surgery for prophylactic reasons are the same as for those who have the surgery because of cancer. In the event of ovary removal, estrogen therapy presents no problem for patients with Lynch syndrome.

Nongynecologic Pelvic Cancers

The reproductive organs are not the only organs hanging out in the pelvis. The bladder, colon, and rectum are also in the neighborhood. It's no surprise that issues associated with bladder and colorectal cancers are often similar to those seen in gynecologic cancers.

Treatment of bladder cancer can range from radiation therapy to extensive surgery in which the bladder, urethra, uterus, and sometimes part of the vagina are removed. In addition to issues associated with vaginal shortening, pelvic nerves and blood vessels are often compromised by bladder cancer surgery. There are very few studies of the sexual issues following bladder cancer, but clearly there is an impact similar to that of surgical treatment of gynecologic cancers.

Colorectal cancer (involving either the colon or the rectum) is the second most common cancer in women. Two-thirds of these cancers originate in the colon. Colon cancer surgery usually does not impinge on other pelvic organs, and in many cases a colostomy is not needed. In general, colon cancer does not have a significantly greater impact on sexual health than any other nongynecologic cancers.

Rectal cancer surgery, on the other hand, often results in impaired sexual function and incontinence due to a shortened vagina or pelvic nerve damage that affects blood flow to the bladder, vagina, and vulva. If radiation is required, there can be radiation effects as well.

Many experienced pelvic surgeons are now able to spare the pelvic nerves when performing rectal cancer surgeries to minimize damage. It's not unusual after rectal cancer surgery to lose the ability to use the rectum, which means an ostomy will be needed as an alternative outlet for a bowel movement. In 25 percent of cases, an ostomy bag is a permanent accessory. Comfortable sexual solutions are discussed in chapter 15.

Advanced Pelvic Cancers

In rare cases, women with advanced pelvic cancers undergo a radical surgery known as pelvic exenteration. This is a lifesaving procedure (not routinely performed) that removes all pelvic organs, including the uterus, cervix, tubes, ovaries, bladder, urethra, and sometimes the colon and vagina. Women who undergo this surgery require ostomies and usually need vaginal reconstruction.

A Word About Lung Cancer

Lung cancer is not a pelvic cancer, or specifically a woman's cancer, but it is the fourth most common cancer in women and the leading cause of death from cancer. Twice as many women die from lung cancer as from breast cancer.

An overwhelming fatigue and chronic shortness of breath precludes sexual activity in many women with lung cancer. This is one of those situations when "scheduling" sexual activity is important in order to make sure you are rested and have just completed a bronchial treatment.

Postmenopause hormone therapy is discouraged in women with lung cancer since there may be an association between hormones and lung cancer recurrence.

The New Normal

While many women are able to resume comfortable and enjoyable vaginal intercourse after cancer, for some women this is a time to find a "new normal" when it comes to sex. Breast stimulation, oral sex, and yes, anal sex, can all be explored. While it may seem daunting, enhancing your sex life after cancer is a good problem to have. It means you have survived and are eager to get your life back. You should not feel guilty about wanting the best quality of life during and after cancer treatment.

If you feel that your oncologist isn't equipped to deal with your specific sexual issues (many have not had specific training in this field), a visit to a sexual health clinic may be well worth it. (And head to the next chapter for plenty of information on finding a clinician.) Don't blame your oncologist—be grateful that he or she has done such a good job with treating your cancer, and focus on the fact that you are now able to live your life to the fullest again!

part six

OTHER PEOPLE

17

FINDING A CLINICIAN WHO WILL ACTUALLY LISTEN

Let's talk vagina

Now that you are an expert on estrogen, vaginal atrophy, long-acting moisturizers, vaginal pH, and orgasms and know what questions to ask your doctor, how do you find one who can actually answer them? How is it that you're such an expert but your doctor may not be? I hate to say this, but an "MD" after the name is no assurance that the person to whom you are about to bare your soul—and your vagina—is an expert in your particular problem.

So, sometimes the savvy consumer has to do a little legwork to find a clinician who is a real expert on sexual health for women. A sexual health expert is not necessarily your gynecologist—or a gynecologist period. This expert is someone who has an interest in this area and is informed about the diagnosis and treatment of the conditions that affect sexual health. So a sexual health expert might be your gynecologist, or an internist, or a family practice doctor, or a urologist. It's also possible that the best clinician to help you with your particular issue may not even be a doctor but a highly trained nurse-practitioner.

I want to provide you with a quick and easy-to-understand

guide to what you should look for to deal with your specific issues. If you understand who you are looking for, what kind of training is necessary for specific titles, how qualified a physician is, and how non-MD clinicians fit into the picture, you will have a better chance of getting the right treatment. Finding the right person to help you isn't always easy, but success is a lot more likely if you know what to look for. This way of deciding on a practitioner not only applies to identifying someone to treat your sexual problems but can be applied to every aspect of your health.

Finding a Doctor
"Doctor": What's in a Title?

A "doctor" is anyone who has a doctorate-level degree. Anyone with "Doctor" in front of his or her name *might* be a physician, but might also be a dentist, podiatrist, psychologist, or English professor. If you are looking for a physician, look for an "MD."

> **MD** *stands for "Medical Doctor." Anyone who has graduated from medical school is allowed to put "MD" after their name. Forever.*
> **DO** *stands for "Doctor of Osteopathy." An osteopath's training is essentially identical to an MD's and should be considered equivalent.*

Licensing

A licensed physician is a physician who is allowed to practice medicine. Each state has its own criteria for granting licenses, but in general, licensure to practice medicine requires only proof of graduation from medical school, at least a year of clinical training, and passing a qualifying exam. To verify that a physician is licensed, go to the Federation of State Medical Boards website (fsmb.org). Please note that licensure is not the same thing as board certification and does not guarantee expertise in a specific field.

Board Certification

Board certification is the gold standard that assures you that a physician is an expert in a specialty or subspecialty. The American Board of Medical Specialties (ABMS) is the medical organization that oversees physician certification by developing standards for the evaluation and certification of physician specialists. To be board-certified, a doctor must complete a residency (post-medical-school training) in his or her specialty that has been recognized by ABMS, followed by rigorous written and oral examinations. If a doctor wants to subspecialize, he or she must then complete fellowship training after finishing residency. For example, to be a board-certified fertility specialist, a medical school graduate must complete a four-year residency in the obstetrics-gynecology specialty, followed by a three-year fellowship in the subspecialty of reproductive endocrinology and infertility.

If that wasn't enough, a specialist or subspecialist has to maintain board certification by taking medical courses and passing tests to prove that he or she is up to date. The criterion in each field is specific to the specialty. Some, but not all, board-certified doctors designate their certification as part of their title. For example, a board-certified gynecologist with the letters FACOG after his or her name is a Fellow in the American College of Obstetricians and Gynecologists. ABMS.org is the site where you can check out whether a physician is board-certified and find out what he or she is certified in.

University Affiliations

It's generally a good sign if a physician has an academic appointment at a medical school. Faculty ranks such as instructor, assistant professor, associate professor, and professor depend on physicians' level of involvement in teaching medical students, their research, and the number and stature of their publications.

If a doctor is not board-certified or has no university affiliation, does this mean he or she is a bad doctor? Of course not! Many non-board-certified physicians are excellent doctors who keep up with advancements in their fields and give very good care. Let's face it, though: if you needed brain surgery, would you go to the brain surgeon who's board-certified, teaches at a medical school, and is current with the field, or would you pick the brain surgeon who finished a residency but failed her boards, took off five years to be an artist, and then returned and has privileges at a hospital that was in such desperate need of a brain surgeon that it didn't require board certification?

By now, I'm sure you get the message.

But vaginal dryness isn't brain surgery. What you need is someone who has an interest in sexual health issues and a knowledge base. Sometimes this expert is a physician, sometimes an internist, sometimes a gynecologist, sometimes a family practice doctor, and sometimes a physician's assistant or nurse-practitioner (more on them later). You may be thinking, *But I'm seeing an expert! If a gynecologist isn't an expert in this area, who is?*

Even in particular fields, doctors have particular areas of interest. A neurologist may be the world's expert on seizure disorders, but not know a lot about stroke. Your ob-gyn may have an incredible expertise about twin pregnancies and preterm labor, but treats women with vaginal atrophy only a few times a year. So how do you know where a doctor's areas of interest lie?

What About Referral Services?

Most hospitals have a physician referral service and will help you find a doctor who is interested in and knowledgeable about your condition. If the hospital you have chosen is well known as a leader in women's health, then that hospital's referral service is usually a great way to find the right doctor. Keep in mind that the people who work in hospital referrals are obligated to make referrals to all the physicians on staff, so if you just call up and say, "Hi, I have a dry vagina. Which ob-gyn is good?" you'll most likely be given the name of whoever is next on the list.

What you need to ask are specific questions that will lead you to the doctor who is most appropriate for you. For example, instead of saying, "I need a gynecologist because sex hurts like hell," you might try, "I'm looking for a board-certified gynecologist who has been in practice for at least five years. I would prefer a woman and would like someone who takes care of a lot of menopausal problems and has identified herself as having an interest or expertise in sexual issues."

You can get a lot of information from physician referral, and it is well worth your time to tell the service exactly what's important to you in a doctor. The referral service will also be able to answer questions about office location and accepted insurance. Frequently, a referral service will help you get an appointment, even if you can't get one just by calling yourself.

Many hospitals also have a "physician finder" section on their website where you can type in a condition to find the physicians who list it as an area of expertise.

Hospital referral services are not the same as the commercial referral agencies that operate independently of hospitals. Take it from me—referral agencies that advertise in magazines, the yellow pages, or on TV are not a great source for good doctors. Participating physicians pay to be part of the service and tell the service what to say. As with any paid advertisement, healthy skepticism is appropriate.

Searching Online for a Doctor

The reason for the increasing popularity of doctor-listing websites is that people are desperate for an easy way to find information about a doctor without actually making an appointment. In our digitally driven society, this seems to be a reasonable desire. After all, wouldn't someone who has already been to that doctor be the best judge of how approachable or knowledgeable he or she is?

Keep in mind that consumer referral lists are no better than asking strangers on the street what they think. Typically, there are no more than a handful of "reviewers" who are rating the doctors. The typical doctor sees thousands of patients a year, and the experience of two or three people is hardly reflective of a typical experience.

More important, you have no idea who is writing these reviews or what their agenda is. A glowing review may be from the wife or mother of the doctor. A scathing review may be from a disgruntled patient or employee, or from the wife or mother of the competing doctor in town. It has become common for "online profile management" companies to post positive reviews for businesses and products for a fee.

Even if reviewers' comments accurately reflect their experience, their comments are usually more about how they were treated at the office than about the skills of the doctor. More than one five-star comment has been posted because the doctor was "really friendly," "had a "great staff," and offered free birth control pill samples.

Professional Societies

Professional societies such as the American Medical Association or the American College of Obstetricians and Gynecologists are all potential sources of referrals. In the case of sexual function, there are a few societies that are particularly appropriate.

North American Menopause Society

The mission of the North American Menopause Society (NAMS), a nonprofit scientific organization, is to promote the health and quality of life of all women during midlife and beyond through an understanding of menopause and healthy aging. To help meet its mission, NAMS developed a certification exam in 2002. Successful completion of the exam provides a doctor with a three-year credential as a NAMS Certified Menopause Practitioner (NCMP). Menopausal medicine has become increasingly complex, so you are lucky if you find a doctor with this level of commitment and competence.

You can pretty much be guaranteed that a NAMS-certified practitioner has not only the interest but also the expertise to evaluate and treat any of your menopausal issues, including the sexual ones. To find a certified menopause practitioner, go to www.meno pause.org.

International Society for the Study of Women's Sexual Health

The International Society for the Study of Women's Sexual Health (ISSWSH) is an interdisciplinary, academic, and scientific organization dedicated to providing the public with accurate information about women's sexuality and sexual health. The organization's website not only is loaded with helpful information and links to resources but provides a list of providers who are experts in sexual health.

Finding Non-MD Clinicians: Advanced Practice Nurses and Physician's Assistants

So, is an MD always the best clinician to help you deal with complex sexual health issues? Sometimes a nonphysician is *more* qualified than many physicians when it comes to diagnosing and treating certain conditions. I am a huge advocate of advanced practice nurses (some are nurse-practitioners and some have other advanced nursing degrees) and physician's assistants. In addition, an advanced practice nurse or physician's assistant is likely to spend more time with you than most physicians. I know this firsthand because I have a fabulous, invaluable advanced practice nurse in my office.

I made the decision to use the words "doctor" and "gynecologist" when referring to a clinician in this book because I am a gynecologist. In addition, most women in this country are still seeing a physician as their primary care practitioner. Also, it would have been cumbersome to use "doctor and/or advanced practice clinician/physician's assistant" throughout the book. To add to the confusion, there are many different degrees that qualify a clinician as an advanced practice nurse.

In general, a clinician designated as a advanced practice nurse has completed the four-year education and clinical experiences necessary to have a bachelor of science degree in nursing, followed by an additional two to three years of a graduate-level nurse-practitioner program (either a master's or doctorate degree) with board certification.

In some states advanced practice nurses work independently of physicians, while in other states partnering with a physician is required for practice. In any case, advanced practice nurses can function as primary care clinicians and diagnose, treat, evaluate, and manage both acute and chronic illness and disease. They also educate and counsel patients on health behaviors and treatment options.

The following are advanced practice nurse degrees:

NP: *Nurse-Practitioner*
DNP: *Doctor of Nursing Practice*
ACNP: *Acute Care Nurse-Practitioner*
ANP: *Advanced Nurse-Practitioner*
APRN: *Advanced Practice Registered Nurse*
ARNP: *Advanced Registered Nurse-Practitioner*
CRNP: *Certified Registered Nurse-Practitioner*
FNP: *Family Nurse-Practitioner*
CNM: *Certified Nurse-Midwife*
RNC: *Registered Nurse-Certified*
MSN: *Master of Science in Nursing*

Certified physician's assistants (PAs) are not nurses but are licensed and certified health care professionals who practice medicine with physician supervision. A PA must complete an undergraduate degree followed by two to three years of PA school that includes learning both science and hands-on clinical skills.

Just like physicians and advanced practice nurses, PAs may choose to specialize in a specific area such as women's health. Advanced practice nurses and physician's assistants are eligible to take the NAMS test and be designated as a NAMS Certified Menopause Practitioner.

Tips for Choosing a Practitioner

After becoming familiar with the background information related to various providers, you can use these practical tips to find someone who can help you.

1. **Ask questions when you make the appointment.** The receptionist who is making the appointment may not have the time or the information that you need. If so, ask to speak to the practice manager. Find out before you make the appointment whether the physician/clinician has an interest in sexual health. You can get very specific. "I have difficulty with painful intercourse. Is this something the doctor treats routinely?"

2. **Check out the medical practice's website.** It's usually pretty obvious if the practice focuses on pregnancy and contraception or issues of midlife women or sexual health issues.

3. **Consider an all-gynecologic practice.** A busy general ob-gyn practice tends to focus on pregnant women. An all-gynecologic practice is likely to have a lot more experience, and a lot more interest, in treating the problems associated with sexuality. In a recent survey of ob-gyns, gynecologists were more likely than obstetrician-gynecologists to communicate with their patients about sexual satisfaction.

4. **Consider a sexual function clinic.** A number of sexual function clinics specialize in women's sexual health. When you search for one in your area, make sure the doctors running the clinic are board-certified in a variety of specialties that treat issues associated with sexual health. Clinics affiliated with a university hospital are often your best bet.

5. **Go to the specialty website.** I admit I'm biased, but I think one of the most reliable ways to find an expert is to check out one of the professional society websites listed in the resources section of this book.

However, even if you do your homework, you may simply not have access to a sexual health expert. You may live in a small town, or your insurance may keep you locked into a particular group of physicians. Or maybe you simply like your doctor and would be happy to have a conversation with him or her, but just don't know how to bring it up. The next section is for you.

Talking to Your Doctor About Sex: If You Don't, They Won't

From what I hear, the typical dialogue during a woman's annual gynecologic visit tends to go like this:

PATIENT: Uh, doctor, I'm having some sexual problems. . . .
DOCTOR: Try a lubricant. So, about your blood pressure. . . .

Actually, this example is a lot longer than most discussions. What typically occurs is *no* discussion at all. Nada. Zip. If you're in that majority, chances are that when you went for your annual exam last year, your doctor didn't even ask you about your sex life, much less offer information on how to make it better! In the 2013 *Revive* survey, two-thirds of women having sexual problems stated they were never asked about it by their gynecologist. Only about 5 percent of doctors across the board initiate a conversation about sexual function and sexual satisfaction. Ob-gyns seem to do a better job than general doctors. According to a recent survey published by the International Society for Sexual Medicine, 65.6 percent of

> Doctor to her 80-year-old female patient: "I said you had acute angina, not a cute vagina!"

ob-gyns *reported* routinely assessing patients' sexual activities. It would be really interesting to poll their patients to see whether 65.6 percent of their patients agreed that their sexual health had been assessed!

Physicians give three reasons for not routinely bringing up sexual health:

1. **Limited time.** It's true that time is limited. There are a lot of issues to be discussed during an annual gynecological visit, and not nearly enough time. By the time you have talked about your elevated cholesterol, your low vitamin D, your overwhelming fatigue, and the swelling in your ankles, there isn't a whole lot of time left to discuss your sex life.
2. **Embarrassment.** This explanation is offered frequently, but I don't buy it. Yes, there are exceptions, but most doctors have no trouble talking about other "embarrassing" things. Have you ever had a doctor change the subject when you brought up your bleeding hemorrhoids?
3. **Lack of knowledge.** Bingo! This reason, more than any other, is probably the culprit. More likely than not, the person you see to check your blood pressure, do your Pap test, and get your thyroid medication doesn't know much about the evaluation or treatment of painful sex.

Now that we have established that your doctor is probably not going to bring up the topic of your sex life, you are going to have to figure out how to bring it up yourself.

Bringing Up the Topic

Studies show that most women don't broach the subject of sexuality with their doctors *ever,* and if they do, it takes an average of two and a half years from the time a woman perceives an issue until she finally gets up the nerve to mention it.

Sometimes women don't bring up sexual health issues because they make the assumption that their issues, such as pain during intercourse, are a "normal part of aging" and should be accepted. It's also not unusual for a menopausal woman to assume that vaginal dryness, like hot flashes and other menopausal symptoms, is temporary. Many are not aware that there are treatments available beyond lubricants. And sadly, too many women don't feel that their discomfort during sex is serious enough to waste their doctor's time talking about. And yes, a woman can be too embarrassed to mention her sex life to a doctor who looks like one of her son's friends or, even worse, golfs with her husband, looks like he hasn't had sex himself in 30 years, or is focused on "more serious" problems.

As one patient said to me during a seminar on sexuality:

The last time I went to the gynecologist I really wanted to discuss the fact that my interest in sex was essentially gone. The only thing my gynecologist seemed to want to talk about was my weight. By the time he told me that I was at risk for dropping dead from a heart attack unless diabetes got me first, it just didn't seem appropriate to bring up my lack of libido.

There's another big reason why women are often reluctant to talk to their doctor about sexual problems. . . .

Your Doctor Doesn't Have a Vagina

Frequently, a new patient will say to me, "I've had the same ob-gyn for 20 years, and I love him, but he's a *man,* so of course there was no way I could talk to *him* about this! I want a woman doctor who will understand."

As a physician, I can tell you that I don't need to have personally experienced vaginal atrophy to help my patient with vaginal atrophy, any more than I need to experience a urinary tract infection to know how to treat it. The gender (and age!) of your clinician really shouldn't matter. *Really.* The exception is the patient who is totally uncomfortable being examined by a man or talking to a man about intimate issues. That patient will be better off with a woman doctor. If you feel somewhat guilty discriminating in this way, consider the number of men who go to women urologists. On the other hand, it would be foolish to go with the less qualified doctor based solely on gender, so keep an open mind.

Many women go to a woman gynecologist because they subconsciously—or even consciously—think that talking to a female gynecologist will be like talking to a girlfriend. While it is generally easier to talk to a girlfriend about sex than to your doctor, you are not looking for a new friend at the doctor's office. You have plenty of people to invite to parties and have lunch with. When choosing your gynecologist, you are looking for someone who has the skills you need and whose judgment you trust. Your doctor need not be your friend, but she *or* he does need to be someone who will talk to you, listen to you, and help you. Sometimes that person is a woman, and sometimes it's a man.

V-A-G-I-N-A, VAGINA!

I've come to the conclusion that one of the reasons women have a hard time talking about sex is that they don't like saying the word "vagina." It's a weird thing. They have no problem saying "bladder," "breasts," or "throat." But when it comes to discussing specifics about our genitals, some ladies just can't spit out the word.

My patients will say things like:

> *"I'm having a problem*—down there."
> *"My* good girl *is itchy."*
> *"My* v-jay-jay *hurts."*
> *"My* huh-huh *(pointing) isn't right."*

One of the many reasons I like Dr. Oz is that he brings the word "vagina" into our living rooms and kitchens on a daily basis.

(The first time I appeared on *The Dr. Oz Show* I asked during the rehearsal if I was allowed to say "vagina," as many television shows won't allow it. I was told, "Are you kidding? We say 'vagina' on this show more often than we say 'hello.'" Love that!)

However, while it's one thing to *say* "vagina," it's another to have a conversation about your vagina. Even with your girlfriends, it's not always so easy. Can you imagine going to lunch with your friend and saying, "Sophie, my vagina is so dry, it is like the Sahara Desert. George and I tried to have sex last night, and it was so painful we gave up. How's your vagina?"

Mention What You'd Like to Discuss When You Make Your Appointment

When you book the appointment, this is a good time to mention that you have an issue you would like to discuss. You can simply say, "In addition to my annual exam, I have some concerns related to pain during sex." It will then be noted as the reason for your visit, making it more likely that your doctor will bring up the issue. Some women find it easier to mention their concerns to the assistant who brings them into the examination room. The assistant lets the doctor know that the patient has brought up a specific topic, and then the doctor is likely to initiate the conversation.

Bring It Up at the Beginning of the Visit

At the time of your visit, immediately say (as in right after "hello"), "I know I need to lose weight, but since we have a limited amount of time, I would prefer to discuss other health concerns today." Then go for it. "My libido is gone, my bladder is leaking, etc." That way the topics you want to cover will be addressed as priorities, not tacked on during the last five minutes of your appointment.

Your doctor may totally surprise you and be very helpful and knowledgeable in this area. He or she will be pleased that you have come armed with a great deal of information as well—which you'll have, of course, after reading this book! More often than not, your doctor will be appreciative that you brought up the topic because he or she simply wasn't aware that it was an issue for you.

If You Have an Issue, Make a Separate Appointment to Discuss It

Often a patient will come for her annual "well woman" visit with 10 or 12 issues she wants to discuss. When I explain that there is not enough time to deal with all the problems in one visit and that another appointment needs to be made, sometimes I get an unhappy patient. I understand. You've taken time off from work, parked, and paid your copay. An additional visit is not only inconvenient but also expensive. But there simply isn't time to adequately address the complexities of these gynecological issues at the time of your annual exam, and they can't—and shouldn't—be quickly tagged onto your routine visit.

Many women are reluctant to make an additional appointment, since their insurance may cover only "well woman" visits and not "problem" visits. But face it, you are having a problem! You deserve and need more time. Your doctor is going to take the time to evaluate and treat the problem if that is specifically why you've made an appointment to see him or her. If it is important enough to you to mention the problem, give yourself permission to go for another appointment.

Consider Seeing a Sexual Health or Menopause Specialist, Even if Your Insurance Doesn't Cover It

While good health care is our right and I believe every man and woman should have access to a doctor who can help them, sometimes the care you need is not available within the limitations of your health care plan. If you really feel that you can't discuss your issues with your current doctor, or if your doctor seems truly clueless or embarrassed when you bring them up, bite the bullet and spend the money to see an expert, even if that person is not covered by your insurance plan.

You spend far more annually on the person who fixes your hair than you will pay to see someone who can fix your vagina. Trust me. Even if you have to do a lot of research or travel a great deal to find the right expert, it is likely that you will need only one or two consultations. And you do not need to end your relationship with your regular gynecologist, whom you can continue to see for routine visits.

Make a List

It's always easier to come up with a list of concerns when you are lying in bed at 3:00 AM than when sitting on an exam table wearing a silly paper gown. So, whether it is an annual exam or a visit with a specialist, make a list of what you are worried about before your visit.

When you see your doctor, you can start by saying, "I have some specific concerns, so I jotted down my questions." If you can't manage to spit it out, just hand the doctor the list. This happens more often than you would think. But keep the list short and specific. For example, "Sometimes when I have intercourse it seems dry. What options do I have?" Don't whip out a three-page list containing every symptom you've ever had in the history of your life, as in: "Four months ago I had a pain in my stomach during sex. It hasn't happened since, but I was wondering what caused it?" Be as clear and concise as possible as you list any symptoms that you've had recently and repeatedly.

If All Else Fails . . .

If you have a hard time talking to your doctor about your sexual issue and you don't have the option of seeing another practitioner, I hope that this book at least will have helped you identify your issues and given you ways to fix them. If you think you need to see a pelvic physical therapist, ask your doctor for a referral. If you need a prescription for a local estrogen, just ask for the one you want. Most likely, your doctor will just give you the referral and the prescription, no questions asked. You're welcome!

18

DATING DANGERS

*Have a positive sexual experience
without testing positive*

After a nasty divorce, 10-plus years of no sex, and then an attempt at intercourse that is beyond painful, you finally fix the issue and, miracle of miracles, meet a fabulous guy. A romantic dinner turns into an even more fabulous evening of amazing slippery sex on his couch. You change your status on Facebook and put your Match .com account on hold. Life is good.

And then, two weeks later, a funny discharge appears and you have a lower abdominal ache. Next comes the nerve-racking visit to the gynecologist, followed by the reality that along with the new relationship has come a new infection.

Every savvy woman needs to keep a few things in mind. If you have a new partner, unless he was a virgin before he met you, avoiding a sexually transmitted infection (STI) is a reality that comes with being sexually active.

And then there's that other sexually transmitted situation that some women need to avoid . . . pregnancy.

Sexually Transmitted Infections Are on the Rise

Any sexually active woman can acquire an infection, but midlife women and women who date midlife men are at much greater risk for STIs than most people appreciate. Most of my patients seem to think that STIs are limited to 20- and 30-year-olds who are hanging out in bars or having random hook-ups. Trust me, it's not as if these nasty bugs demand to see proof of age before infecting someone.

The primary risk factors for acquiring a sexually transmitted infection at any age are being unmarried, being sexually active, and having a new sexual partner. Over 50 percent of women over the age of 40 who have never been married or are divorced or widowed are in this category. There are over 50 sexually transmitted diseases, and the midlife woman is not spared. Women bear the consequences more than the guys since STIs are more easily passed from man to woman than from woman to man. If exposed, a woman is twice as likely as a man to contract hepatitis B, gonorrhea, or HIV. To add to the issue, women are less likely to have symptoms than men, which means diagnosis is often delayed or missed altogether.

A lot of women are reassured by the fantasy that the typical 50-year-old guy is "low-risk," especially if he just ended his 30-year marriage. And that's true if he and his wife were monogamous. But let's get realistic. A lot of marriages end because someone wasn't monogamous. It's also not unusual for a newly single person to go maybe just a little overboard with making up for years spent in an unhappy marriage.

So many times my patients say, "I'm not worried . . . he's a *really nice guy*." I've got news for you. Sometimes the nice guys are the ones most likely to have an infection. Face it: creepy guys usually have a harder time getting someone to sleep with them.

There's another reason why women who are postmenopause are at particular risk. Women with low estrogen levels and genital dryness have an elevated likelihood of acquiring an infection since vaginal tissue is thinner and more likely to tear during intercourse, allowing infection an easy portal. That's why the age group in which STI rates are rising most rapidly is adults at midlife and beyond. The Centers for Disease Control and Prevention (CDC) reports that cases of syphilis and chlamydia rose 43 percent among US adults age 55 or older between 2005 and 2009. High-risk HPV is also on the rise.

One solution is to stay home, watch *Sex in the City* reruns, and stick to self-stimulation. A better solution is to know your enemy so you can protect yourself. Here's a summary of the major bugs out there.

HPV

There are one hundred types of human papilloma virus (HPV), most of which are harmless. HPV is currently the most common sexually transmitted infection and is responsible not only for cervical cancer but also for vulvar, vaginal, anal, bladder, and some head and neck cancers. Did I mention genital warts?

HPV isn't new; evidence suggests that ancient Greeks and Romans also suffered from problems related to HPV. There are 20 million documented cases of HPV in the United States each year, but the numbers are likely to be much higher since many people with HPV have no symptoms and don't know they have it. While the highest prevalence of HPV is in 20- to 24-year-old women, who account for 45 percent of infections, a 2007 study in the *Journal of the American Medical Association* found that 27 percent of women between the ages of 25 and 39 had HPV. A 2004 study in the *Journal of Infectious Disease* focused on women up to the age of 85 and found that new infections occurred in *every age group*. While the lowest incidence of new HPV was in the over-45 age group, among those women there was still an infection rate of 12.4 percent. Currently, 80 percent of adults will have been exposed to HPV by the time they are 60. So, no matter how old you are, even if you're a 75-year-old great-grandma, you may be at risk.

While precancer or cancer related to HPV is the most serious consequence of exposure, the most likely consequence of exposure is a crop of genital warts, also known as *Condylomata accuminatum*. Warts are upsetting. *Really upsetting.* It doesn't matter if you are 24, 54, or 84. No one likes getting bumps all over her vagina that look ugly, are irritating, and need to be burned, lasered, or cut off multiple times. While it takes me only a couple of minutes to treat a cluster of warts with topical acid, I spend a lot more time trying to calm down a distressed, usually angry woman who has discovered a nest of "love bumps" all over her genitals.

Consider Sylvie's story:

At 74, I had been a widow and not sexually active for over 15 years. As a birthday present, my son gave me a vacation on the QEII. *During our transatlantic crossing, I met Hymie, and the attraction was instant. Such a happy ending . . . that is, until two months later when a garden of warts developed all over my genitals. This was a souvenir that I could have lived without. I refused to have anything more to do with Hymie and have been alone ever since, because I don't want to tell another man that I have an STD.*

Sylvie was my patient almost 15 years ago, and I will never forget how upset she was, how betrayed she felt, and how the STI kept her from ever initiating another relationship. It was very sad and, potentially, very unnecessary.

Condoms help prevent the transmission of HPV, but they don't guarantee protection since transmission is possible through skin-to-skin contact, known as "outercourse." Gardasil, a vaccine for women ages 9 to 26, guards against the four most common types of HPV. Gardasil is not FDA-approved for women older than 26, not because it is ineffective or dangerous, but because the FDA has determined that the "cost benefit" is not enough to make it worthwhile. Your doctor may be willing to vaccinate you (I vaccinate anyone who requests it), but in addition to sticking out your arm, you will need to stick out your checkbook since insurance won't cover the cost.

Fortunately, most HPV infections clear up on their own, have no consequences, and require no treatment. Your best bet to avoid acquiring HPV is to use a condom. It's also a good idea to do a thorough visual inspection before you turn off the lights. He will just think you are fascinated with his amazing package.

Herpes

Back in the 1970s, herpes became known as "the gift that keeps on giving" owing to the high recurrence rates years after the initial infection. Originally it was thought that if no sore appeared, herpes could not be passed on. While the risk of spreading herpes is highest during outbreaks, the virus is always present in the urinary and genital tract. Even during periods when no sores are visible, there is always the possibility of asymptomatic shedding when the virus can be transmitted between sexual partners. Once a sore does develop, the virus has been present and infectious for days *before* you could see anything.

The result? Infection is often transmitted unknowingly to susceptible partners. In fact, 70 percent of herpes infections can be linked to sexual contact when the "giving" partner had no symptoms.

There are two types of herpes. The first, herpes simplex virus type 1, is most commonly the cause of the oral herpes that is responsible for cold sores on the mouth and lips. The second is herpes simplex virus type 2, which is generally the cause for genital herpes. However, type 1 and type 2 can both be the cause of genital infection as a result of oral sex when there is a cold sore on the mouth of the "giver."

The symptoms of genital herpes are generally most severe during the initial episode and get less severe in recurring episodes. During the first breakout, multiple blisters appear in the genital area and may continue to spread, with new lesions appearing for up to seven days. It is also possible to get blisters on other areas besides the genitals, such as your mouth and lips, during this time. Painful urination, swollen lymph nodes in the groin, and flulike symptoms are all part of herpes. Symptoms generally go away within two to three weeks. The virus will then go into the symptom-free latent stage and lie dormant in a bundle of nerves at the base of the spine, where it remains inactive.

Recurrences are usually much milder than the first outbreak. Some women experience pain, itching, or tingling in the legs, hips, or buttocks before a recurrent outbreak.

If you have no visible ulcers but believe that you may have been exposed, a blood test will detect if you are one of the 20 to 30 percent of sexually active adults who are asymptomatic carriers of herpes. Antibody responses to the virus take some time to build up in your body, usually about three to four months after the initial episode. So a herpes blood test may still have a negative result if you recently became infected. In other words, if you notice the funny sore on his penis after you have sex and get tested the next day, it is too soon to know if you were infected.

Once your blood test is positive for herpes, it will remain positive for life. It is also important to know that your herpes blood test will be positive if you have had a cold sore on your lip.

While there is no cure for herpes, suppressive therapy (taking an antiviral medication every day) not only reduces the likelihood of an actual outbreak but also decreases the chance of asymptomatic transmission. Once an attack begins, starting antiviral therapy as soon as possible will lessen the duration and severity of the symptoms.

If you are not already a carrier of the herpes virus, how do you avoid acquiring herpes? Abstain if your partner has any oral or genital lesions. If no sores are present, a condom should be used to prevent infection by asymptomatic viral sharing. If your partner is a carrier of the herpes virus, he or she should take a daily dose of an antiviral pill (available by prescription), such as acyclovir, valcyclovir, or famciclovir. Be assured, however, that you cannot get herpes by using his toilet, towels, or bedsheets or from sipping out of his wineglass.

If you are the one with herpes, you should take a daily dose of antiviral medication and insist on a condom to protect your partner, unless he already has it.

Gonorrhea

Gonorrhea has been, and still is, one of the most "popular" infections contracted during sexual intercourse. Roughly 700,000 people are infected in the United States every year. The bacteria, officially called *Neisseria gonorrhea,* can be passed on through the mucous membranes of the mouth, throat, anus, urethra, and vagina. It is not in sperm, which is why ejaculation is not necessary to infect someone.

As with almost every other sexually transmitted infection, many people with gonorrhea have no symptoms at all, which is why carriers unwittingly spread the infection before they know they have it. Symptoms that indicate a possible gonorrhea infection include burning during urination, sore throat, abnormal discharge, vaginal itching, bleeding between periods, and infection of the uterus, fallopian tubes, and ovaries. It's important to get screened for gonorrhea regularly. Your doctor can test for it from a cervical swab or a urine test.

If you are not aware that you have gonorrhea, you may end up with gonnococcal arthritis or a joint infection. You can also get a pelvic infection, which can be serious enough to require hospitalization and maybe even surgery. Gonorrhea treatment is a onetime antibiotic treatment with either a shot or a pill.

Chlamydia

Chlamydia is the most common sexually transmitted bacterial infection. Four million cases of *Chlamydia trachomatis* occur every year. The bacteria can be passed on through the mucous membranes of the mouth, throat, anus, urethra, and vagina, and ejaculation is not necessary to spread it. Contrary to popular belief, chlamydia cannot be transmitted via inanimate objects such as a toilet seat. (Are you feeling better about public toilets yet?)

Some people with chlamydia have no symptoms at all, but there are several symptoms that indicate a chlamydia infection:

- Abnormal discharge, abdominal pain, or bleeding between menstrual periods
- Pain during intercourse
- In women, an infection of the urethra causing symptoms similar to a urinary tract infection, including a frequent urge to urinate, burning during urination, and low abdominal pain
- Pelvic inflammatory disease

Chlamydia can be detected by a urine test, with a cervical swab, or with a self-administered vaginal swab. It is easily treated with an oral antibiotic.

Hepatitis

Hepatitis is simply inflammation of the liver. There are multiple types of hepatitis, but the form of this virus that is most commonly spread by engaging in unprotected sexual intercourse is called hepatitis B. This virus can survive outside of the body for a long period of time, so personal items such as toothbrushes and razors can also carry it.

A vaccine is available to protect against hepatitis B and can also be administered after exposure. Signs of hepatitis include right-sided abdominal pain, nausea, vomiting, fatigue, and the whites of the eyes turning a rather unattractive shade of yellow (the most characteristic sign). If your blood test screens positive for hepatitis, you will be referred to a specialist who treats liver disease.

HIV

HIV, or human immunodeficiency virus, weakens the body's immune system, which makes it difficult to fight a multitude of infections and cancers. When the infection is in its most advanced stages, it is called AIDS (acquired immune deficiency syndrome). Without treatment, HIV can cause extreme illness and death. While this is probably the infection that my patients are most concerned about, it is also the infection I diagnose most rarely. Not to minimize the importance of HIV transmission, but the statistics are relatively low for transmission in a heterosexual or lesbian relationship. Having said that, the consequences of this virus are grave, and therefore screening and prevention are critical.

It is possible to have HIV without having any symptoms. Even without symptoms, the illness can be passed on through sexual contact or exposure to contaminated needles. The CDC recommends at least one screening blood test in every sexually active woman, and repeat tests in the event of a new partner. When a test is positive, it is confirmed with another test. One can be tested for HIV at any time, but it is suggested to have a repeat test done at 6, 12, and 24 weeks after suspected exposure.

Syphilis ... Not Just of Historical Interest

When Christopher Columbus discovered America, among the gifts he brought from the Old World was one of the oldest known sexually transmitted diseases . . . syphilis. Al Capone, Adolf Hitler, Scott Joplin, Ludwig von Beethoven, and Abraham Lincoln are all included on the list of famous people alleged to have had this infection, caused by bacteria known as *Treponema pallidum*.

Today, when I suggest to someone that they consider a blood test for syphilis as part of an STI screen, they look at me like I just escaped from the 19th century. Syphilis rates were sky-high in the 1940s but dropped precipitously when penicillin became available for treatment. In 2001 the incidence started to creep up again, but it seems to have leveled off since 2010.

Many people are unaware of the sore that erupts in early syphilis, or they assume that it is nothing to worry about. This painless open sore is called a chancre (pronounced "shanker") and is often found in the genital area, anus, or mouth, but it can be found wherever the bacteria entered the body. After the initial phase, four to ten weeks can go by without symptoms until the second stage occurs; then a rash, fever, or enlarged lymph nodes appear. Secondary syphilis is highly contagious through direct contact with the mucous membranes. If still unrecognized and untreated, tertiary syphilis, the most serious form, can develop one to 30 years later, resulting in neurologic or other life-threatening problems.

Once someone is infected with the organism that causes syphilis, it is *highly* contagious. While most people are aware that the infection is passed on by intercourse, kissing or touching an active sore on the lips, breasts, or genitals can also transmit it.

How to Protect Yourself from STIs
I Use Condoms, I Have Nothing to Worry About, Right?

Wrong. The reality is that condoms are not foolproof. First of all, the HPV and herpes viruses are not in semen but live on skin, so intercourse is not necessary to transmit them. Since a condom covers only the penis, short of strapping on a hefty bag to cover a man's scrotum, anus, and surrounding skin, there is no such thing as total protection.

In general, my patients are very responsible and hyper-aware that infection can be prevented by being vigilant about condom use. In spite of that, studies (and my experience talking to my very responsible, hyper-aware patients) show that single women in midlife who have two or more sexual partners rarely report consistent condom use.

Here's why: Older women are generally dating (surprise!) older men. The older a guy gets, the more difficulty he's going to have getting and maintaining an erection under the best of scenarios. Add a few glasses of wine and a condom, and it's game over. The reality for many men over the age of 60 is that putting on a condom often puts an end to the party, and if a woman wants to get anything accomplished, she often has no choice but to forgo any extra distractions. Since contraception is no longer much of an issue, and a good man is hard to find, but a hard man is just about impossible to find, she usually puts up less of a fight.

So while my patients all *intend* to use condoms, they often don't, since the situation can be "lose the condom or lose the guy." In addition, many of these men and women became sexually active during a time when STIs were not such a heavily discussed issue, so while they intellectually are aware of the risk, emotionally they really don't put themselves in the category of someone who might catch an STI. (This is where the "he's a really nice guy" rationalization comes into play.)

I'm not going to tell you what to do, but I can tell you that I see and treat a lot of infections in women who decided to skip the condom "just this once." But you can also take matters into your own hands! The female condom has not yet caught on, but it is a very viable option. The FC2 condom (formerly known as the Reality Female Condom) is a nonlatex (the same material that's used for surgical gloves), very soft, thin sheath that lines the vagina and not only covers the cervix and vaginal walls but also shields the outside of the vagina. An FC2 condom can be bought over the counter and prevents both infections and pregnancy. No special fitting is needed: one size fits everybody. There is a ring on the outside of the condom that prevents it from getting pushed inside the

> ## Dr. Streicher's SexAbility Survey
>
> Single women were asked what they would do if a new partner was not able to maintain an erection with a condom.
>
> - 47.2 percent said, "Break up. It's not worth chancing a sexually transmitted infection."
> - 38.2 percent said, "I'd have sex, but not intercourse."
> - 14.6 percent said they would forget the condom and hope for the best. (After all, he's a really nice guy.)

vagina during intercourse and also provides protection during oral sex. And as a bonus, many women report that the ring stimulates the clitoris and enhances arousal.

It goes without saying that you should not depend on the man to come prepared. You should have an assortment of male condoms on hand. Be sure they are all marked "extra-large."

Saran Wrap Is Not Just for Food

When HIV first became a health hazard, there was a lot of buzz about using dental dams as protection during oral sex. Dental dams are small sheets of latex that are intended for dentists to use, but they can also be placed on the outside of the vagina during oral sex. But have you ever seen dental dams in a store? Have you ever actually spoken to someone, other than a dentist, who uses dental dams? Neither have I.

It's actually easy to make your own version of a dental dam. Simply take an unlubricated condom (one he's not using!) and cut off the tip. Then cut through one side of it to make a square of latex, which can then be stretched over your vulva.

Another popular alternative to dental dams is plastic wrap, as in the plastic wrap that is intended for food storage. That's right. Many women stretch a piece of plastic wrap over their vulva to prevent any diseases that lurk on his (or her) tongue from infecting their vulva or vagina. I have even been told that the wrap increases sensation. So the next time you are in your grocery aisle and the lady in front of you has just put a jumbo box of plastic wrap in her cart, consider that it may not be for her leftovers.

But buyer beware: plastic wrap intended for food has never been tested for this other purpose, and there is concern that products intended for microwave use may be too porous to keep out HIV and other infectious bugs. You are probably better off cutting open a condom or using a female condom.

A Few Other Tips for the Savvy Dater

One recurrent theme here is that the majority of these infections have no symptoms in their earliest stages. That's why screening is so important. And no, screening for STIs is *not* done automatically when you go to your doctor, nor is it part of a Pap test. So, if your doctor doesn't mention this, you need to ask. You don't need to go into lengthy explanations about the guy you slept with though you probably shouldn't have, or about the indiscretion with your coworker. Simply say, "I would like a screen for sexually transmitted infections today." If your doctor doesn't tell you what he or she usually screens for, ask.

If you are having any symptoms, or know that a sexual partner had an infection, by all means mention it. Your doctor will not be shocked. *Really.* If for whatever reason you prefer not to mention it to your doctor, Planned Parenthood and your local board of health clinics will perform confidential screening.

If you are diagnosed with a sexually transmitted infection, it is important to inform all your current or recent sexual partners, so that they can also be treated. Even if the guy is a jerk you never intend to see again, consider the next woman he might sleep with and do her a favor.

Preventing Pregnancy! Are You Kidding?

Young women are well aware that a possible consequence of having sex is pregnancy. It's the woman who is perimenopausal who often thinks she does not need to worry about inadvertently conceiving. And that may be true. If it has been more than 12 months since your last menstrual period, you have had a hysterectomy or tubal ligation, you're using reliable contraception, you've been infertile before, or your guy has had a vasectomy, you can skip this section. But if you are not in any of those groups, read on.

Roughly 40 percent of pregnancies in the United States are unintended. Not surprisingly, the highest rate of unintended pregnancy is among women aged 24 and younger. Surprisingly, the second-highest rate is among women over 40. In fact, unplanned pregnancies in women over 40 have recently increased because so many women in that group assume they are no longer fertile.

Creep Alert

I know this will shock you, but . . . not every guy is 100 percent honest. (Gasp!) Just because a guy says he's been "fixed" doesn't always mean he's been fixed. I have had two patients who conceived after having sex with a boyfriend who insisted that no protection was necessary.

Most of my patients assume that the further they are on the other side of 40, the less the need for contraception. It's correct that fertility dramatically declines as time marches on: just ask any 40-year-old who is trying to get pregnant. But "declines" is not the same as "disappears." While pregnancy is a lot less likely after 40, it can, and does, happen.

Doctors Know That . . .

. . . 75 percent of pregnancies in women over 40 are unplanned.

Think about it: Geena Davis was 48. Madonna was 44. Jane Seymour was 45. At first glance, you would think that these are the ages at which these celebrities won an Oscar, not the age at which they had a baby. Of course, most midlife pregnancies are a result of in vitro fertilization, using a donor egg from a younger woman. But some women do spontaneously conceive in their forties. While the number-one predictor of fertility is age, there is a significant variability in ovarian aging: some women are infertile at 35, while others are still going strong at 45. That's why contraception is still needed, unless an unplanned pregnancy would not be the end of the world.

Genetics definitely plays a role here. Even if you have nothing in common with your mother, her hormonal pattern is frequently predictive of when you are genetically destined to wind down your fertility. If your mom went through menopause late, you are likely to do so as well—which usually means you will be fertile longer.

The best test of fertility is to become pregnant. Short of that, here are the indicators of your current fertility and of how long you will be fertile:

Clockwork periods: *While regular menses are not a guarantee of ovulation or fertility, it is a pretty good indicator that your ovaries are pumping out estrogen, releasing an egg, and then producing progesterone. Obviously, if you are on the pill, regular periods don't count.*

Blood hormone levels. *Measuring your blood FSH (follicle-stimulating hormone) level is helpful. A low FSH level correlates with good ovarian function and high estrogen levels. A midrange level means things may be winding down, and very high levels usually indicate that the ovaries are out of business. But FSH levels do not steadily decline; they fluctuate from month to month, particularly as women get older. An FSH level tells you where you are hormonally on the day you take the test; it does not predict how long you will stay at that level. Until FSH has been above 30 IUs per milliliters for 12 months, a woman should still consider herself at risk for pregnancy.*

Anti-Müllerian hormone. *Anti-Müllerian hormone (AMH) is the newest way, and probably the best way, to evaluate a woman for ovarian reserve—that is, how good your eggs are and how long they will continue to be functional. AMH is secreted by cells from follicles in the ovary. Follicles are only present if healthy eggs are still around. AMH declines with age as the "good" egg pool declines, and it's completely gone after menopause. Unlike other hormones used to measure fertility, AMH doesn't vary through the cycle and can even be measured in women who are taking birth control pills. While AMH blood level is a reliable way to know what your ovarian reserve is, there is no consensus as to what the lowest level is that indicates you don't* *need contraception. In general, if AMH is above 0.5, there is good ovarian reserve and contraception is needed.*

Fortunately, if you are a midlife woman still at risk of pregnancy, you have a lot of options.

Contraceptive Options at Midlife

Barrier contraception is still the go-to method for most women. Yes, I'm referring to condoms. Readily available, easy, and safe, condoms are a tried-and-true method that works. The bonus is that they also protect against sexually transmitted infections if that is an issue. The main limiting factor is that some men don't want to use them.

Diaphragms seem primitive, but they still have a place. A side bonus for the midlife woman is that the diaphragm sometimes gives a little support to the urethra and helps with incontinence! There are other barrier methods, such as the female condom, the cervical cap, and the vaginal contraceptive sponge, but like condoms, they all need to be used correctly and consistently. I'm a big fan of long-acting, set-it-and-forget-it methods, such as intrauterine devices and Nexplanon.

Hormonal Contraception

Many women think that the pill is not an option for the over-35 crowd, but contrary to popular belief, healthy, normal-weight women who are nonsmokers can safely use hormonal contraception, such as the pill or vaginal ring, up to age 55. The newest pills contain minuscule amounts of estrogen compared to earlier birth control pills and therefore have a much lower risk of complications such as blood clots or stroke.

In addition to preventing pregnancy, hormonal contraception has a number of noncontraceptive benefits that are particularly relevant to woman over 40. These include less pain with periods, lighter periods, and, best of all, a significant decrease in ovarian and uterine cancer. In addition, taking a low-dose birth control pill is an excellent way to regulate the erratic periods and crazy mood swings that are part of the perimenopausal hormonal roller coaster. The downside is that in a small but very real percentage of women, hormonal contraception can cause vaginal dryness and decreased libido. For more detailed information on birth control options, refer back to chapter 12.

Good to Go!

So now that you are ready to have safe sex (and are not too freaked out, I hope, by the possibility of acquiring an infection), it's time to have *fun sex*. Confidence is a huge part of that equation. Not a day goes by that I don't see a midlife patient who is reentering the dating scene after a long hiatus and feeling more than a little trepidation. Childbirth and time (and gravity!) are not always kind to women's thighs and butts, and many women express at least some insecurity about the appearance of their middle-aged body. That's understandable, since many women who reenter the dating scene are not only 20 years older than the first time around but at least 20 pounds heavier.

If you are feeling less than confident about the appearance of your body, there are a few things to keep in mind:

- The guy you are dating is likely to be the same age as you, or even a few years older, and he won't look like his 20-year-old self either! His six-pack will probably have morphed into a not so attractive one-pack.
- Older guys don't have great eyesight.
- There is no such thing as owning too much beautiful lingerie. Wear it even if you are not planning a sexual encounter.
- Candlelight is essential. Not only is it incredibly romantic, but everyone looks more attractive.

So turn out the lights! But not before you read chapters 19 and 20.

part seven

TAKING YOUR NEW SEXABILITY
TO THE NEXT LEVEL

19

VAGINAL VANITY

Why some opt for an upgrade

Throughout history, women have adorned or altered their appearance to appear more attractive and desirable. Today we curl, roll, set, perm, and straighten our hair. We paint our fingernails and toenails. We tattoo our faces and bodies. We wear jewelry around our necks, on our fingers, and in our ears. Never mind the clothes we purchase, design, or create to adorn our bodies.

The genitals are no exception to this rule of adornment. Hair removal, piercings, tattoos, and yes, even surgery are all things that many women choose to do in the interest of making their private parts more attractive. It's interesting to note that some women spend an inordinate amount of time and energy "enhancing" the appearance of their external genitalia when the average guy would probably flunk even the simplest quiz regarding the appearance of his partner's parts. Face it, how many guys even notice when you make a major change to the hair on your *head*? These enhancements usually say more about how *we* want to look than about any preferences the men in our lives seem to have.

The Bare Necessities: What You Should Know Before Grooming Your Pubes

Changing trends in hairstyles are not limited to the hair on your head. As a gynecologist, I get a firsthand view of what's trendy when it comes to pubic hair. Today less is more, and many of the women I see alter their pubic hair in some way, whether it's just a trim or complete removal.

But sparse pubic hair wasn't always the style. During the 15th century, abundant pubic hair was a sign of not only sexuality but also good health. Someone with a Brazilian in 1450 hadn't just been to the beach but more likely had a sexually transmitted disease. Syphilis was the STD du jour back then, and the only treatment was mercury injections, which had the nasty side effect of making hair fall out. All of it. If you were lucky enough to escape syphilis, you probably contracted pubic lice. And without the option of stocking up on anti-lice shampoo from the corner drugstore, you would simply shave everything off. Enter the merkin: a pubic hair wig that men and women pasted on to hide their vulvar baldness due to syphilis or lice.

Why Do We Have Pubic Hair?

Before central heating, pubic hair was what kept the genitals warm. The obvious evolutionary advantage here is that people with warm genitals are more likely to take their clothes off, and men are more likely to maintain an erection. Evolutionarily, the other function of pubic hair was to draw attention to the genitals. (Evidently it is not just the modern man who seems to need a map to ensure he is heading in the right direction.) The natural oil in hair also provides skin lubrication and decreases friction during intercourse. I've seen some pretty nasty "rug burn" from rubbing while bare.

Why Do Women Choose to Remove It?

Today's styles range from full bush to completely hairless. While most hairstyles follow the fashion of the day, some women remove public hair for religious reasons. Others say that baldness increases sensation during sex and that they feel it is more "hygienic." But most simply prefer the way it looks when they have little pubic hair. Pubic hair spilling out the sides of a bathing suit is a major *Glamour* "don't." But I'm a gynecologist, not a stylist, so I'm going to focus on the medical aspects.

What Is the Best Way to Remove Pubic Hair?

If you do choose to lose the pubes, a multimillion-dollar industry has evolved around pubic fashion, giving you no shortage of options. Waxing, shaving, electrolysis, clipping, chemical depilatories, and laser removal are all at your disposal.

Keep in mind that, with the exception of clipping, red bumps commonly result no matter what method you choose, particularly in African American women. Professional waxing and electrolysis result in the least amount of irritation, allergy, or complications, but these methods can be expensive . . . not to mention painful. Some women use a topical anesthetic (Emla cream, available by prescription) to reduce the agony.

In spite of what seems to be the proliferation of waxing salons on practically every corner, the overwhelming majority of women simply shave their pubic hair and consider the task no different than shaving the hair on their legs or in their armpits.

My only word of warning is this: before choosing a method of permanent hair removal, such as electrolysis, keep in mind that next year the bush may be in style again and you may be forced to invest in a modern-day merkin!

Hairstyles

Let me tell you, when it comes to pubic hairstyle, I have seen it all:

Natural: *Full bush, forest*
Trimmed: *hair shortened in length, but not removed or shaped*
Shaped: *Removal of the hair that would be sticking out of a bathing suit, but otherwise left alone*

"Fancy" shapes: *Hearts, arrows, and initials*
Landing strip: *a thin "runway" right down the middle*
Brazilian: *Bare and bald, "Hollywood Bare"*

From both my observation and research, how women choose to style their pubic hair seems to be associated with age, socioeconomic status, religion, race, and yes, sexual behavior. The 20- to 30-year-old crowd is the most likely to go bald (intentionally anyway), and the more disposable income they have the more they tend to go to a waxing salon, as opposed to doing it on their own at home. For the record, most women I see are either au natural or somewhat shaped.

Complications of Hair Removal

Burns from wax that is too hot, ingrown hairs, and chafing are all possible consequences of hair removal. While many women tell me that they shave because it feels "cleaner" and more hygienic, the truth is that hair removal may increase the risk of some skin infections. In surgery, any shaving is done just minutes before the surgeon makes a skin incision since it has been shown that shaving the day before surgery increases the chance of wound infection.

A study released in March 2013 suggested that the irritation from hair removal may be responsible for an increased vulnerability to acquiring vulvar molluscum contagiosum, a common sexually transmitted virus that causes a skin eruption.

But if hair removal goes wrong? Not to worry! Consider this:

"Botched Brazilian? Misbehaved shave? Kitty Carpet™ 'reusable downstairs toupee' to the rescue!" This is an actual product! I can't make this stuff up!

And accidents can happen. One of my patients, Emily, decided to wax her pubic hair the day before her son's bar mitzvah. For those of you who are not Jewish, let me tell you that there is no tradition that requires the mother of the bar mitzvah boy to have groomed pubic hair. The wax was way too hot, and Emily ended up with second-degree burns on her vulva. She may well be the only mother of a bar mitzvah boy who has ever attended her son's service wearing a skirt and no underpants.

> According to *The Journal of Urology,* self-inflicted cuts and infections from grooming pubic hair accounted for 1,089 ER visits between 2002 and 2012.

Embellishments
Hair Dye

Botox and face-lifts are not the only way women camouflage their true age. Pubic hair dye is alive and well in more salons and pharmacies than you know. (Yes, that's what's going on behind those closed doors!) For you do-it-yourselfers, Smart Bikini Colour and Betty Beauty ("for the hair down there") comes in an array of colors. For example, Smart Bikini comes in hot chocolate, cool blond, amber flame, intense red, and for those really special occasions, carmine pink.

But beware! Terri, a 48-year-old attractive blonde, called my office frantically one afternoon and insisted on an emergency appointment. When she walked in the door, it was obvious she was in a lot of pain. A quick exam revealed that her vulva was blistered, bright red, and so swollen she was unable to pee. She admitted that she had been dying her pubic hair to match the hair on her head. "My husband doesn't know I'm not a real blonde," she explained. Midway through the dye job, she got distracted and left it on too long.

I inserted a catheter, applied a burn salve, gave her some pain medication, and sent her home. Four weeks later, I saw her for a follow-up visit and was not surprised to see that she was now a brunette—top and bottom.

Genital Piercing

Now, I happen to love a bauble as much as the next girl, but the idea of genital jewelry has never really appealed to me. Having said that, many women don't limit the holes in their body to their ears.

Female genital piercing has been around for thousands of years, although exactly how long, is difficult to say since plenty of myths seem to be woven into histories of piercing.

Piercing in modern Western culture became fashionable with the punk movement and among some gay and S&M subcultures, but now this fashion has become quite mainstream.

Why do women pierce their genitals? Well, it's clearly not to show off a gift from a lover, since no one gets to see it except the lover—that would be kind of like getting a gift of a beautiful diamond ring that you only get to wear to bed.

Clitoral hood piercing is by far the most popular such adornment. I've also seen piercings of the inner and outer labia. The very brave actually pierce the clitoris, but bleeding and nerve damage often result.

Many women who pierce their genitals do so not for the sake of appearance but to improve sexual stimulation. Since for many women orgasms occur only with clitoral stimulation, a clitoral hood piercing increases the chance of having an orgasm during vaginal intercourse. In surveys, some women reported having their first orgasm only after getting pierced. (Those women evidently do not own vibrators.)

While you might assume that the woman who has a pierced nose, pierced tongue, and 12 holes in her ears is the most likely to also have a pierced clitoral hood, that is far from the case. Many women who have a genital piercing don't have any other piercings but are just trying to spice up their love lives. Some critics believe that genital piercing is motivated by masochism—after all, what could seem more masochistic than driving a needle through the most sensitive part of your anatomy? But evidently, if pain is what you're after, genital piercing isn't really what you want because it doesn't really hurt that much, no more than piercing an ear or a navel—or so I am told.

The Risks of Genital Piercings

Most physicians oppose piercing anywhere but the earlobe. Not just because a ring through the nose looks just fine on a pig but really unattractive on a human, but because of the possibility of a complication. For starters, even "professional" piercers are often unregulated and therefore not required to know anything about anatomy or sterile technique. It is therefore no surprise that every year a significant number of labial piercings end disastrously owing to serious infections, bleeding, nerve damage, or scarring. If equipment isn't being sterilized at a piercing studio, the procedure could also pass on any number of diseases, including hepatitis, HIV, and other STDs. The Red Cross has a 12-month waiting period before accepting a blood donation from someone who has been pierced, sending a clear message about the increased risk of infection. Is it worth potentially losing your labia—or your life for that matter—to make a fashion statement?

If you decide to forge ahead, at a minimum, make sure the piercer is a member of the Association of Professional Piercers to ensure that he or she is trained in sterile technique and knows basic first aid. Make sure the piercer wears gloves, uses a fresh needle, and cleans the area with antiseptic. To minimize the chance of infection, choose stainless steel, niobium, or titanium jewelry. Avoid sex, pools, hot tubs, and tight clothing until the piercing has healed. And avoid telling your mother—*forever*.

The ultimate complication I am aware of was a case that was presented at a sexual medicine conference of a woman who was receiving oral sex. She evidently made a sudden movement and her clitoral hood piercing got caught in her lover's teeth (brace yourself ladies!), causing her clitoris to partially tear off. Thankfully, doctors were able to reattach the tissue. I suspect she did not reattach her jewelry.

Vajazzling: A Special Gift for the Woman Who Has Everything

If you have never heard of Vajazzling (yes, it's a verb), visit http://www.vajazzling.com to expand your clearly limited education. Vajazzling is defined as "the act of applying glitter and jewels to a woman's bikini area for aesthetic purposes." You will find information on this site so that you too can "start Vajazzling your business," "treat yourself to a Swarovski experience," and learn "how to stand out against competitors" by learning to apply hearts, stars, and other designs to your vulva. You will even discover a tutorial on combining a tattoo with Vajazzling for added effect. No pubic hair required.

Tattoos

Vulvar tattoos, while not as mainstream as hair removal, are accepted by many teens, young adults, and yes, midlife women. Tattoos on the vulva present the same issues as tattoos on other parts of the body, including infection, scarring, and regret. The only thing less fun than getting a tattoo on the pubic area is removing a tattoo on the pubic area. However, unlike the tattoo on your arm, there is always the option of letting your pubic hair grow over RALPH—I WILL LOVE YOU FOREVER once Ralph is out of the picture.

A study published in the *Journal of Sexual Medicine* in 2012 looked at sexual behavior and vulvar "modification" and found that women who had tattoos and piercings were more likely to have intercourse at an early age, more likely to have frequent intercourse, and more likely to have oral sex than women without embellishment.

Cosmetics

I would be willing to bet that when your mother gave you your first lipstick, she did not mention that there was also makeup for your other lips. My Own Pink Button is a cosmetic to pink up your labia and clitoris, which is evidently something that some women feel makes them more attractive.

For those who aren't interested in making their genitals pinker but feel compelled to make their genitals lighter, there is Pink Daisy Labia Bleaching Cream and Biofade vulvar bleaching cream. I can't imagine why someone would purchase those products, but evidently someone is doing just that.

Extreme Makeover: Vagina Edition

It's one thing to glue a few crystals on your mons or dye your pubic hair pink for kicks. It's quite another thing to undergo plastic surgery to change the appearance of your genitals. Along with the "less is more" pubic hair trend comes the ability to clearly see what things look like, and as with every other part of the body, women tend to be really critical of their appearance.

When I first went into practice, I never had a single patient request cosmetic genital surgery. Now it is a request I get at least once a week. While many women are motivated by the perception that surgery will result in improved sexual pleasure, others simply don't like the appearance of their genitals. A desire for improved "self-esteem" is often expressed, and there is no question that comfort with one's genitals is associated with sexual confidence and enjoyment. It is not unusual for women to have surgery in midlife, when they find themselves between relationships and want to "reinvent" themselves.

In general, there are two categories of genital plastic surgery—external or internal.

External Genital Procedures

The most common form of external plastic surgery that women undergo is a labioplasty, or surgery to the labia. Usually, women choose this procedure when they perceive their labia minora to be too long, too thick, or asymmetrical. Some women, when reassured that their labia are slightly longer than average but perfectly normal, still want a "trim" based on their idea of what is attractive. Some women are reluctant to let their partners see them since they think their labia are "too floppy," and therefore they avoid being sexually intimate.

Some women do have excessively long labia, a condition referred to as labial hypertrophy. Labial hypertrophy is defined as labia that are longer than four centimeters and extend well beyond the labia majora. When measuring labia, in case you are so inclined, you should spread the labia outward (like a butterfly) and measure from the base to the tip of the triangle. While many women want surgery solely for cosmetic reasons, some women with excessively long labia have difficulty with vaginal irritation, urine spraying in all directions, and discomfort during sports or sex.

Dr. Streicher's SexAbility Survey

When asked how they felt about their labia,

45.5 percent of women said, "I don't think about my labia."
11.5 percent said, "I wish they were shorter."
35.4 percent said, "I love my labia just the way they are."
7.6 percent said, "I have a labia?"

When the men weighed in and were asked what they thought about their wife's/partner's labia,

31 percent said, "I don't think about her labia."
2.5 percent said, "I wish they were shorter."
57.1 percent said, "I love her labia just the way they are."
8.9 percent said, "She has a labia?"

Both gynecologists and plastic surgeons perform labioplasty, but not *every* gynecologist or plastic surgeon does the procedure. If you are interested, not only do you need to ask your doctor if he or she performs this procedure, but how often and using what technique. Some simply trim the labia. Others take out a wedge of tissue in order to keep an anatomically correct shape and labial edge. Some women desire clitoral hood reduction as well.

As with any cosmetic procedure, in order to get the result you have in mind, you need to clearly communicate with your doctor! Furthermore, I strongly advise that your discussion with your doctor include a mirror so that you point to exactly what you want changed.

Most women who undergo labioplasty are very satisfied with the results and are glad they went through with it, even if it means a month of no sex, bike riding, or tight clothes.

Women who requested labioplasty in one study gave the following motivations for the surgery:

Aesthetic dissatisfaction (87 percent)
Discomfort in clothing (64 percent)
Discomfort in playing sports (26 percent)
Uncomfortable sex (43 percent)

Internal Genital Procedures

Labial shortening isn't the only vaginal cosmetic procedure that women request. Vaginal tightening surgery, also known as "vaginal rejuvenation," is increasingly popular and includes procedures that are *designed* to reduce the size of the opening of the vagina, or the introitus, and in some cases bring together lax musculature along the length of the vagina to make things tighter during intercourse.

Women who have had many children, large children, or vaginal tears at the time of delivery often are left with a relaxed or scarred introitus. A vaginal opening that gaps due to childbirth usually has no effect on sexual function and response. Nevertheless, some women find a gaping vaginal opening aesthetically displeasing or less sexually satisfying and want the vaginal opening to be tightened. This procedure, called perineoplasty, involves making a small incision at the bottom of the vaginal opening, taking out a small V-shaped segment of skin, and restoring the opening of the vagina to a prepregnancy appearance. While I am occasionally asked to do a perineoplasty, the majority of the time I do this as part of a more extensive surgery, such as repair of a dropped bladder or rectum or an incontinence procedure.

The goal of this type of surgery is to restore normal anatomy without making things *too* tight. Some women are curious if physicians need to know the measurement of the penis in their life prior to surgery. The answer is no; I neither ask for measurements nor take measurements. Surgeons simply use a "standard" guide to determine the size: if two fingers can fit with a bit of "wiggle room," the opening will be just fine for most any penis.

Every ob-gyn has had the experience of the witty guy who requests "an extra stitch to tighten things up for me" while still in the delivery room or during a pre-op consultation. The only appropriate response, of course, is for the obstetrician to look piercingly at the guy's crotch and inquire just how small he needs it.

Tightening of the actual vaginal walls (removal of excess internal tissue) is not generally performed for cosmetic purposes, but only if there is pelvic relaxation or prolapse of the bladder or rectum. Some experts will surgically tighten pelvic floor muscles, but most experts believe that pelvic physical therapy (as opposed to surgery) is a far more appropriate way to enhance sexual satisfaction if the vagina is perceived as being "too loose." While using a local vaginal estrogen product has not been proven to "tighten" vaginal walls, it stands to reason that the increased blood flow, increased lubrication, and thickening of the tissue might make a difference.

Dr. Michael Goodman, a leading expert in female genital plastic surgery, has done extensive research into the motivations, complications, and outcomes of genital cosmetic surgery. According to one of his large studies, women's motivations for genital plastic surgery include:

To look better
To enhance self-esteem
To feel more normal
"I feel discomfort" (with sex, sports, clothes, etc.)
Chafing
"I feel loose," "I feel large," etc.
To increase friction, enhance sex
Pleasure
To increase partner's sexual pleasure
At the urging of sexual partner

Dr. Goodman's research shows that self-esteem and sexual satisfaction are very dependent on a woman feeling comfortable with the appearance of her genitals. "Every published study on outcomes after female plastic genital surgery," he says, "shows that *in the hands of an experienced genital plastic/cosmetic surgeon,* 95% of women undergoing external cosmetic procedures were happy with the results and 85–90% of women undergoing vaginal tightening reported enhancement of sexual function. A single study examining men's experience showed that less than 80% of these women's male partners noted enhanced sexual experience."

While I have not personally done research in this area, I can tell you anecdotally that my patients who have chosen to have surgery are pleased with the results and express increased confidence and sexual satisfaction.

A few years ago a woman came to see me escorted by her husband, who requested a vaginal tightening. At my insistence, he reluctantly did not accompany her during the examination. Her vagina and vulva were completely normal, and I asked her why she wanted the procedure. She explained that "he wanted it" and she wanted "whatever he wanted."

I declined to do the surgery and explained to him that she was completely normal and that any "tightening" would result in pain during intercourse. As he stormed out my office door he angrily said, "You must think I'm a real pencil dick!"

I agreed.

It goes without saying that no woman should ever be pressured into undergoing surgery by a partner.

With all of these genital surgical procedures, as in any surgical procedure, there is always the risk of a complication such as infection or bleeding. There is always the risk that you won't be happy with the results. Unlike shaving, hair dye, or Vajazzling, there's no going back if you go under the knife. Be sure before you proceed, and be sure you have a surgeon who is experienced.

What Are the Strangest Things Gynecologists Have Seen?

I am asked this question at cocktail parties on a regular basis: "What is the most unusual vaginal adornment, piercing, hairstyle, or tattoo that you've ever seen?"

After more than 20 years in clinical practice, I've seen my share of strange and wondrous things when women come in for their regular exam. Here's a sampling from my practice as well as other doctors':

- A "mange-moi" tattoo on the mons, right next to the clitoris, with a picture of the Rolling Stones logo
- A little square of hair left on the mons that looked like a Hitler mustache

- Sparkly "hair" spray
- Tattoos of "kissing" lips on the mons
- A tattoo on the mons of little eyes looking out
- A chain between a clitoral piercing and a labial piercing
- A tattoo of an ice cream cone on the pubic area
- A tattoo on the inner thigh consisting of an arrow pointing to the introitus and the words ENTER HERE

20

TOYS YOU DON'T WANT TO SHARE WITH YOUR CHILDREN

How toys can add pleasure and novelty to your sex life

Sex toys are not for lonely deviants—they are . . . well, for you. And if you are a woman who has never entered the wonderful world of vibrators, dildos, and erotica, it's time to enhance your SexAbility and take the plunge.

You may think that this is a strange and slightly unorthodox recommendation coming from an academic, board-certified gynecologist, but it makes perfect sense considering that, historically, vibrators were not sexual items that women bought for themselves but *medical* devices used by doctors as treatment methods.

The History of Vibrators
It all started in the 1800s. But first, we have to go back much further. To ancient Greece.

Hyster, the ancient Greek word for "uterus," eventually became the root word for many medical terms describing conditions that plague women. Originally the word "hysteria" dated back to

300 BC when Hippocrates (of Hippocratic Oath fame) described hysteria as suffocation or madness of the womb resulting from sexual deprivation or lack of orgasms.

During Victorian times, the word "hysterical" had nothing to do with finding something really funny or becoming uncontrollably emotional—it was all about problems stemming from the uterus being "sick." Specifically, an American gynecologist theorized that a "sick womb" could cause both physical and psychological disturbances such as anxiety, depression, sleeplessness, pelvic heaviness, fainting, nervousness, edema, shortness of breath, disinterest in sex, and, in its most severe form, insanity. Some women were accused of having hysteria if they didn't obey their husbands or if they rejected traditional "womanly" roles.

This concept continued well into the late 1800s, when nearly every ailment that might befall a woman, including tuberculosis and heart and lung disease, was at some point blamed on a "sick, wandering" uterus. Women were advised to placate their "angry" uterus by having babies, being submissive, not educating themselves, not expressing their opinions, and most important, letting the men run the show. The medical diagnosis of hysteria was practically epidemic.

Every Disease Needs a Cure

It wasn't long before treatments to restore uterine health were proliferating. Many "hysterical" women were sent off for "rest cures" in which they were submitted to isolation and sensory deprivation for extended periods of time. If they weren't hysterical at the beginning of the "cure," they were generally truly hysterical by the end.

The other popular cure for hysteria was to stimulate a woman to orgasm. The rationale was that an orgasm, or paroxysm, would cause the "sick uterus" to be restored to health, which in turn would improve the general health of the woman.

Ideally, this orgasm would be produced by intercourse in the marriage bed. Single women who suffered from hysteria were told to marry. Married women were told to spend more time in bed with their husband.

Not every case of hysteria responded to more sex, and some hysterical women didn't have a husband. Desperate cases called for desperate measures, so the doctor was obligated to elicit orgasm by massaging a woman's genitals in his office. As you can imagine, this therapy, while wildly popular, was *exhausting* for the poor physician, especially when women would return week after week for additional treatments.

History does not indicate that the doctor personally experienced any sexual pleasure himself. Manually massaging a woman to orgasm was burdensome and tedious. It sometimes took an hour or more, and since women were rarely "cured," weekly or, in extreme cases, daily treatments were necessary. Aside from being exhausting, this treatment regimen was not particularly lucrative because it took so much time.

"Necessity is the mother of innovation," and by the mid-1800s a number of innovative devices were invented so that the doctor no longer had to use his hand to "treat" hysterical women. The first of these devices, in 1843, was the French Water Jet Massage treatment. (Evidently hysterical women lived all over the world!) The hysterical woman would sit in a chair and a jet of water would be directed at her clitoris until orgasm was reached. Water systems never became popular, but while "effective," they were expensive, cumbersome, and not practical for most doctors' offices since a special water chamber with pipes and a warmer was required. So the search for easier methods continued.

Keep in mind that in the mid-1860s electricity had not yet been harnessed for power. Before electricity, steam was the source of power, not just for trains but also—you guessed it—for vibrators. In 1869 a hysterical woman would lie facedown on a "Manipulator Table" (with a hole conveniently cut out to expose her pelvic region) in order to have her genitals "massaged" by a steam-operated paddle.

Electricity to the Rescue

It was in 1880, when inventors were trying to find new uses for the recently discovered electricity, that the first electric vibrator became part of the treatment option for doctors who were exhausted from manually manipulating women.

The first electromechanical device to emerge was the Weiss Model. Over the next 15 years, more than 12 electric models were invented to increase the efficiency of inducing orgasm. By the late 1880s, electrical devices were commonplace, and electric vibrators were routinely used in physicians' offices to treat primarily middle- and upper-class white Victorian women.

Time is money, and one of the advantages of the electric vibrator was how fast it could do the job. Manual massage required not only skill but time. An electric vibrator induced orgasm in less than four minutes—sometimes quicker! Electrical treatment of hysteria was effective, efficient, and extremely lucrative, since severe cases required multiple treatments a week.

The First Half of the 20th Century: The Vibrator Comes Home

During the Victorian era, masturbation was frowned upon. Women were discouraged from horseback riding or even traveling on trains, since the motion might elicit "excitement." Using vibration for medical purposes, however, was in a different category, and in the early 1900s, ads for home devices began to pop up in women's magazines, such as *The Women's Home Companion* and *Home Needlework Journal*. Again, these ads emphasized that vibrators were to improve health and treat medical problems. They were never advertised or meant to be used as sexual devices.

Vibrators really hit the mainstream when they made it into the 1918 version of eBay . . . the Sears, Roebuck catalog. For the first time vibrators were marketed not just to wealthy white women but to the mainstream.

Buried in the middle of a page filled with small electrical appliances meant for the home, the ad read:

Aids That Every Woman Appreciates
Portable Vibrator. Neat, compact vibrator with 3 applicators.
Very useful and satisfactory for home service.
Complete with attachments for churning, mixing,
beating, grinding, buffing, and operating a fan
$5.95

This was quite the luxury item considering that a sewing machine sold for $8.95. Since the portable vibrator could also be used for churning, mixing, grinding, buffing, and operating a fan, however, it was actually quite the bargain!

By 1920 hysteria was no longer a popular diagnosis, and vibrators disappeared from doctors' offices. Ads for vibrators were no longer seen in the "respectable" press. For the first time vibrators showed up as "sexual devices" in early porn films. In 1952 the American Psychiatric Association dropped "hysteria" as a medical term, and an era officially came to an end.

Around 1969 the vibrator reemerged in advertisements in women's magazines, where it was touted as a "beauty aid" or a "personal body massager" to be used "anywhere."

The 1970s: The Medical Community Weighs In

In direct opposition to the Victorians' attitude toward vibrators, the mid-twentieth-century medical community declared that vibrators were not only not medically beneficial but actually harmful. During the 1970s, a number of journals published articles with the same themes:

- Vibrators are harmful
- Normal women don't need or use vibrators

- Vibrators are used by only a small number of dysfunctional women
- Women who use vibrators are in danger of becoming "vibrator-dependent"

In 1953 Alfred Kinsey reported that fewer than 1 percent of women used vibrators. In the early 1990s, attitudes began to shift, and a 1992 National Health and Social Life Survey revealed that, while only 2 percent of women had purchased vibrators, 17 percent were "interested." Interest turned into practice, and in 2003 a study showed that 16 percent of women were using vibrators. By 2004 almost half of American women had at least tried one.

Fast-forward to today. Vibrators are commonly used and recommended by enlightened doctors for sexual health. In 2009 the largest scientific study of vibrator use was conducted by the Indiana University of Sexual Research and published in the *Journal of Sexual Medicine*. In that study, 2,056 women between the ages of 18 and 60 were questioned about personal vibrator use. Fifty-two percent of them reported not only that they had used a vibrator but that their sexual satisfaction had increased as a result.

And far from being something that is used only for masturbation, vibrators were used by couples 80 percent of the time.

Why and When I Recommend Vibrators

As a physician and sexual health expert, I recommend the use of a vibrator in a number of situations and medical conditions.

To Reach Orgasm

Many of my patients have never had an orgasm. Ever. They expect to have an orgasm during intercourse, and when it doesn't happen, they not only are at a loss but often feel like there is something wrong with them. It was Sigmund Freud who set the stage for the notion that women should expect to have vaginal orgasms, and this myth was propagated until the more realistic (and scientific) Kinsey reported in 1953 that clitoral stimulation is unlikely to happen during intercourse. In their estimate, only 30 percent of women are able to achieve an orgasm with intercourse.

More recent scientific studies show that 30 percent is probably a gross overestimation and that only about 5 percent of women are able to reach orgasm with vaginal intercourse. This is not to say that a vibrator is always required to reach orgasm for everyone else, since clitoral stimulation to elicit orgasm can occur with digital, oral, or other stimulation. But for many normal women, the intensity of a vibrator provides the only way they are able to climax.

To Enhance Arousal

As women age and hormones decline, very often so does clitoral and vaginal sensation. Many women after menopause find that achieving an orgasm becomes a lot more difficult. Just as Victorian doctors found fingers to be inefficient and tedious, many modern women find that a vibrator is the best way to intensify sensation. In addition, many medical conditions, such as diabetes, cardiovascular disease, and multiple sclerosis, cause nerve damage that results in a need for more intense stimulation to achieve the same effect (see chapter 15).

To Spice Up a Stagnant Sex Life

Face it. Spending years with the same partner can get a little boring. As I mentioned earlier in the book (and have said on *The Dr. Oz Show*), "If you have cornflakes for breakfast every day for 30 years, you get to the point where you don't even want breakfast anymore. If one day a chocolate chip pancake shows up on your plate, suddenly breakfast is a lot more appealing." Sometimes a vibrator is as good as a chocolate chip pancake.

Partner Issues

This is actually one of the most common reasons why women buy and use a vibrator. Many women have no partner, or they have a partner who is physically incapable of intercourse. Sometimes men who suffer from erectile dysfunction avoid intimacy, knowing that they can't "deliver." They are thrilled and relieved to find a way to pleasure their partner *without* intercourse.

Use It or Lose It

Multiple scientific studies have shown that women who are sexually active, with or without a partner, have less vaginal atrophy, even when their estrogen levels are very low. Women who regularly are having intercourse with a dildo or penis (twice a week, ideally), with consistent stretching of the vaginal walls and increased vaginal blood flow, have better tissue elasticity and less pain if they resume intercourse. Even if intercourse never again occurs, vaginal tissues are healthier when "used."

When Intercourse Is Off the Table

Vaginal atrophy cannot be reversed instantaneously, and it is important to keep sexual stimulation alive and well while "repair" is in progress. Some women with severe atrophy, despite everything, are simply not able to have comfortable sexual intercourse. Most find it is not an issue if they are able to experience intimacy and satisfying orgasms with clitoral stimulation.

Likewise, some women are not able to have intercourse because of medical conditions such as vaginismus or radiation or because they're recovering from surgery. Just because a woman can't have intercourse doesn't mean she can't have sexual stimulation and reach orgasm. The vibrator makes it easier, with or without a partner.

Types of Sex Toys

Sex toys fall into two basic categories: those that are inserted into the vagina (and sometimes rectum), and those that are used for external stimulation. Some toys do both. They come in multiple lengths, diameters, materials, and colors. Most vibrators are battery-operated or rechargeable. There are even vibrators with a USB port so that it can be recharged on your computer. Explain that to your boss at work!

Internal Toys

A traditional internal toy is four to eight inches in length and shaped like a penis. A nonvibrating toy is called a dildo. A vibrating toy stimulates only the vaginal walls and sometimes the G-spot. This is the type of toy that well-meaning men often buy for their partners, thinking that what women want is something that is exactly like a penis only always hard and constantly shaking.

External Toys

Since most women are unable to have an orgasm without clitoral stimulation, it makes sense that external clitoral stimulators are the preferred toy. External vibrators come in a variety of shapes and sizes. Many are small enough to slip into your pocket or purse for a "quick fix."

The Best of Both Worlds

The cameo appearance of the Pearl Rabbit on the hit TV show *Sex in the City* probably had the biggest impact on normalizing the use of the vibrator.

Women who had *never* had an orgasm became, thanks to the Rabbit, multi-orgasmic. In no time the Rabbit became the most popular adult toy and a popular gift. Nothing says Valentine's Day like a pink Rabbit and a heart-shaped box of chocolates.

The Rabbit is a multi-area, multi-action stimulator toy. Essentially, it is a penis-shaped vibrator that provides internal G-spot stimulation. The spinning "pleasure beads" (the pearls), located at the bottom of the shaft, stimulate the inside of the vaginal opening. Finally, there is a protruding "rabbit's head" that vibrates while the rabbit ears "tickle" the clitoris. The speed and intensity of the vibrations can be controlled with either a hand-held control or a speed control at the base of the toy. Be prepared to buy lots of batteries.

Partner Toys

While any toy can be used with a partner, some toys are specifically designed for a couple to use. My favorite is the Pleasure Commander, a small, vibrating bullet on a stretchy silicone band that goes around the base of the man's penis, allowing the woman to get clitoral stimulation during intercourse. The "Commander" gets to control the speed and intensity of the bullet with a remote control. The guy gets the pleasure of thinking that your happy reaction is from his penis. Many men also find that the ring around the base of the penis increases stimulation. Everybody wins!

Dr. Streicher's SexAbility Survey

When I proposed to the women surveyed, "If you die unexpectedly, you are not worried about your children finding your vibrator collection because . . ."

- 42.7 percent said, "I don't care, I'll be dead."
- 4.7 percent said, "My best girlfriend has the key to my house and knows where it is."
- 7.7 percent said, "I told my partner (husband) how to dispose of them after he calls 911."
- 44.9 percent said, "What vibrator collection? I didn't know I was supposed to have a vibrator collection!"

There are also partner control vibrators in which a guy can control your clitoral stimulation from 50 feet away. The vibrator can be discreetly tucked away in specially designed panties. So next time you are at a meeting and one of your coworkers seems to be smiling just a little too much, look around and see if there is a guy with a remote control and a twinkle in his eye sitting across from her.

Why Do So Many Vibrators Have Ears and Noses?

The Rabbit, the Hungry Bear, the Pearl Panther, the Diving Dolphin, and yes, Hello Kitty. What's with all the animals? Certainly a vibrator can have things sticking out to stimulate all the right places without bringing an entire zoo into your bedroom. Evidently, many of the original vibrators were made in Japan, where the manufacture of sex toys resembling genitals was prohibited by law. Today, in the states where it is still illegal to sell sex toys, an animal-shaped vibrator can legally be marketed and sold as an animal "novelty" that just happens to vibrate and be shaped like a penis. This is great information for your next cocktail party.

Shopping for a Vibrator

So now that you're convinced that every woman should have at least one vibrator, if not an assortment, where do you go to buy a toy? What do you buy? How do you know what will work? It's not like shopping for a new bra—you can't take an assortment into the dressing room and find the one that fits.

I'm still waiting for "Vibrators Are Us" to become a franchise, but in the meantime, there are many places to pick one up—that is, unless you live in Alabama, Georgia, or Louisiana, where it is against the law to buy or sell a vibrator. Evidently, in those states, only men have a constitutional right to have an orgasm. Texas used to outlaw vibrators too, but in 2008 the Texas law was overturned after Joanne Webb, a married mother of three and a schoolteacher, faced up to a year in prison for selling a vibrator to two undercover cops posing as a married couple at a private party.

So where do you get these toys? No, you don't have to go to a questionable neighborhood wearing a disguise and dark glasses. Today you can buy a vibrator in your corner drugstore, online, or even in the grocery store. Recently I even saw vibrators being sold at an airport gift shop, presumably not to be used during takeoff or landing.

The best and biggest assortments of vibrators, not to mention salespeople who aren't embarrassed to help you and answer your questions, can be found in erotica boutiques. Most major cities have perfectly respectable erotica stores intended to give normal women the opportunity to shop comfortably. In addition to toys, most of these stores have fabulous sexy lingerie along with a great selection of erotic books and tapes. They also generally stock better lubricants than your local drugstore. The staff are usually knowledgeable and very happy to help. Go with your partner or a pal. It's easier and more fun than going alone. You can always say you're buying a gift for "a friend."

Now, if you read this chapter first, it's time to go back and read the rest of the book. I won't tell.

resources

Bookstores and the Internet are wonderful places where you can browse, buy, and become informed, but they can also provide information that is quite frankly confusing, misleading, or just wrong.

If you want to read more about the history of sexual medicine or perhaps learn more about a specific medical condition (beyond the sexual issues!), I have personally checked out the following resources and can vouch for them as trustworthy. I may not agree with every piece of information found in these publications and on these sites, but they are generally good sources of accurate information.

This is also the place to find out more information on many of the products and devices mentioned in the book. Although I have been compensated for my time to educate women on behalf of a few of these companies, *no one paid to be mentioned in this book or included in this resources section*. Also, please check out my website, DrStreicher.com, for more resources, links, and updates.

To help you find what you need, the resource chapter is organized as follows:

General Medical Information
Domestic Violence and Sexual Abuse Support
Relationships

Online Female-Friendly Erotica Shopping

SexAbilitators (Products and Websites)

> Vaginal Lubricants/Moisturizers
>
> Accessories
>
> Vibrators
>
> Dilators
>
> Pelvic Floor Strengthening Devices
>
> Pelvic Physical Therapy
>
> Sexual Ergonomics

History of Sexual Health

Finding a Clinician

Specific Medical Conditions

> Arthritis
>
> Cancer
>
> Depression
>
> Diabetes
>
> Disabilities
>
> Endometriosis
>
> Epilepsy
>
> Heart Disease
>
> Hereditary Cancer
>
> Hysterectomy
>
> Incontinence
>
> Inflammatory Bowel Disease
>
> Interstitial Cystitis
>
> Kidney Disease
>
> Lung Disease
>
> Menopause
>
> Orgasms
>
> Osteoporosis
>
> Parkinson's Disease
>
> Sexual Pain
>
> Vulvar/Vaginal Health

General Medical Information

Websites
UpToDate
www.uptodate.com

This outstanding website is authored by physicians and has summaries of the latest information on every medical condition.

National Institutes of Health (NIH), US National Library of Medicine
http://www.nlm.nih.gov/hinfo.html

A service of NIH that provides information about medical conditions and drugs.

US Department of Health and Human Services (HHS)
www.healthfinder.gov

This HHS website provides links to health and human services resources and information produced by the US government and partner organizations.

Everyday Health
www.everydayhealth.com

This site provides articles about the latest health news as well as general information and recommendations for specific health conditions.

American Congress of Obstetricians and Gynecologists (ACOG)
http://www.acog.org/For_Patients

The ACOG website provides information from leading experts in women's health care and gynecologic conditions.

National Institutes of Health (NIH), National Center for Complementary and Alternative Medicine (NCCAM)
www.nccam.nih.gov

NCCAM was developed within NIH to provide information on complementary and alternative medicine.

US Food and Drug Administration (FDA)
http://www.fda.gov/ForConsumers/ConsumerUpdates/ucm050803.htm
At its web page "FDA 101: Dietary Supplements," the FDA offers consumer information and suggestions about the use of dietary supplements, including herbal preparations.

US Food and Drug Administration (FDA)
http://www.fda.gov/drugs/guidancecomplianceregulatory information/pharmacycompounding/ucm183088.htm
On this web page, the US watchdog agency explains its oversight of pharmacy compounding of custom-made prescription drugs, including bio-identical hormone therapy.

Books

Arlene Weintraub, *Selling the Fountain of Youth*. Basic Books, 2010.

Domestic Violence and Sexual Abuse Support

Websites
National Domestic Violence Hotline
www.ndvh.org
This 24-hour hotline provides information on both local shelters and the nationwide service providers available for victims, friends, and family.

Rape, Abuse, and Incest National Network
www.RAINN.org
The nation's largest anti-sexual-violence organization has thou-

sands of trained volunteers available 24/7. If you call 1-800-656-HOPE, a computer notes the area code and first three digits of your phone number, then instantaneously connects you to the nearest RAINN member center.

Books

Wendy Maltz, *The Sexual Healing Journey: A Guide for Survivors of Sexual Abuse*. HarperCollins, 2012.

Relationships

Books

Andrew Cherlin, *The Marriage Go-Round*. Vintage, 2010.

Helen Fisher, *Why We Love*. Henry Holt, 2004.

Gregory Godek, *1001 Ways to Be Romantic*. Source Books, 2000.

John Gottman and Joan DeClaire, *The Relationship Cure*. Three Rivers Press, 2001.

John Gottman and Nan Silver, *The Seven Principles for Making Marriage Work*. Three Rivers Press, 2001.

Barbara Keesling, *Talk Sexy to the One You Love*. HarperCollins, 1996.

Howard Markman, Stanley Scott, and Susan Blumber, *Fighting for Your Marriage*. Jossey-Bass, 2001.

Barry and Emily McCarthy, *Rekindling Desire: A Step-by-Step Program to Help Low-Sex and No-Sex Marriages,* rev. ed. Brunner-Routledge, 2013.

Ester Perel, *Mating in Captivity: Reconciling the Erotic and the Domestic*. HarperCollins, 2006.

Joan Price, *Naked at Our Age: Talking Out Loud About Senior Sex*. Amazon Digital Services, 2011.

David Schnarch, *Passionate Marriage*. Henry Holt & Co., 1997.

Pepper Schwartz, *Prime: Adventures and Advice About Love, Sex, and the Sensual Years*. HarperCollins, 2007.

Pepper Schwartz, with Janet Lever, *Getaway Guide to the Great Sex Weekend*. World Wide Romance Press, 2012.

Pepper Schwartz, with Christiane Northrup and James Witte, *The Normal Bar: The Secrets of Happy Couples*. Random House/Harmony, 2013.

Online Female-Friendly Erotica Shopping

Erotica Shops
Babeland: www.babeland.com
G Boutique: www.boutiqueg.com
Good for Her: www.goodforher.com
Good Vibrations: www.goodvibrations.com
Kitty's Toy Box (LGBT-friendly): www.Kittystoybox.com
Middle Sex MD: www.middlesexmd.com
Pure Romance: www.pureromance.com
DrStreicher.com

SexAbilitators (Products and Websites)
All of the erotica shops listed above sell many of the following lubricants, moisturizers, vibrators, and dilators.

Vulver/Vaginal Lubricants/Moisturizers
Here are a few products to get you started, but always remember to check ingredients to know what you are getting!

Silicone-Based
Pink, Pjur, System Jo Silicone, Swiss Navy Silicone, Replens Silky Smooth

Water-Based
Liquid Silk, Pink Water, Maximus, Pre-Seed (fertility-friendly),
Sliquid H2O, Yes Water-Based, Wet Naturals

Hybrids (Both Silicone- and Water-Based)
Sliquid Silk Intimate Hybrid, Wet Synergy

Long-Acting Vaginal Moisturizers
Replens Long-Acting Vaginal Moisturizer (www.replens.com)

Vulvar Soothing Cream
Neogyn Vulvar Soothing Cream (www.neogyn.us)

Accessories
Condoms
    Female condom: FC2
    Non-latex condoms: Trojan Supra Bareskin Condoms
    Non-lubricated condoms: Trojan ENZ non-lubricated condoms
(to use for dental dams or to add your own lube)

Handy Harness Velcro Glove
http://ergoerotics.com/pleasure/26-handy-harness.html
    Don't worry, this accessory to hold a vibrator comes in both
right- and left-handed varieties!

Waterproof Throw Blanket
http://ergoerotics.com/86-waterproof-throw-blanket.html

Sheets with Velcro to Stabilize Limbs
http://www.sportsheets.com

EROS Clitoral Therapy Device
http://eros-therapy.com

The Love Swing
http://www.loveswing.com

Comeclose Collision Ring
www.comeclose.co.uk

Lubricant Delivery Device
Lube Shooter (no website but available at erotica shops)

Pillows/Bolsters
Many styles and decorator colors are available at both ergoerotics
(http://ergoerotics.com/7-position) and Liberator (http://www
.liberator.com/wedge.html).

To Buy a Merkin...
MaxWigs (www.maxwigs.com).
Kitty Carpet (in black, blond, or pink!)

Vibrators

A wide assortment of vibrators can be found at all of the erotica
shops listed on page 420 (not to mention your corner drugstore).
In addition, if you are willing to splurge, check out:

Lelo (www.lelo.com): INA 2, Mia 2 Lipstick Vibrator with
USB, SIRI

Jimmyjane (www.jimmyjane.com): Hello Touch, Form 2, 4,
or 6

We-Vibe (www.we-vibe.com): A couple's vibrator—We-Vibe
2, 3, or 4, Thrill

Crave (www.lovecrave.com): Duet 8GB Lux, Solo

Thrill (We-Vibe 2, 3, or 4; Thrill couples vibrators)

Vaginal Dilators

DrStreicher.com

Cool Water Cones: www.coolwatercones.com

Soul Source: www.soulsource.com

Middle Sex MD: www.middlesexmd.com

Pure Romance (www.pureromance.com): Tapered silicone dilators

Pelvic Floor Strengthening Devices

InControl Medical (www.incontrolmedical.com): InTone

Pour Moi (www.pourmoi.com): Apex, Intensity

Pelvic Physical Therapy

Section on Women's Health (SOWH) of the American Physical Therapy Association (APTA)

http://www.womenshealthapta.org

Herman & Wallace Pelvic Rehabilitation Institute

www.hermanwallace.com

International Pelvic Pain Society

www.pelvicpain.org/providers/find-provider.aspx

Sexual Ergonomics

Ergoerotics

www.ergoerotics.com

This site has information on innovative adjustment devices, educational materials, patient forums, additional resources, and even private consultations. It also provides books and videos to demonstrate positions and the best use of devices like pillows and bolsters to optimize comfortable intercourse and oral and manual stimulation.

History of Sexual Health

Books

Winfield Scott Hall, PhD, *Sexual Knowledge*. John Winston Co., 1916.

Shere Hite, *Hite Report on Female Sexuality*. Macmillan, 1976.

Alfred C. Kinsey et al., *Sexual Behavior in the Human Female*. W. B. Saunders Co., 1953.

Rachel Maines, *The Technology of Orgasm: "Hysteria," the Vibrator, and Women's Sexual Satisfaction*. Johns Hopkins University Press, 1999.

William Masters and Virginia Johnson, *Human Sexual Response*. Little, Brown and Co., 1966.

Marie Stopes, *Married Love*. G. P. Putnam, 1918.

Samuel-Auguste Tissot, *Onanism, Treatise on the Diseases caused by Masturbation, Self Pollution and Other excesses* (1758).

Finding a Clinician

In addition to the resources listed here, check your local hospitals or universities for sexual health clinics.

American Board of Medical Specialties (ABMS)

www.abms.org

This organization oversees physician certification by developing standards for the evaluation and certification of physician specialists. Go to the ABMS website to find out whether a physician is board-certified.

Federation of State Medical Boards (FSMB)

www.fsmb.org

Go to this website to verify that a physician is licensed.

American Congress of Obstetricians and Gynecologists (ACOG)

http://www.acog.org/About_ACOG/Find_an_Ob-Gyn

This site will help you find a board-certified gynecologist.

International Society for the Study of Women's Sexual Health (ISSWSH)

www.isswsh.org

This website will help you find a sexual medicine specialist.

Society for Sex Therapy and Research (SSTAR)

www.sstarnet.org

The SSTAR website will point you toward therapists who are trained in sexual function.

American Association of Sex Educators, Counselors, and Therapists (AASECT)

www.aasect.org

Therapists trained in sexual function can also be found using the AASECT website.

North American Menopause Society (NAMS)

http://www.menopause.org/for-women/find-a-menopause -practitioner

NAMS will help you find a certified menopause practitioner.

Specific Medical Conditions

Arthritis

American College of Rheumatology
http://www.rheumatology.org/default.aspx
Arthritis Foundation
www.arthritis.org

Cancer

American Cancer Society (ACS)
www.cancer.org

ACS is a nonprofit organization dedicated to cancer prevention, detection, and treatment.

CancerCare
www.cancercare.org/index.php

CancerCare provides free professional support services to anyone affected by cancer—people with cancer, caregivers, children, loved ones, and the bereaved.

Centers for Disease Control and Prevention (CDC), National Breast and Cervical Cancer Early Detection Program
www.cdc.gov/cancer/nbccedp

The CDC's early detection program provides access to breast and cervical cancer screening services.

Foundation for Women's Cancer
www.thegcf.org

This site provides updated news and information on cancer, as well as resources for finding doctors and clinical trials, survivor stories, a bookstore, and other links.

National Institutes of Health (NIH), National Cancer Institute, Cancer Information Service
www.nci.nih.gov

A nonprofit organization within NIH, the Cancer Information Service provides extensive cancer information for health care providers and the public on types of cancer, treatments, screening and testing, clinical trials, risk factors, and statistics.

National Comprehensive Cancer Network (NCCN)
www.nccn.com

NCCN is a not-for-profit organization whose website provides cancer news, treatment summaries, and links to cancer treatment centers.

Depression
American Psychiatric Association
http://www.psychiatry.org/mental-health
American Psychological Association
http://www.apa.org
International Foundation for Research and Education on Depression
http://www.ifred.org

Diabetes
American Diabetes Association (ADA)
www.diabetes.org

Disabilities
SexualHealth.com
www.sexualhealth.com

This is a comprehensive online source for disability and sexuality information.

Mitchell Tepper
http://mitchelltepper.com

Disabled himself, sexologist Dr. Mitchell Tepper provides expert advice on sexual health, disabilities, and medical conditions.

Queers On Wheels
http://disqueers.tripod.com

Queers On Wheels is an organization that serves the physically disabled GLBTQ (gay, lesbian, bisexual, transgender, or queer) community by providing literature, classes, workshops, and networking.

Life Center: Rehabilitation Institute of Chicago
http://lifecenter.ric.org

Books

Gary Karp, *Disability and the Art of Kissing* (available on the author's website, Lifeonwheels.net)

Miriam Kaufman, Corey Silverberg, and Fran Odette, *The Ultimate Guide to Sex and Disability: For All of Us Who Live with Disabilities, Chronic Pain, and Illness.* Amazon Digital, 2007.

Ken Kroll and Erica Levy Klein, *Enabling Romance: A Guide to Love, Sex and Relationships for People with Disabilities,* No Limits Communications, 2001.

Endometriosis

Endometriosis Association
www.endometriosis.org
Endometriosis Foundation of America
www.endofound.org

Epilepsy

Epilepsy Foundation
www.epilepsyfoundation.org
National Institutes of Health (NIH), National Institute of Neurological Disorders and Stroke
www.ninds.nih.gov/disorders/epilepsy/detail_epilepsy.htm

Heart Disease

American Heart Association
www.americanheart.org

Hereditary Cancer

National Society of Genetic Counselors (NSGC)
www.nsgc.org

This site will help you locate a genetic counselor who specializes in cancer risk.

US Equal Employment Opportunity Commission (EEOC)
http://www.eeoc.gov/laws/types/genetic.cfm

This EEOC web page on genetic information discrimination provides information about the laws that prevent employers or health insurers from using genetic testing results in decisions about eligibility, rates, or coverage.

Myriad
www.myriad.com

Myriad is the company that developed testing to detect the presence of genes for hereditary cancers, such as the BRCA gene. The website provides a great deal of information about testing and risk reduction.

Bright Pink
www.brightpink.org

This organization works on behalf of *young* women who are at genetic risk for breast and ovarian cancer.

Facing Our Risk of Cancer Empowered (FORCE)
www.facingourrisk.com

This organization is dedicated to providing information about hereditary cancers.

Hysterectomy

American Association of Gynecologic Laparoscopic Surgeons (AAGL)
www.aagl.org

AAGL provides information about minimally invasive surgery such as laparoscopic and robotic-assisted surgery, hysterectomy, and myomectomy.

Books

Lauren Streicher, *The Essential Guide to Hysterectomy: Advice from a Gynecologist on Your Choices Before, During, and After Surgery.* Rowman and Littlefield, 2013.

Incontinence

American Urogynecology Association (AUGS)
www.mypelvichealth.org

Women's Health Foundation (WHF)
http://womenshealthfoundation.org
The WHF is a nonprofit organization dedicated to improving women's pelvic health.

The Total Control Program
www.totalcontrolprogram.com
The Total Control program is a comprehensive pelvic fitness and wellness program designed by leading experts in the fields of urogynecology, physical therapy, and fitness.

National Association for Continence (NAFC)
www.nafc.org
Education and support for health care professionals and the general public is provided by this nonprofit organization with a focus on prevention, diagnosis, treatment, and management solutions for incontinence.

Inflammatory Bowel Disease

American Society of Colon and Rectal Surgeons (ASCRS)
www.fascrs.org
American Gastroenterological Association (AGA)
www.gastro.org

Crohn's and Colitis Foundation of America (CCFA)
www.ccfa.org

Interstitial Cystitis
Interstitial Cystitis Network (ICN)
www.ic-network.com

Kidney Disease
National Kidney Foundation
www.kidney.org
American Association of Kidney Patients (AAKP)
www.aakp.org

Lung Disease
American Lung Association
www.lungusa.org
Alpha-1 Foundation
www.alphaone.org

Menopause
North American Menopause Society
www.menopause.org
American Congress of Obstetricians and Gynecologists, Pause
The ACOG Guide to Midlife Health: www.pause.acog.org

Orgasms
Books

Betty Dodson, *Orgasms for Two: The Joy of Partnership.* Random House, 2002.

Betty Dodson, *Sex for One: The Joy of Self Loving.* Crown, 1996.

Julia Heiman and Joseph LoPiccolo, *Becoming Orgasmic: A Sexual and Personal Growth Program for Women.* Prentice-Hall, 1988; Piatkus, 2010.

Barry R. Komisaruk, Carlos Beyer-Flores, and Beverly Whipple, *The Science of Orgasm*. Johns Hopkins University Press, 2006.

Osteoporosis

National Osteoporosis Foundation
www.nof.org

Information for health care providers and the public on the bone-thinning disease osteoporosis is available on this site from a nonprofit US organization.

Parkinson's Disease

National Parkinson Foundation
www.parkinson.org
American Parkinson Disease Association
www.apdaparkinson.org
National Institute of Neurological Disorders and Stroke
www.ninds.nih.gov/disorders/parkinsons_disease/detail_parkinsons_disease.htm
Parkinson's Disease Foundation
www.pdf.org
Worldwide Education and Awareness for Movement Disorders
www.wemove.org

Sexual Pain

International Pelvic Pain Society
www.pelvicpain.org
Vaginismus: Helping Women Overcome Sexual Pain
www.vaginismus.com

Books

Andrew Goldstein, Caroline Pukall, and Irwin Goldstein, *When Sex Hurts: A Woman's Guide to Banishing Sexual Pain*. Perseus Books, 2011.

Vulvar/Vaginal Health

International Society for the Study of Vulvovaginal Disease (ISSVD)

www.issvd.org

National Vulvodynia Association (NVA)

www.nva.org

Center for Vulvovaginal Disorders (CVVD)

www.cvvd.org

CVVD is Dr. Andrew Goldstein's center, with offices in Washington, New York, and Annapolis, which is devoted to sexual pain, sexual dysfunction, vulvar pain, vulvodynia, lichen sclerosus, decreased libido.

Books

Debby Herbenick and Vanessa Schick, *Read My Lips: A Complete Guide to the Vagina and Vulva*. Rowman and Littlefield, 2011.

Elizabeth G. Stewart and Paula Spencer, *The V Book: A Doctor's Guide to Complete Vulvovaginal Health*. Bantam Books, 2002.

acknowledgments

It's been quite the journey from a simple blog about vaginal lubricants to a comprehensive female sexual health book.

It was almost ten years ago that Michele Weldon, an assistant professor at the Medill School of Journalism at Northwestern University, introduced me to my first agent when I didn't even know I needed an agent to publish what started out as *Taking the Hysteria Out of Hysterectomy,* and ultimately became *The Essential Guide to Hysterectomy.*

This time around, I decided to self-publish what I affectionately referred to as my "dry giney book" in order to get it out fast. (I am by nature an impatient person and considered 50 million dry vaginas to be a national emergency.) Susy Schultz, a talented writer and cofounder of Chicago's Association for Women Journalists, was kind enough to look at an early manuscript, and Susan Mango Curtis, an assistant professor at the Medill School of Journalism at Northwestern University, provided an early cover design that didn't make it to the final book, but was wonderful nonetheless.

My plan to self-publish flew out the window after I spent an afternoon with the indomitable Yfat Reiss Gendel, who convinced me that this book was too big and too important to self-publish and offered to represent me. I am probably the only author in history who *needed* to be persuaded to be represented by one of New York's top literary agents. Of course, if Scott Yonover had not introduced me to Yfat, none of this would have happened.

Carrie Thornton, my editor at HarperCollins, saw my vision and realized that this topic was valuable enough to take a chance on. She kept me on track, didn't make me delete too many things, and was a pleasure to work with. I appreciate that that is not the case with every editor! Billie Fitzpatrick was also an integral part of the team.

My involvement with NAMS and ISSWSH introduced me to a phenomenal group of sexual health and menopause experts. I am grateful to every single colleague whose articles, lectures, and personal conversations educated me. I particularly would like to thank Andrew Goldstein, MD; Steve Goldstein, MD; Sheryl Kingsberg, PhD; Michael Krychman, MD; Stacy Lindau, MD; Marla Mendelson, MD (cardiology); Leah Millheiser, MD; David Portman, MD; Jan Shifren, MD; and Jim Simon, MD.

In addition, acknowledgment goes to Debra Herbenick, PhD, MPH, whose work at Indiana University was the basis of many studies cited throughout the book, along with Heather Howard, PhD, MPH, who introduced me to the world of sexual ergonomics.

I had the pleasure of meeting Rachel Maines and personally discussing her research and historical information from her book, *The Technology of Orgasm*.

Thanks also to my friend, the prolific writer and sociologist, Pepper Schwartz, PhD, who conducted the survey to end all surveys about sexual behavior for her book *The Normal Bar*.

No sexual health expert can do what he or she does without the pelvic physical therapists of the world. I want to thank my personal "magician," Dr. Judith Florendo, who not only takes care of my patients, answered dozens of questions, and reviewed the manuscript, but also allowed me to shadow her so I could get a glimpse into what really happens during a pelvic floor physical therapy session.

To Suzy Ginsberg, my dear friend and PR agent extraordinaire, who has made it her life's mission to educate women about their bodies, and specifically about having a healthy vagina. Thank you, Suzy, for not only introducing me to magazine editors and TV producers but also for insisting we dash into Bergdorf Goodman and Henri Bendel for quick shopping fixes in between meetings.

To John Reilly, a dear friend and extraordinary photographer who jumped in at the eleventh hour to shoot a new photo for the cover.

An enormous, heartfelt thank-you goes to my partners and dearest friends, Shari Goldman Snow and Jane Blumenthal, for always understanding when I was out of the office writing, traveling, or speaking. And who along with Drs. Michelle Baer, Christie Beyer, and Kristy Tough DeSapri, took care of my patients when I wasn't around.

Ultimately, *everything* that really matters I have learned from my patients. Until I see what works and what doesn't, information from articles, book, or lectures doesn't count. And yes, the stories and anecdotes throughout the book are true. Sometimes it's a combination of more than one patient's story, but it's all stuff that has happened. My patients often tell me, "You should write a book about the things you see." And now I have.

I may be the first author to thank an inanimate object, but I credit my treadmill desk with the fact that not only did I not gain 50 pounds while writing this book, but that I never had the neck or back pain that are the scourge of many authors who spend hours hunched over a desk. In case you are wondering, I walked 1,050 miles.

And then there's my family.

My brothers, Paul, Michael, and Ian, who I would like as friends even if they were not my brothers. They cheered me on every step of the way (probably to make up for giving me a hard time as a kid) and proudly exhibit my books even though it is a little strange for a guy to display *The Essential Guide to Hysterectomy* and *Sex Rx* on his living room coffee table).

My terrific stepdaughters, Jessie and Julian, got a lot more than they bargained for when their dad brought me into the family. Thanks for being such good sports about all the vagina talk at the dinner table.

My daughters, Rachel and Danielle, are what every mother hopes and dreams of when she has children. They have grown up into bright, lovely, interesting, accomplished young women. Their love and support has kept me going.

Rachel, a talented writer, gets total credit for the tantric sex sections, the religion section, and many of the witty chapter titles and subtitles, including When Your Vagina Is in a Phunk and "I'd like to buy a vowel—the key to getting the big O back." Thanks, Rach!

And to Jason, my everything. This book could not, would not, have happened without you. Every day you were there to encourage me, cook for me, and, most important, love me no matter how tired, cranky, or distracted I was. And we are not even talking about the foot rubs. I love you so much and can't imagine life without you.

index

acquired vestibulodynia, 131, 242
adenomyosis, 155–156, 160
adhesions, 156–157, 170
adrenaline, sexual response and, 37
age issues. *See also* menopause
    adolescents and endometriosis,
        150
    aging and libido, 181–182
    aging and sexual frequency, 26
    estrogen use and, 283–284
    sexual dysfunction in young women, 2
    sexual response and, 42
AIDS, 375
alcohol use
    libido and, 182–183
    orgasm and, 209
allergies
    avoiding irritants, 131–132, 143–144
    sex-related, 140–141
aloe vera, 89
alternative therapies. *See also* pelvic
        physical therapy
    diet and, 136, 192, 237
    "natural" drugs, 115–117, 198
    nonhormonal prescription
        pharmaceuticals, 217–219
    supplements and PMS, 237
amantadine, 218
American Board of Medical Specialties
    (ABMS), 353

American College of Obstetrics and
    Gynecology, 114, 353
American Physical Therapy Association,
    99
American Urology Association,
    158
anal sex, 44–45
anatomy. *See* clitoris; medical
    examinations; ovaries; pelvic
    physical therapy; penis; uterus;
    vagina; vestibule; vulva
androgens, 175–177, 240
androstenedione, 175–177
anesthetics
    for physical therapy, 98, 106
    for pubic hair removal, 389
anorgasmia, 205–206
antidepressants
    for hot flashes, 291–292
    libido and, 179–180, 188, 195
    monoamine oxidase inhibitors
        (MAOIs), 180, 218
    orgasm and, 209, 218
    selective serotonin reuptake inhibitors
        (SSRIs), 179–180, 188, 209,
        238
Anti-Müllerian hormone (AMH),
    381–382
Apex, 100–101, 255
ArginMax, 220

arousal
  defined, 31, 32, 34
  effect of hormones and
    neurotransmitters on, 38
  impaired, 35
  orgasm and, 202, 206
  vibrators for, 408
arthritis, 320
Association of Professional Piercers, 393
atherosclerosis, 303
atrophic vaginitis, 68–69
atrophic vestibulodynia, 134–135
Avner, Lindsay, 343

baby oil, 81
bacterial vaginosis (BV)
  atrophic vaginitis compared to, 68–69
  complications of, 68
  defined, 63
  petroleum jelly and, 80–81
  preventing problems of, 67, 68
  yeast infection compared to, 63–65
balls/beads, for pelvic physical therapy,
    101
barrier contraception methods. See birth
    control; condoms
Basson, Rosemary, 32–33
Becoming Orgasmic (Heiman), 215
Benzocaine, 144
benzoic acid, 89
Betty Beauty, 391
bicycle riding, 211
bimanual exam, 48
bio-adhesive products, 86, 87
Biofade, 395
biofeedback, 97–98, 313–314
bio-mimetic plant-derived estrogen,
    116
biopsy, 128, 137
birth control. See also birth control pills
  barrier contraception methods, 382
  dating and pregnancy prevention,
    397–383
  for endometriosis, 152–153
  female condom (FC2), 141, 377–378
  hormonal contraception and libido,
    178, 238–247
  progestin-only contraception, 153
  religious beliefs about, 152

birth control pills
  cancer and, 335, 342–343, 344
  continuation rate, 245
  at midlife, 382–383
  for PMS, 238
  systemic estrogen compared to, 287
  vaginal discomfort and, 70
bisexuality, defined, 31–32
black cohosh, 280
bladder. See also urinary incontinence
  cancer, 345–346
  interstitial cystitis, 157–159
  menopause and, 262
bleaching cream, for genitals, 395
bleeding. See also menstruation
  after biopsy, 128
  prior to gynecologic exam, 50
  vaginal dilators and, 106
blood clots, 284–286
blood flow/supply. See also heart health
  heart disease and, 303
  menopause and, 260
  orgasm and, 203, 208
blood sugar, 308–309
board certification, of physicians, 353
bodily fluids, for lubrication, 81
Body Bouncer, 108
body image
  breast cancer and, 334
  cosmetic alteration and self-esteem, 399
  dating and sex, 383
  libido and, 184, 189–190
  postpartum sex and, 253
  sexual inhibition and, 28
bolsters, 108
bone health, 294
boredom, with relationship. See
    relationship issues
Boteach, Rabbi Shmuley, 80
Botox, 98
bowel health
  colon cancer, 344, 345–346
  Crohn's disease and ulcerative colitis,
    315–317
  fecal incontinence, 96, 107, 315
  prolapse and, 165
brain
  cognitive decline and estrogen,
    294

multiple sclerosis and neuromuscular conditions, 318–320

neurotransmitters, 36–40, 132, 174–177

orgasm and headaches, 224–226

orgasm and stimulation, 203, 205

sexual response and, 36–40

BRCA1/BRCA2, 339–344

breast cancer

estrogen and, 273, 274–275, 284

genetic risk for, 339–344

specific problems of, 329–339

breast-feeding, postpartum sex and, 251, 255

Breast Journal, 330

Bremelanotide, 197

Bright Pink, 343

Brisdelle, 179, 291, 333

British Medical Journal, 23–24

Buddhists, beliefs about sexual behavior, 27–28

bupropion, 188, 195, 218

buspirone, 188, 218

CA125, 336, 342

calendula, 89

calories, burned during sex, 20

cancer, 323–347

birth control pills and, 335, 342–343, 344

bladder, 345–346

breast, 273, 274–275, 284, 329–334

cervical, 334, 337–338

chemotherapy, 324–326

colon, 344, 345–346

estrogen alternatives and, 274–275

estrogen therapy and, 273, 284

fallopian tube, 335–336

genetic risk, 339–344

HPV and, 370

hysterectomy and orgasm, 211

lung, 346

ovarian, 246, 334, 335–336

ovarian cysts and, 159

pelvic radiation, 327

progestin and, 288

rectal, 344, 345–346

screening, 336, 340–341

seeking medical advice about, 323–324, 346–347 (*see also* physicians)

stem cell transplants, 327–328

sterilization and, 246

surgery for, 328–329 (*see also individual types of cancer*)

uterine, 288, 334, 335

vaginal, 339

vulvar, 138, 338

Candida albicans, 63

capsaicin, 80, 133

carbomer, 89

Catholics

beliefs about sexual behavior, 27

contraception and, 152

Center for Vulvar Vaginal Disorders (New York), 145

cervix

anatomy of, 56, 58

cervical cancer, 334, 337–338

orgasm and, 207

orgasm and surgical removal of, 210–211

cetyl alcohol, 89

chemotherapy, 324–326

chlamydia, 373–374

chorhexidine deglutinate, 89

Church of Latter-Day Saints, beliefs about sexual behavior, 27

Cialis. *See* phosphodiasterase (PDE5) inhibitors (Viagra, Cialis)

citric acid, 90

cleansers, pH balance of vagina and, 62

clitoris

anatomy of, 52

clitoral hood piercing, 392

clitoral orgasm *versus* vaginal orgasm, 204–205

clitoral phimosis, 138

clitoral stimulators, 410, 411

orgasm and pain, 224–225

stimulation of, and orgasm, 202, 203, 206–207, 215–216

Clobetasol, 139

CLOSER Study, 178

coital alignment technique, 216

collagen, 22–23

colon cancer, 344, 345–346

Comeclose collision ring, 170

communicating, with physicians, 1–2, 9–13, 323–324, 346–347, 360–366, 397

compounding pharmacies, 113–115, 289
conception, using lubricants and, 82–83
condoms. *See also* birth control
    allergies and, 141
    female condom (FC2), 141, 377–378
    lubricants used with, 77, 78, 81
    sexually transmitted diseases and,
      376–378, 382
cones, for pelvic physical therapy, 101, 109
congenital vestibulodynia, 133–134
contraception. *See* birth control
Cool Water Cone dilators, 144
cosmetic alteration, 387–401
    extreme examples, 400–401
    genital cosmetic (make-up) products,
      395
    genital piercing, 392–393
    pubic hair dye, 391
    pubic hair grooming, 388–391
    self-esteem and, 399
    tattoos, 394
    vaginal plastic surgery, 53–54,
      395–400
    Vajazzling, 394
Cowan, Robert, 225
creams, vaginal estrogen, 266–267, 271,
    272–273
Crohn's disease, 315–317
Cromolym, 133, 141
cultural issues
    contraception and, 152
    genetic risk of cancer and, 340
    orgasm and, 207–208
    sexual behavior, 25
Cymbalta, 333
cystitis, interstitial cystitis compared to,
    158
cysts, ovarian, 159

dating. *See* safe sex
deep dyspareunia, 148–170
    adenomyosis, 155–156
    adhesions, 156–157
    diagnosing, 148–149
    dyspareunia compared to, 124–125,
      126
    endometriosis, 149–155
    interstitial cystitis, 157–159
    ovarian cysts, 159

    post-hysterectomy issues and, 167–170
      (*see also* hysterectomy)
    uterine prolapse, 164–167
dental dams, 378
Depo-Provera, 243, 245
depression
    antidepressants, 179–180, 188, 195,
      209, 218, 291–292
    dopamine and, 20–21
    libido and, 179–180
    postpartum depression (PPD), 254–255
    sexual dysfunction and, 318
    systemic estrogen and, 295–296
dermatologic (skin) conditions, 137–143
desire. *See also* libido
    defined, 31, 32
    effect of hormones and
      neurotransmitters on, 38
desquamative inflammatory vaginitis
    (DIV), 142–143
devices, sexual. *See* pelvic physical
    therapy; toys
Devrom, 317
DHEA, 194–195, 217, 275, 277, 333
diaphragms, 382
diazepam suppositories, 98
diazolidinyl urea, 90
diet
    foods as aphrodisiacs, 192
    PMS and, 237
    vulvar pain and, 136
dilation and curettage (D&C), 162–163
dilators. *See* vaginal dilators
dildos, 410
dimethicone, 90
discharge. *See also* dyspareunia; pH
    balance
    diagnosing vaginal discomfort and,
      65–66
    as normal, 56
doctors. *See* physicians
DO degree, defined, 352
dopamine, 20–21, 37, 174, 218
dopamine agonists, 195
douche, 62, 70
Dr. Oz Show, The, 192, 363–364, 408
Dry Babe, 334
Duavee, 289
Duke University, 24

duloxetine, 333
dyspareunia, 123–147
  allergies, 140–141
  causes of, 126, 128–129
  as chronic, 145–146
  deep dyspareunia compared to, 124–125,
    126 (see also deep dyspareunia)
  defined, 35, 124–126
  dermatologic (skin) conditions,
    137–143
  dryness and, 143
  exams for, 126–128
  partner support and, 146–147
  superficial dyspareunia, 124–126
  tips for healing, 143–145
  vagina size and, 146
  vaginismus, 125
  vestibulodynia, 129–137, 242
  vulvodynia, 129–137
  vulvovestibulodynia, 129–137, 145–146

Effexor, 333
electrical stimulation, 98, 313–314
Elmiron, 159
Emla, 389
endometrial cancer, 331. See also uterus
endometriosis, 149–155, 160
endorphins, 20, 37, 333
erectile dysfunction (ED). See also
    phosphodiasterase (PDE5) inhibitors
    (Viagra, Cialis)
  as acceptable topic, 13–14
  tobacco and, 209
Ergoerotics.com, 108
EROS Clitoral Therapy Device, 222,
  309–310
erotica stores, 413
Essential Guide to Hysterectomy, The
  (Streicher), 59, 149, 163
Essure, 246
Estring, 267–268
estrogen. See also local estrogen therapy;
    systemic estrogen therapy; individual
    types of cancer
  atrophic vaginitis and, 69
  atrophic vestibulodynia, 134–135
  in birth control pills, 240, 242
  collagen formation and, 22–23
  libido and, 175–177

  natural production of, 259–260
  orgasm and, 208–209, 216–217
  PMS and, 237
  postpartum sex and, 251
  progestin used with, 288–289
  safety of, 281–286, 287–288
  selective estrogen receptor modulators
    (SERMs), 274–275, 289, 329
  sexual response and, 36, 38, 39
  vaginal atrophy and, 87
  for vaginal discomfort, 70
excitement stage, of sexual response, 32
exercise, for hot flashes, 333–334
external genitalia, anatomy of, 48, 50–55

FACOG, defined, 353
fallopian tube cancer, 335–336
fantasizing, during sex, 212–213
fecal incontinence, 96, 107, 315. See also
  bowel health
Federation of State Medical Boards, 352
female condom (FC2), 141, 377–378
female sexual dysfunction (FSD),
  defined, 35–36
female superior position, 216
Feminine Forever (Wilson), 281
Femprox, 219
Femring, 264–265
fibroids, 160–163
financial issues, of medication, 117–119
flatulence, 317
flavored lubricants, 79–81
flibanserin, 112, 196
follicle-stimulating hormone (FSH) level,
  381
Food and Drug Administration
  class labeling, 266
  lubricants and moisturizers, 84, 85, 87
  medication approval and, 110–111, 113,
    193–194, 196–197
  warnings by, 332 (see also individual
    names of products)
French Water Jet Massage, 404
Freud, Sigmund, 204, 407
fungal infection, 63–65

gabapentin, 132
Gardasil, 370–371
Gardnerella vaginalis, 61, 64, 66

generalized vulvodynia, 135–136
genetic risk
  birth control pills and, 242
  endometriosis, 150
  fertility and, 381
  hereditary breast and ovarian cancer syndrome (HBOC), 339–344
  lichen sclerosus, 138
  Lynch syndrome, 343
  osteoporosis, 294
  PMS, 237
genital dryness (GD)
  as acceptable topic, 15
  menopause and, 261–262, 276–277
  systemic estrogens for, 292–293
genital piercing, 392–393
ginseng, 90
glans, 52
glycerin, 77, 90
Goldstein, Andrew, 145–146
gonadotropin-releasing hormones (GnRH), 153–154
gonorrhea, 373
Goodman, Michael, 399
graduated vaginal dilators, 102–106
Grafenberg, Ernst, 57
G-spot, 57
gynecologic exam. *See* medical examinations
gynecologic practice, choosing, 359. *See also* physicians
gynecologists. *See* physicians

Hall, Winfield Scott, 41
Handy Harness Glove, 109
happiness, sexual activity and, 23
Hart's Line, 127, 129
Harvard University, 35
Headache Program, Stanford University, 225
headaches, orgasm and, 224–226
heart health
  heart disease, 302–307
  heart disease and estrogen, 293–294
  sex for, 21
Heiman, Julia, 215
hepatitis, 374
hereditary breast and ovarian cancer syndrome (HBOC), 339–344

hereditary nonpolyposis colorectal cancer (HNPCC), 344
hereditary risk. *See* genetic risk
Herman & Wallace, 99
herpes, 371–373
heterosexuality, defined, 31–32
Hite, Shere, 204
Hite Report on Female Sexuality (Hite), 204
HIV, 375
home testing kits, for vaginal discomfort, 66
homosexuality, defined, 31–32
hormones, 235–256. *See also* estrogen; menopause; progestin; testosterone
  follicle-stimulating hormone (FSH) level, 381
  hormonal contraception and libido, 178, 238–247
  hormonal contraception for endometriosis, 152–154
  hormone therapy for orgasm, 216–217
  infertility, 247–248
  libido and, 175–177, 181–182, 193–198
  for multiple sclerosis, 319–320
  oxytocin, 22, 37–38
  postpartum sex, 251–256
  premenstrual syndrome (PMS), 235–238
  prescribed, 110–119 (*see also* local estrogen therapy; systemic estrogen therapy)
  progesterone, 237, 284
  progestin, with estrogen, 288–289
  pubic hair and, 51
  sex during pregnancy, 249–251 (*see also* pregnancy)
  sexual response and, 36–40
hot flashes. *See also* systemic estrogen therapy
  breast cancer and, 332–334
  prescriptions for, 179–180, 290–291
  sleep and, 293
Howard, Heather, 106–107
human fibroblast lysate cream, 88
human papilloma virus (HPV), 369–371
hyaluronic acid, 90
hydration products, 86
hydroxyethyl cellulose, 90

hygiene
 douche and, 62, 70
 prior to gynecologic exam, 49–50
 for vaginal dilators, 106
hymen, 54–55
hyperplastic dystrophy, 140
hypertonic pelvic floor, 97
hypoactive sexual desire disorder
  (HSDD). *See also* libido
 causes, 174–182
 defined, 18, 172–173
 help for, 186–192
 lifestyle issues and, 182–185
 medication for, 192–198
hysterectomy
 for endometriosis, 154–155
 The Essential Guide to Hysterectomy, 59,
  149, 163
 for fibroids, 162
 history of, 166
 orgasm and, 210–211
 pain after, 168–169
 pelvic physical therapy following,
  170
 radical, 337
 sex after, 167–168
"hysteria," 402–407
hysteroscopic myomectomy, 162
hysteroscopy, 162–163

implanted birth control, 245
incontinence
 fecal, 96, 107, 315
 orgasm and, 226
 urinary, 311–315
Indiana University, 213–214
Indiana University of Sexual Research,
  407
Indiana University School of Public
  Health, 248
infection. *See also* pH balance; sexually
  transmitted infections (STIs)
 fear of, 28
 sex as prevention for, 21
infertility, 247–248
inflammatory vestibulodynia, 131
injectable birth control, 245
insomnia. *See* sleep
Intensity, 221–222

intercourse. *See also* birth control;
  sexually transmitted infections
  (STIs)
 orgasm and positions for, 206–207,
  215–216 (*see also* orgasm)
 pain during (*see* deep dyspareunia;
  dyspareunia)
 pH balance of vagina and, 62, 71–72
 prior to gynecologic exam, 49–50
internal genitalia, anatomy of, 48–50
International Society for the Study of
  Women's Sexual Health (ISSWSH),
  106, 357
Internet searching, for physicians,
  355–356
InterStim, 223
interstitial cystitis, 157–159
InTone, 313–314, 315
intrauterine devices (IUDs), 244–245
 uterine cancer and, 335
 vaginal progestins used with estrogen,
  288–289
introitus, 54–55, 397
iso-osmotic lube, 83

Jews
 beliefs about sexual behavior, 26
 genetic risk for cancer, 340
 kosher lubricant products for, 80
Johnson, Virginia, 32, 204
joint mobilization, 97
Journal of Hypertension, 306
Journal of Sexual Medicine, 57, 79, 147, 241,
  242, 394, 407
Journal of the American Medical Association,
  22, 304, 369

Kaufman, Miriam, 322
Kegel exercises, 99–100, 255
Kinsey, Alfred, 407, 408
Kinsey Institute, 42, 204
kitchen products
 for lubrication, 81
 as protection, 378
Kosher Sex (Boteach), 80
K-Y Liquibeads Vaginal Moisturizer, 85

labial hypertrophy, 396
labia majora, 53

labia minora, 53–54, 242, 396–397
  Hart's Line, 127, 129
  plastic surgery, 53–54, 395–400
labiaplasty, 396–397
lactobacilli, 61, 62, 71, 260
lactoferrin, 88
lactoperoxidase, 88
latex allergy, 141
Lela, 85
Liberator foam wedge, 108
libido, 171–198
  "cycle of sex" and, 171–172
  desire, 31, 32, 38
  hormonal contraception and, 238–247
  hypoactive sexual desire disorder
    (HSDD), causes, 174–182
  hypoactive sexual desire disorder
    (HSDD), defined, 172–173
  improving, 186–192
  improving, with medication, 192–198
  lifestyle issues and, 182–195
  sleep and, 184, 190
  systemic estrogen and, 296
licensing, of physicians, 352
lichen planus, 142
lichen sclerosus, 137–139
lichen simplex chronicus, 140
Lindau, Stacy, 17
local estrogen therapy
  breast cancer treatment and, 331, 332
  diabetes and, 309
  products, 265–269, 271, 272–273
  progestin with, 289
  systemic estrogen compared to,
    264–265, 285–286, 288–289,
    292–293
  "tightening" vaginal walls and,
    398–399
long-acting vaginal moisturizers, 86–88
longevity, 23–24
Love Sex Again (Streicher), 2, 4–5
lubrication, 75–91
  applying, 82
  birth control pills and, 241–242
  cancer treatment and, 326 (see also
    cancer)
  choosing products for, 75–76
  conception and, 82–83
  heart disease and, 305

infertility and, 248
ingredients in lubricants and
  moisturizers, 77, 83, 87, 89–91
lubricants, specialty, 79–81
lubricants, types, 76–79, 85
lubricants and orgasm, 220
for menopause symptoms, 264,
  276–279
moisturizing products compared to
  lubricants, 83–88
natural, 56
superficial dyspareunia and dryness,
  143 (see also dyspareunia)
for vaginal atrophy, 292–293
with vaginal toys, 77
vulvar creams compared to lubricants,
  88–89
lung cancer, 346
Luvena, 87–88
Lybrido, 197
Lybridos, 197
Lynch syndrome, 344
Lyrica, 132
lysozyme, 88

Magic Banana, 101–102
Manipulator Table, 404
marijuana, orgasm and, 210
Married Love (Stopes), 199
Masters, William, 32, 204
masturbation. See also toys
  orgasm and, 214–215
  pelvic physical therapy and, 108–109
  sexual response and, 31–32, 41–43
MD degree, defined, 352
medical conditions, 299–322. See
    also cancer; deep dyspareunia;
    dyspareunia; medical examinations;
    pain
  arthritis, 320
  Crohn's disease and ulcerative colitis,
    315–317
  diabetes, 307–310
  heart disease, 302–307 (see also heart
    health)
  impact of, on sexual health, 299–301
  incontinence, fecal, 96, 107, 315
  incontinence, urinary, 22, 95, 107,
    226, 255, 311–315

libido and, 180, 182, 190
metabolic syndrome, 310
multiple sclerosis and neuromuscular
    conditions, 318–320
obesity as, 310–311
orgasm and, 208
physical disabilities, 320–322
sexual dysfunction and psychiatric
    disease, 318 (see also depression)
surgery and, 317–318
medical examinations. See also physicians
to diagnose infection, 65–66
diagnosing pain during intercourse,
    126–128
gynecologic exam, described, 47–50
menopause symptoms and, 263
by pelvic physical therapists, 96–98
medication, 110–119. See also local
    estrogen therapy; lubrication;
    systemic estrogen therapy
antidepressants, 179–180, 188, 195,
    209, 218, 291–292
compounding pharmacies, 113–115, 289
cost of, 117–119
for deep dyspareunia issues, 151–154
for hot flashes, 291–292
to improve libido, 192–198
libido affected by, 178–180, 181,
    187–188
"natural," 115–117
nonhormonal prescription
    pharmaceuticals, 217–219
nonsteroidal anti-inflammatory drugs
    (NSAIDS), 151–152
"off label" prescribing, 112, 194, 197
orgasm and, 217–220
pain during intercourse and, 128,
    132–133, 139, 140, 141, 142–143,
    144–145 (see also dyspareunia)
pelvic physical therapy and, 98, 106
research and, 110–112, 196–197
for vaginal discomfort, 66, 68, 70–71
    (see also pH balance)
vaginal discomfort caused by, 62
men. See also partners; relationship issues
anatomy of, 104, 146, 170, 398
erectile dysfunction (ED), 13–14, 209
    (see also phosphodiasterase (PDE5)
    inhibitors (Viagra, Cialis))

male physicians, 362–363
pharmaceutical research and, 111–112
menopause, 257–276. See also hot flashes
atrophic vestibulodynia and, 134–135
from chemotherapy, 326
diagnosing problems of, 263
estrogen production and, 259–260
external physical changes during,
    261–262
hot flashes, 179–180, 290–291, 293,
    332–334
libido and, 175, 177–178, 187
life expectancy and, 262–263
local estrogen alternatives, 274–276
local estrogen therapy compared to
    systemic, 264–265, 285–286,
    288–289, 292–293
lubrication and, 264
orgasm and, 208–209
pH balance of vagina and, 62
severity of issues from, 276–279
sexual health after, 2
specialists, 365–366
surgical, 168, 343–344
vaginal atrophy, 258–259
vulvar dystrophies and, 137
menstruation
fertility indicators, 381–382
menstrual cramps, 20
pain during (see adenomyosis;
    endometriosis)
pH balance of vagina and, 61, 69–70
merkin, 388
metabolic syndrome, 310
methyl paraben, 90
mineral oil, 90
Mirena, 244–245
moisturizing products, 83–88, 277. See
    also lubrication
monoamine oxidase inhibitors (MAOIs),
    180, 218
mons pubis, 50–51
morcellation, 162
More, 115
Mormons, beliefs about sexual behavior,
    27
multiple sclerosis, 318–320
muscles, strengthening. See pelvic
    physical therapy

Muslims, beliefs about sexual behavior, 26–27
myofascial (tissue) release, 97
myomas, 160
myomectomy, 162
My Own Pink Button, 395

National Bureau of Economic Research, 23
National Health and Social Life Survey, 407
National Sleep Foundation, 184
National Survey of Sexual Health and Behavior (Kinsey Institute), 42
"natural" drugs, 115–117, 198
Neogyn Vulvar Soothing Cream, 88–89, 144–145
neuromuscular conditions, 318–320
neuropathy, 308
neurotransmitters
    libido and, 174–177
    neurologic drugs, 132
    sexual response and, 36–40
neutraceuticals, 219–220
New England Journal of Medicine, 17, 167, 182
Nexplanon, 243, 245
nitric oxide, 37
non-physician clinicians. See also pelvic physical therapy
    advanced practice nurse degrees, 358
    finding, 357–360
nonsteroidal anti-inflammatory drugs (NSAIDS), 151–152
norepinephrine, 37, 132
Normal Bar, The (Schwartz, Witte), 16, 40–41, 42
"normal" sexual response, 40
North American Menopause Society (NAMS), 273, 289, 331, 356, 359
Northwestern University Medical School, 41
nurse-practitioners, finding, 357–360
nursing, postpartum sex and, 251, 255
Nuva ring, 243

obesity, 20, 165, 189–190, 310–311
obstetrician-gynecologists (OB-GYN), all-gynecologic practice versus, 359

Obstetrics and Gynecology, 79
Odette, Fran, 322
odor
    fecal, 317
    vaginal, 67, 71
"off label" prescribing, 112, 194, 197
oil-based lubricants, 78–79
Onania (Tissot), 43
oral contraception. See birth control pills
oral estrogen. See systemic estrogen therapy
oral sex. See also sexually transmitted infections (STIs)
    dental dams, 378
    herpes and, 371–372
    vaginal odor and, 71
orgasm, 199–231
    clitoral versus vaginal, 204–205
    defined, 31, 32, 201
    devices for, 221–224
    effect of hormones and neurotransmitters on, 39
    faking, 213–214
    heart disease and, 303, 304–305, 306
    historic views of, 199–200
    hormone therapy for, 216–217
    intercourse positions and, 215–216
    lubricants and, 220
    masturbation and, 214–215
    neutraceuticals, 219–220
    nonhormonal prescription pharmaceuticals, 217–219
    normal patterns of, 200–201
    orgasmic disorders, 205–206
    pain from, 224–227
    persistent genital arousal disorder (PGAD) and, 227–231
    during pregnancy, 250
    problems attaining, 35, 206–211
    relationship and psychological aspects of, 207–208, 212–214
    selective serotonin reuptake inhibitors (SSRIs) and, 179–180
    sexual response cycle and, 202–203
    vibrators for, 407–408
ospemifene, 274–275, 277, 332
osteoporosis, 294
Ostrzenski, Adam, 57

ovaries
  anatomy of, 58, 59
  hormones produced by, 176
  ovarian cancer, 246, 334, 335–336, 339–344
  ovarian cysts, 159
  surgical removal of, 337
oxytocin, 22, 37–38
Oz, Mehmet, 192, 363–364, 408

pain. *See also* medical conditions; medication
  endorphin release and, 20
  during intercourse (*see* deep dyspareunia; dyspareunia)
  libido issues and, 177, 186 (*see also* libido)
  from orgasm, 224–227
  pain-free/pain-reducing products, 87
paraffin, 90
Paraguard, 244
paroxetine, 291–292, 333
partners
  lack of, 25–26
  sex toys used by, 411 (*see also* toys)
  sexual orientation and, 31–32
  support of, 146–147, 400
Pearl Rabbit, 410–411
pectin, 90
pelvic exenteration, 346
pelvic floor dysfunction (PFD), 94
Pelvic Organ Prolapse (POP), 164–167
pelvic physical therapy, 92–109
  for adhesions, 157
  after hysterectomy, 170
  benefits of, 94–96
  determining need for, 92–93
  home strengthening devices, 100–102
  for incontinence, 313, 315
  for interstitial cystitis, 159
  Kegel exercises and, 99–100
  orgasm and, 221
  pelvic floor anatomy and, 93–94
  physical therapists for, 96–99
  for posterior vestibulodynia, 135
  for prolapse, 167
  sexual ergonomics, 106–109
  vaginal dilators, 102–106
pelvic radiation, 327

penis
  Comeclose collision ring for, 170
  size, 104, 146, 398
Pentosan polysulfate, 159
perimenopause. *See also* menopause
  pH balance of vagina and, 62
  vulvar dystrophies and, 137
perineoplasty, 398
perineum, 54
persistent genital arousal disorder (PGAD), 227–231
pessary, 167
petroleum jelly, 80–81
Pfizer, 14
pharmaceutical drugs. *See* medication
pH balance, 60–72
  bacterial vaginosis (BV) and, 63–65
  changes to, 61–62
  defined, 60–61
  diabetes and, 309
  maintaining, 69–71
  medical diagnosis and, 65–66
  menopause and, 262
  myths about vaginal discomfort, 72
  preventing problems of, 67, 68
  self diagnosis and, 64–65
  sexual activity and, 62, 71–72
  yeast infections and, 63–65, 77
phosphodiasterase (PDE5) inhibitors (Viagra, Cialis)
  libido and, 188, 196
  medical research and, 14
  for women, 217–218
  for women, with cancer, 327
  for women, with heart disease, 306
physical disabilities, 320–322. *See also* medical conditions
physical therapists, 96–99. *See also* pelvic physical therapy
physicians. *See also* surgery
  board certification, 353
  cancer and advice about sexuality by, 323–324, 346–347 (*see also* cancer)
  degrees, 352
  discussing sexual health with, 1–2, 9–13, 323–324, 346–347, 360–366, 397
  finding, 351–352
  history of vibrators and, 402–407

physicians (*cont.*)
    licensing of, 352
    online searches for, 355–356
    professional societies, 356–357
    referral services, 354–355
    training of, 2
    university affiliation of, 353–354
physician's assistants (PAs), 358–359
piercing, of genitals, 392–393
pillows, 108
Pink Daisy Labia Bleaching Cream, 395
plateau, defined, 31, 32
Pleasure Commander, 411
polycarbophil, 87, 90
polysorbate 60, 90
posterior vestibulodynia, 135
postpartum depression (PPD), 254–255
postpartum sex, 251–256
Pourmoi.com, 222
pregabalin, 132
pregnancy
    fear of, 28
    infertility, 247–248
    postpartum sex, 251–256
    preventing, 379–383 (*see also* birth
        control; sexually transmitted
        infections (STIs))
    prolapse and, 165
    sex during, 249–251
Premarin, 116, 266, 281
premenstrual dysphoric syndrome
    (PMDD), 236–237
premenstrual syndrome (PMS), 235–238
prescriptions. *See* alternative therapies;
    lubrication; medication
Pre-Seed, 83, 248, 326
Preside Study, 35
privacy, 29
Pro B, 71
probiotics, 61, 62, 71, 260
professional societies, for finding
    physicians, 356–357, 360. *See also*
    individual names of professional societies
progesterone
    estrogen taken with, 284
    PMS and, 237
progestin
    in birth control pills, 240, 243
    in injectable/implanted birth control, 245

in IUDs, 244
    with local estrogen therapy, 289
    progestin-only contraception, 153
    with systemic estrogen therapy, 288
prolactin, 21–22, 36, 38, 177
prolapse, uterine, 164–167
prophylactic surgery, for genetic risk
    factors, 339–340, 342
propylene glycol, 77, 90–91
provoked vestibulodynia, 131
pruritus vulvae, 140
pubic hair, 50–51, 53, 261, 388–391
pudendal neuralgia, 136–137
PUF (Pelvic Pain and Urgency/
    Frequency) symptom scale, 158

Rabbit, 410–411
radical hysterectomy, 337
Ramin, Cathryn, 115
rape, 28
Reader's Digest, 281
rectal cancer, 344, 345–346
Red Cross, 393
referral services, for physicians, 354–355
relationship issues. *See also* partners
    libido and, 183, 185, 189, 191–192
    orgasm problems and, 207–208, 212–214
    postpartum sex and, 253
    seeking information about, 45–46
    sexual behavior and, 25
    sexual response and, 45–46
religion
    contraception and, 152
    genetic risk of cancer and, 340
    kosher lubricant products, 80
    sexual behavior and, 26–28
Remote Butterfly, 109
remote control, for sex toys, 109, 322, 411
Rephresh, 68, 71
Replens, 69, 71, 87
resolution stage, of sexual response, 32, 39
Revive (2013 survey), 10, 360
Ruby Remote 3-Speed, 109
rugae, 260

safe sex, 367–383
    chlamydia, 373–374
    gonorrhea, 373
    hepatitis, 374

herpes, 371–373
HIV, 375
HPV, 369–371
importance of, 367–368
pregnancy prevention, 379–383
protection, 376–378
risk of sexually transmitted infections, 368–369
screening for sexually transmitted infections, 379
syphilis, 375–376
scar tissue, adhesions compared to, 156
Schwartz, Pepper, 16, 40–41, 42, 185
screening
for cancer, 336, 340–341
for sexually transmitted infections, 379
Sears, Roebuck catalog, 405–406
selective estrogen receptor modulators (SERMs), 274–275, 289, 329
selective serotonin reuptake inhibitors (SSRIs), 179–180, 188, 209, 238
self-esteem, 28
self-sexuality, 31–32, 41–43. *See also* masturbation
semen, allergy to, 140–141
sensate focus treatment, 215
serotonin
libido and, 174
sexual response and, 36, 38
serotonin and norepinephrine reuptake inhibitors (SNRIs), 180, 333
SexAbilitation, defined, 4
SexAbilitators
defined, 3
home strengthening devices, 100–102
Kegel exercises and, 99–100
sexual ergonomics, 106–109
vaginal dilators, 102–106
SexAbility. *See also* sexual response
defined, 1–6
SexAbility Screen, 5–6
SexAbility Survey
contraception, 243
hysterectomy, 163–164, 168, 169
labia, 396
libido, 175
lubricants, 82
oral sex and vaginal odor, 71
orgasm, 201, 211

pelvic physical therapy, 93, 102
pubic hair, 53
sexual health discussions between patient and doctor, 11
sexually transmitted infections, 377
sexual response, 34
tattoos, 394
sex-hormone binding globulin (SHBG), 175–177
sexual abuse, 28
sexual assault, 28
sexual dysfunction. *See also* deep dyspareunia; dyspareunia; libido; lubrication; pH balance
non-physical factors contributing to, 24–29
pervasiveness of, 18, 173
in young women, 2
sexual ergonomics, 106–109
sexual experience, orgasm and, 206
sexual frequency
benefits of, 18–24, 279
statistics, 15–17
vibrators and, 409
sexual function clinics, 359
"sexual health facilitators," 321–322
sexual health specialists, 365–366
Sexual Knowledge (Hall), 41
sexually transmitted infections (STIs)
chlamydia, 373–374
genital piercing risk, 393
gonorrhea, 373
hepatitis, 374
herpes, 371–373
historic treatments for, 388
HIV, 375
HPV, 369–371
importance of safe sex, 367–368
prevention, 376–378
risk of, 368–369
screening for, 379
syphilis, 375–376
sexual neutrality, 33–34
sexual orientation, 31–32
sexual response, 30–46
brain and, 36–40
female sexual dysfunction (FSD) and, 35–36
masturbation and, 41–43

sexual response (*cont.*)
  "normal," 40
  receptivity and, 30–34
  relationship issues and, 45–46
  sexual orientation and, 31–32
  types of sexual activity and, 40–41, 43–45
Shifren, Jan, 35, 173
silicone-based lubricants, 77–78, 83, 85
Silk-E Vaginal Moisturizer, 86
Silverberg, Corey, 322
Singer, Helen, 32
skinning vulvectomy, 338
Skyla, 244–245
sleep
  hot flashes and, 293
  insomnia and libido, 184, 190
  libido and, 184, 190
  postpartum sex and, 253
  sex for improved sleep, 21–22
  sleep patterns and schedule, 29
Slightest Touch Electro Sex, 222
Smart Bikini Colour, 391
sodium benzoate, 91
sorbic acid, 91
sorbitol, 91
speculum, 48–49
sperm viability, lubricants and, 82–83
spooning, 216
Sports Sheet, 109
Stanford University, 225
stellate ganglion block, 292
stem cell transplants, 327–328
sterilization, 245–246, 247
steroids, 139
stimulation, orgasm and, 202, 203
stomas, 316–317
Stopes, Marie, 199
Streicher, Lauren. *See also* SexAbility
    Survey
  The Essential Guide to Hysterectomy, 59,
      149, 163
  Love Sex Again, 2, 4–5
strengthening devices, for pelvic floor
    muscles, 100–102
stress, 28, 184, 188–189
stress incontinence, 311–315
superficial dyspareunia
  after hysterectomy, 169
  defined, 124–126

surgery
  adhesions from, 156
  body image and, 334
  for cancer, 328–329 (*see also individual
      types of cancer*)
  for fibroids, 162–163
  hysterectomy, for endometriosis,
      154–155
  for nongynecologic pelvic cancers,
      345–346
  orgasm and, 210–211
  orgasm-enhancement claims about,
      223
  plastic surgery for genitals, 395–400
      (*see also* cosmetic alteration)
  prophylactic surgery for genetic risk
      factors, 339–340, 342
  radical hysterectomy for cervical
      cancer, 337
  sex after, 317–318
  shaving before, 390
  skinning vulvectomy, 338
  for uterine cancer, 335
Symmetrel, 218
syphilis, 375–376
systemic estrogen therapy, 280–296
  benefits of, 290–296
  breast cancer treatment and, 331
  hot flash symptoms and, 290–291 (*see
      also* hot flashes)
  local estrogen therapy compared
      to, 264–265, 285–286, 288–289,
      292–293
  Premarin, 116, 266, 281
  progestin used with estrogen, 288–289
  safety of, 283–286, 287–288
  uses of, 280–281
  Women's Health Initiative on, 281–283

tablets, vaginal estrogen, 268–269, 271
taboo topics, 9–29
  benefits of having sex, 18–24
  difficulty of discussing sexual health,
      1–2, 9–13, 323–324, 346–347,
      360–366, 397 (*see also* non-physician
      clinicians; pelvic physical therapy;
      physicians)
  erectile dysfunction (ED) as acceptable
      topic, 13–14

factors contributing to sexual dysfunction, 24–29

frequency of sexual activity and, 15–17

genital dryness (GD) as acceptable topic, 15

sexual dysfunction pervasiveness and, 18

tamoxifen, 329

tampons, 63, 70

tantric sex, 200, 224

tattoos, genital, 394

tension-free vaginal tape (TVT), 314

testosterone

birth control pills and, 240–241

libido and, 175–177

orgasm and, 208–209, 216–217

sexual response and, 36, 38, 39

for women, 112, 193–194, 197, 275–276

time issues, scheduling sex and, 188–189

Tissot, Samuel-Auguste, 43

tobacco

libido and, 182–183

orgasm and, 209

prolapse and, 165

tooth decay, 23

Total Control Programs, 313

toys, 402–413

history of vibrators, 402–407

orgasm and, 214–215, 223

pelvic physical therapy with, 104, 108–109

recommendations for vibrators, 407–409

shopping for, 412–413

types of sex toys, 409–412

transdermal estrogen, 285–286

transdermal progestogens, 114

tubal interruption (tubal ligation), 245–246, 247, 336

ulcerative colitis, 315–317

Ultimate Guide to Sex and Disability, The (Kaufman, Silverberg, Odette), 322

university affiliation, of physicians, 353–354

University of Chicago, 301, 330

University of Florida, 182

University of Michigan, 252

University of Washington, 185

urethra, 54

urinary incontinence

orgasm and, 226

pelvic physical therapy and, 95, 107

postpartum, 255

during sex, 226

sex for, 22

stress incontinence, 311–315

urge incontinence, 312, 314–315

urine, irritation from, 144

uterine artery embolization, 163

uterine leiomyoma, 160

uterus. *See also* hysterectomy

adenomyosis, 155–156

anatomy of, 58–59

endometriosis, 149–155

fibroids, 160–163

hyster terminology and, 402–403

uterine cancer, 288, 334, 335

uterine prolapse, 164–167

Vagifem, 268–269, 331

vagina

anatomy of, 55–56, 58

clitoral orgasm *versus* vaginal orgasm, 204–205

discussing sexual health with clinicians, 1–2, 9–13, 323–324, 346–347, 360–366, 397

long-acting vaginal moisturizers, 86–88 (*see also* lubrication)

menopause changes to, 260 (*see also* menopause)

pH balance of, 60–72

plastic surgery for, 395–400 (*see also* cosmetic alteration)

postpartum healing, 256

sexual response and, 39

size of, 146 (*see also* dyspareunia; vaginal dilators)

vaginal cancer, 339

vaginal intercourse alternatives, 43–45

vaginal rejuvenation, 397–400

vaginal atrophy

breast cancer and, 330–331

discussing with physicians, 365

estrogen for, 87

"genital dryness" (GD) and, 15

vaginal atrophy (*cont.*)
    libido and, 178
    from menopause, 258–259
    vibrators and, 409
vaginal DHEA, 275, 277
vaginal dilators
    Cool Water Cone dilators, 144
    estrogen and, 278–279
    pelvic physical therapy techniques,
        102–106
    surgery recovery and, 328–329
vaginal toys. *See* toys
vaginismus, 94, 125
vagus nerve, 203, 207
Vajazzling, 394
vasectomy, 247
venlafaxine, 333
vestibule
    anatomy, 54
    biopsy, 128
    vestibular pain and birth control pills,
        242
    vestibulectomy, 133, 134
    vestibulodynia, 129–137, 145–146, 242
Viagra. *See* phosphodiasterase (PDE5)
        inhibitors (Viagra, Cialis)
vibrators
    animal-shaped, 412
    history of, 402–407
    orgasm and, 214–215, 223
    pelvic physical therapy with sex toys,
        104, 108–109
    recommendations for, 407–409
    shopping for, 412–413
    types of sex toys, 409–412
Vielle, 223

vitamin E, 91
V Magic, 88
vulva
    anatomy, 50
    biopsy, 128
    vulvar cancer, 138, 338
    vulvar creams, 88–89
    vulvar dystrophies, 137–143
    vulvar moisturizer/lubricants, 85–86
    vulvar skin, 52
    vulvar tattoos, 394
    vulvodynia, 129–137
    vulvovaginal atrophy, 261
    vulvovestibulodynia, 129–137,
        145–146

warming lubricants, 80
water-based lubricants, 76–77
Webb, Joanne, 412
weight issues, 20, 165, 189–190, 310–311
Weiss Model, 405
Wellbutrin, 188, 195, 218
Wet, 80
Wet wOw, 220
Wilson, Robert, 281
Witte, James, 16, 40–41
Women's Health Initiative, 281–283
wrinkles, 22–23, 295

Yale University, 211
Yaz, 238
yeast infection, 63–65, 77, 308
Yohimbe, 218

Zestra, 219
Zyban, 195, 218